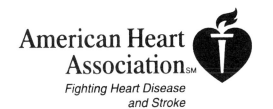

American Heart
Association sm

*Fighting Heart Disease
and Stroke*

Monograph Series

ATRIAL ARRHYTHMIAS
State of the Art

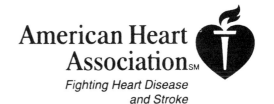

American Heart
Association℠

*Fighting Heart Disease
and Stroke*

Monograph Series

ATRIAL ARRHYTHMIAS
State of the Art

Edited by

John P. DiMarco, MD, PhD

*Director, Clinical Electrophysiology Laboratory
Department of Internal Medicine
Division of Cardiology
University of Virginia Health Sciences Center
Charlottesville, Virginia*

Eric N. Prystowsky, MD

*Director, Clinical Electrophysiology Laboratory
St. Vincent Hospital, Indianapolis, Indiana;
Consulting Professor of Medicine
Duke University Medical Center
Durham, North Carolina*

Futura Publishing
Company, Inc.
Armonk, NY

Library of Congress Cataloging-in-Publication Data
Atrial arrhythmias : state of the art / edited by John P DiMarco.
   Eric N. Prystowsky.
         p.   cm. — (American Heart Association monograph series)
      Includes bibliographical references and index.
      ISBN 0-87993-604-5 (alk. paper)
      1. Atrial arrhythmias.   I. DiMarco, John P.   II. Prystowsky,
   Eric N.   III. Series.
      [DNLM: 1. Atrial Fibrillation—physiopathology.   2. Atrial
   Fibrillation—therapy.   WS 330 A88151 1994]
   RC685.A72A883   1994
   616.1'28—dc20
   DNLM/DLC
   for Library of Congress   94-23566
                                                                  CIP

Copyright © 1995

Published by
Futura Publishing Company
135 Bedford Road
Armonk, New York 10504

LC #: 94-23566
ISBN #: 0-87993-604-5

Every effort has been made to ensure that the information in this book is as up to date and accurate as possible at the time of publication. However, due to the constant developments in medicine, neither the author, nor the editor, nor the publisher can accept any legal or any other responsibility for any errors or omissions that may occur.

Printed in the United States of America on acid-free paper.

Preface

Atrial fibrillation is the most commonly encountered sustained arrhythmia in medical practice. It can occur in virtually all forms of cardiac disease but also can affect patients without structural cardiac abnormalities. Atrial fibrillation is not an acutely life-threatening arrhythmia, but its presence is associated with significant long-term morbidity, including congestive heart failure and stroke, and increased mortality.

Until recently, there has been little change in our concepts of the mechanisms responsible for atrial arrhythmias and in therapy for patients with this disorder. However, in recent years, investigators from many disciplines have shown a rekindled interest in the study of atrial fibrillation and new concepts are rapidly emerging. In October 1993, the Councils on Clinical Cardiology, Basic Science, Cardiovascular Disease in the Young, and Stroke of the American Heart Association sponsored a two-day conference to focus attention on atrial arrhythmias. Experts from North America and Europe from the fields of cardiology, epidemiology, neurology, pediatrics, and basic science reviewed the current state of knowledge concerning atrial fibrillation, presented intriguing new observations, and exchanged ideas with their colleagues. This book is a summary of the proceedings of that conference.

The editors wish to thank the participants in the symposium and the staff members of the American Heart Association who made this conference possible. We hope this book will allow the reader a comprehensive review of exciting new developments in this field.

John P. DiMarco, M.D., Ph.D.
Eric N. Prystowsky, M.D.

Contributors

Masood Akhtar, MD Mt. Sinai Medical Center, Milwaukee WI

Maurits Allessie, MD Professor, Department of Physiology, University of Limburg, Maastricht, The Netherlands

D. Woodrow Benson Jr, MD, PhD Director, Division of Cardiology, Children's Memorial Hospital, Chicago, IL

Zalmen Blanck, MD Milwaukee Heart Institute, Sinai Samaritan Medical Center, Milwaukee, WI

Penelope Boyden, PhD Associate Professor, Department of Pharmacology, College of Physicians and Surgeons of Columbia University, New York, NY

Douglas A. Cameron, MD, FRCP Division of Cardiology, Toronto Hospital, Toronto, Ontario, Canada

A. John Camm, MD, FRCP Professor of Clinical Cardiology, Department of Cardiological Sciences, St George's Hospital Medical School, London, England

James H. Chesebro, MD Associate Director, Cardiovascular Institute, Mt. Sinai, New York, NY

Sanjay Deshpande, MD Milwaukee Heart Institute, Sinai Samaritan Medical Center, Milwaukee, WI

Anwer Dhala, MD Milwaukee Heart Institute, Sinai Samaritan Medical Center, Milwaukee, WI

John P. DiMarco, MD, PhD Director, Clinical Electrophysiology Lab, Department of Internal Medicine, University of Virginia Health Science Center, Charlottesville, VA

Kenneth A. Ellenbogen, MD Medical College of Virginia, Richmond, VA

Valentin Fuster, MD, PhD Cardiovascular Institute, Mt. Sinai Medical Center, New York, NY

Arthur Garson Jr, MD, MPH Department of Pediatric Cardiology, Duke Univerity Medical Center, Durham, NC

Bernard J. Gersh, MD Associate Professor of Medicine, Georgetown University Medical Center, Washington, DC

Augustus O. Grant, MD, PhD Duke University Medical Center, Durham, NC

Jerry C. Griffin, MD InControl Incorporated, Redmond, WA

Jonathan L. Halperin, MD Mt. Sinai Medical, New York, NY

Robert G. Hart, MD University of Texas Health Science Center, San Antonio, TX

Richard N.W. Hauer, MD, PhD, Director, Clinical Electrophysiology, University Hospital, Utrecht, The Netherlands

Mohammed Jazayeri, MD Milwaukee Heart Institute, Sinai Samaritan Medical Center, Milwaukee, WI

Mark E. Josephson, MD Beth Israel Hospital, Harvard-Thorndike EPS Institute, Oklahoma City, OK

George Klein, MD Cardiac Investigation Unit, University Hospital, London, Ontario, Canada

K. Konings, MD University of Limburg, Maastricht, The Netherlands

James E. Lowe, MD Professor of Surgery, Department of Surgery, Duke University Medical Center, Durham, NC

Kevin M. Monahan, MD Beth Israel Hospital, Boston, MA

Carlos A. Morillo, MD Veteran's Administration Medical Center, Richmond, VA

Francis D. Murgatroyd, MRCP St. George's Hospital Medical School, London, England

Andrea Natale, MD Milwaukee Heart Institute, Sinai Samaritan Medical Center, Milwaukee, WI

Douglas L. Packer, MD Mayo Foundation, St. Mary's Hospital, Rochester, MN

Edward L.C. Pritchett, MD Professor of Medicine, Department of Medicine, Duke University Medical Center, Durham, NC

Eric N. Prystowsky, MD Duke University Medical Center, Durham, NC; Northside Cardiology, Indianapolis, IN

Dan M. Roden, MD Division of Clinical Pharmacology, Vanderbilt Univerity School of Medicine, Nashville, TN

Michael R. Rosen, MD Professor of Pediatrics, Department of Pharmacology, College of Physicians and Surgeons of Columbia University, New York, NY

Yoram Rudy, PhD Professor, Department of Biomedical Engineering, Case Western Reserve University, Cleveland, OH

Mark J. Seifert, MD Beth Israel Hospital, Boston, MA

Daniel E. Singer, MD Director of Clinical Epidemiology, Massachusetts General Hospital, Boston, MA

Madison S. Spach, MD Division of Pediatric Cardiology, Duke University Medical School, Durham, NC

Jasbir Sra, MD Milwaukee Heart Institute, Sinai Samaritan Medical Center, Milwaukee, WI

Robert W. Wald, MD Mt. Sinai Hospital, Toronto, Ontario, Canada

Albert L. Waldo, MD The Walter H. Pritchard Professor of Cardiology and Professor of Medicine, Case Western Reserve University, Cleveland, OH

Menashe B. Waxman, MD Toronto General Hospital, Toronto, Ontario Canada

David W. Whalley, MD Royal North Shore Hospital, New South Wales, Australia

M. Wijffels, MD University of Limburg, Maastricht, The Netherlands

Raymond Yee, MD, FRCPC, FACC University Hospital, London, Ontario, Canada

Douglas P. Zipes, MD Professor of Medicine, Indiana University of Medicine, Krannert Institute of Cardiology, Indianapolis, IN

Contents

Chapter 1

The Epidemiology of Atrial Fibrillation and Atrial Flutter

Bernard J. Gersh, MD

Introduction

Atrial fibrillation is a common arrhythmia (perhaps the most common rhythm disturbance after extrasystoles), affecting approximately 1 to 1.5 million patients in the United States and a source of considerable morbidity and mortality.[1-3] Among patients in the United States hospitalized with arrhythmia as a primary diagnosis, atrial fibrillation was the most frequent, accounting for approximately 1 million hospital days in 1989 (Fig 1). [4,5] Moreover, atrial fibrillation is by far the leading cause of embolic stroke, being responsible for approximately 75000 strokes per year.[6-8] Since the incidence and prevalence of atrial fibrillation and its impact on the risk of stroke are markedly age-dependent,[3] it is evident that the socioeconomic and medical implications of atrial fibrillation will assume increasing importance among the burgeoning population of the elderly in this and other countries. The significance of atrial fibrillation extends beyond its direct impact on morbidity and mortality. The associations between atrial fibrillation, age, and cardiovascular disease (overt and subclinical) may lead us to new insights into the interactions among aging, risk factors, and the cardiovascular system.

This discussion of the epidemiology of the atrial arrhythmias will focus on atrial fibrillation and atrial flutter and their independence or coexistence. Nonetheless, a role for other forms of supraventricular tachycardia in the genesis of atrial fibrillation is recognized (Fig 2). Moreover, the era of the implantable cardioverter

From DiMarco JP, Prystowsky EN (eds): *Atrial Arrhythmias: State of the Art*. Armonk, NY, Futura Publishing Company, Inc., © 1995.

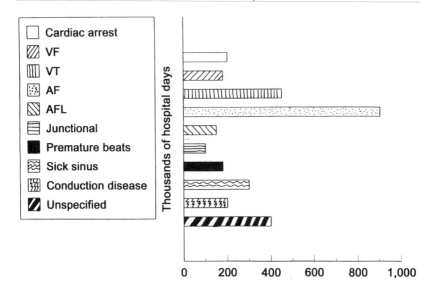

FIGURE 1. *Estimated number of hospital days with arrhythmia as the principal diagnosis derived from the Commission for Professional and Hospital Activity data (United States 1990). Reproduced with permission from References 4 and 5. VF = ventricular fibrillation; VT = ventricular tachycardia; AF = atrial fibrillation; AFL = atrial flutter.*

defibrillator has drawn attention to the frequent coexistence of atrial fibrillation with ventricular arrhythmias and its attendant implications for therapy.

Incidence and Prevalence

There are serious limitations to the ability of most current databases to accurately determine the incidence and prevalence of atrial fibrillation.[9]

1. The majority are based on the sampling of a 12-lead electrocardiogram at specified time intervals or during symptomatic episodes. The frequency of *paroxysmal* atrial fibrillation, in which many of the episodes are asymptomatic, could lead to a systematic underestimate of the prevalence of atrial fibrillation[10] (E.L.C. Pritchett, personal communication). The natural history of atrial fibrillation is probably biphasic, with the development of *chronic* atrial fibrillation preceded in a substantial (but unestablished) pro-

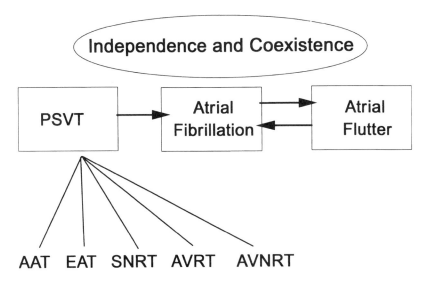

FIGURE 2. *Proposed interrelationships between paroxysmal supraventricular tachycardia, atrial fibrillation, and atrial flutter. PSVT = paroxysmal supraventricular tachycardia; AAT = intra-atrial tachycardia; EAT = ectopic "automatic" atrial tachycardia; SNRT = sinus node reentry tachycardia; AVRT = atrioventricular reentry tachycardia; AVNRT = atrioventricular nodal reentry tachycardia.*

portion of patients by a period of paroxysmal, recurrent episodes (Table 1).[11]

2. An additional issue leading to underrepresentation of the frequency of atrial fibrillation in published studies is the use of drugs or cardioversion, which suppress the frequency of recurrences and mask their symptoms during episodes.[9]

3. The development of transient (or nonrecurrent) atrial fibrillation during acute precipitating circumstances, eg, alcohol use, infections, thyrotoxicosis, or cardiothoracic surgery, is another source of inaccuracy in the determination of the true incidence and prevalence of atrial fibrillation.

Inconsistencies in Definitions

There is no consensus among classifications, and the terminologies used to characterize the clinical syndromes of atrial fibril-

TABLE 1. Multivariate Correlates of the Prevalence of Atrial Fibrillation in the Cardiovascular Health Study: Multivariable Stepwise Models

Age (7 years)	Demographic
History of congestive heart failure History of rheumatic heart disease History of Stroke	Clinical cardiovascular disease
Mitral Stenosis or aortic insufficiency on echocardiography Left atrial dilatation on echocardiography Treated hypertension	Subclinical cardiovascular disease Risk Factors

Cause or consequence?
Adapted from Reference 9, Table 2.

lation differ among studies. Atrial fibrillation is variably described as paroxysmal, transient, recurrent, established, or chronic. Definitions of "lone" atrial fibrillation are discussed elsewhere (see below).

Incidence

After 30 years of follow-up in the Framingham Study, of the 5209 men and women 30 to 62 years old who entered into the study, 7.2% had developed chronic atrial fibrillation.[7,8] The incidence is strikingly age-dependent; this becomes particularly evident after the age of 50 years (Fig 3).[12] Chronic atrial fibrillation is slightly but significantly more frequent in men than in women, but the relationship to age is present in both sexes. There is a paucity of epidemiological data on paroxysmal atrial fibrillation, but in the Framingham study, the incidences of paroxysmal and chronic atrial fibrillation are approximately similar (Fig 3).[12]

Prevalence

Several studies from North America, Great Britain, and Iceland suggest a prevalence of chronic atrial fibrillation of approximately

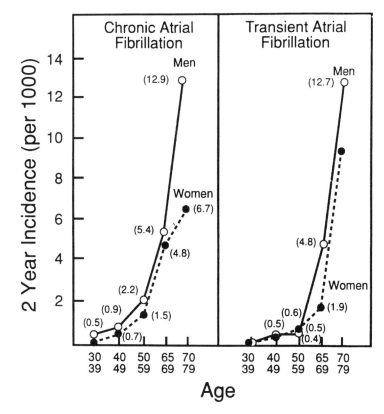

FIGURE 3. *Two-year incidence of chronic and transient atrial fibrillation by age and gender from the Framingham Study. Reproduced with permission from Reference 12.*

0.5% to 1% of the population.[7,8,13-15] In two studies confined to patients >60 years old, the prevalence ranged from 2.3% to 5% at entry, but this increased to 5% to 9% after 5 to 15 years of follow-up.[16,17] In a geriatric hospital population of 1171 patients, the prevalence was 15%.[8]

The most current data emanate from the National Heart, Lung, and Blood Institute–sponsored Cardiovascular Health Study (CHS) of 5201 men and women >60 years old in four communities in the United States.[9] The prevalence of atrial fibrillation on entry into the study in 1989 is illustrated in Fig 4. Among CHS participants, 4.8% of women and 6.2% of men had atrial fibrillation at the time of the

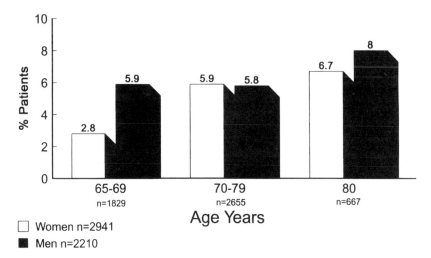

FIGURE 4. *Prevalence of atrial fibrillation (%) by age and gender in the Cardiovascular Health Study (adapted from Reference 9).*

baseline examination, but the increase in prevalence with age reached statistical significance only in women. The prevalence was 9.1% in men and women with clinical evidence of cardiovascular disease, 4.6% in individuals with "subclinical" disease (see below), and only 1.6% in patients with neither clinical nor subclinical disease.

Pathogenesis

Most patients with atrial fibrillation have underlying structural heart disease, and in a recent series of 246 patients undergoing direct-current cardioversion for chronic atrial fibrillation, valvular heart disease was the most common underlying abnormality (Fig 5).[18] In contrast, among 161 patients in a European multicenter registry with paroxysmal atrial fibrillation, a diagnosis of "lone" atrial fibrillation accounted for the majority of cases.[19] Other predisposing conditions, which have perhaps been underemphasized in the large epidemiological or multicenter studies, include the growing patient population with previously surgically repaired congenital heart disease. In a 30-year follow-up study from the Mayo Clinic of patients undergoing atrial septal defect repair, the prevalence of atrial fibrillation both preoperatively and at late follow-up increased with the

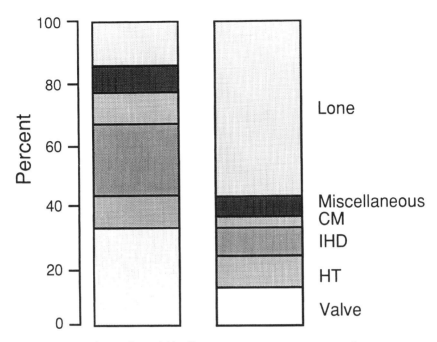

FIGURE 5. *Etiology of atrial fibrillation (AF) in 246 patients undergoing DC cardioversion for chronic atrial fibrillation and 161 patients with paroxysmal atrial fibrillation. Reproduced from Reference 4 with permission of* The Lancet *and Dr Camm. Data adapted from References 60 and 61. CM = cardiomyopathy; IHD = ischemic heart disease; HT = hypertrophy.*

age at operation, but this was very low in patients less than approximately 20 years old at time of operation.[20] Moreover, late postoperative atrial fibrillation in this series was strongly associated with late deaths due to stroke.[20] Other conditions associated with atrial fibrillation include diabetes,[1] mitral valve calcification,[21] mitral valve prolapse, cardiac surgery, and recent acute myocardial infarction.[1,2]

Framingham Study

In the Framingham Study, the presence of cardiovascular disease increased the risk of developing chronic atrial fibrillation approximately threefold to fivefold (Fig 6).[1,12] Rheumatic heart disease and congestive heart failure are traditionally accepted to be the

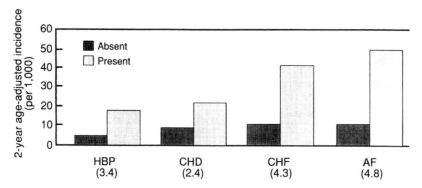

FIGURE 6. *Incidence of stroke in men and women 50 to 89 years old in the Framingham Study stratified by the presence or absence of a cardiovascular abnormality. Atrial fibrillation (AF) is associated with a 4.8-fold increased risk of stroke. HPB = high blood pressure; CHD = coronary heart disease; CHF = congestive heart failure. Reproduced with permission from Reference 1.*

most frequent risk factors, but in the present era, they have been superseded by hypertension and coronary artery disease, particularly in association with left ventricular hypertrophy and congestive heart failure, respectively.[1]

Cardiovascular Health Study

The CHS is an invaluable source of information in regard to current practice, in that the baseline examination performed in 1989 included two-dimensional and Doppler echocardiography and noninvasive evaluations of the peripheral vasculature for features of premature or early atherosclerosis.[9,22,23] Patients were characterized according to demographic variables, the presence of traditional risk factors for cardiovascular disease, the presence of overt cardiovascular disease, and a definition of "subclinical" cardiovascular disease. The latter referred to either echocardiographic evidence of valvular disease, left atrial dilation, left ventricular dysfunction, or regional wall motion abnormalities, an increase in left ventricular mass, or evidence supporting a diagnosis of atherosclerotic disease based on ultrasonography of the carotid arteries or an ankle-arm blood pressure index of <0.9.[23] According to this classification, 57% of patients with atrial fibrillation had clinical cardiovascular disease, 35% had subclinical disease (especially valvular/atrial disease), and only 8% had neither clnical nor subclinical disease.[9]

Independent associations with the prevalence of atrial fibrillation (either causal or consequential) are listed in Table 2; these include advanced age, treated hypertension, evidence of overt coronary artery disease, and variables reflecting subclinical disease.[9] Surprisingly, in the multivariate analysis, neither diabetes, an abnormal left ventricular ejection fraction, left ventricular regional wall motion abnormalities, nor a history of coronary artery disease was identified as an independent risk factor. In contrast, in the Framingham study, diabetes increased the risk by twofold to threefold, with a more powerful impact noted among women.[12]

In epidemiological studies of patients with coronary artery disease, atrial fibrillation is a frequent accompaniment of acute myocardial infarction ($\approx$15%),[24,25] but in the Coronary Artery Surgery Study (CASS) registry of patients undergoing angiography, primarily for a diagnosis of angina or other chest pain syndromes, the prevalence of atrial fibrillation was only 0.6%.[26] Autopsy studies, which inherently introduce a selection bias toward patients with severe disease or recent myocardial infarction, have also documented a high proportion of patients with atrial fibrillation.[24] The strong association between atrial fibrillation and coronary artery disease among autopsy studies or in clinical studies of patients with acute myocardial infarction, in contrast to the weaker association

TABLE 2. Baseline Characteristics and Outcomes in Three Studies of "Lone" Atrial Fibrillation

	Olmsted County <60 years	Olmsted County >60 years	Framingham 55% aged >70 years
Hypertension	Excluded	Excluded	32%
Risk of stroke	Not increased	Not increased	(relative risk 4.1)
Risk of stroke/ transient ischemic attack	Not increased	Increased	

Adapted from References 50, 51, and 56.

documented in patients with more stable coronary disease, suggests that atrial fibrillation in the setting of coronary artery disease is a marker of more severe disease.[24]

Impact on Mortality

Over a 22-year period in the Framingham study, the development of atrial fibrillation approximately doubled the cardiovascular mortality, the rate of sudden death, and death due to all causes.[12] Seven other studies comprising 2889 patients with atrial fibrillation and a control population, with a follow-up ranging from 8 months to 15 years, implied that chronic atrial fibrillation is associated with an approximate doubling of mortality rates (mortality ratio ranging from 1.6 to 2.0)[8,13–17,26]

The poorer prognosis among patients with atrial fibrillation is readily explicable on the basis of the undisputed increased risk of stroke and other embolic phenomena, in addition to the association between atrial fibrillation, advanced age, and other comorbid conditions including congestive heart failure, valvular heart disease, hypertension, and coronary artery disease. Moreover, atrial fibrillation may be a marker for other manifestations of cardiovascular or peripheral vascular disease, which in themselves increase mortality. There is speculative but intriguing evidence that atrial fibrillation lengthens the QT interval (corrected for a specific heart rate); theoretically, this could increase the vulnerability of such patients to malignant ventricular arrhythmias.[2,27] Nonetheless, this mechanism, although plausible, requires extensive further study before a definitive link with sudden cardiac death can be established.

Several studies have addressed the impact of atrial fibrillation on the prognosis of patients with heart failure.[28–39] Comparisons between studies are hampered by a small sample size in individual studies and differences in the severity and pathogenesis of heart failure between series.[28] Not surprisingly, the results are controversial, with the majority of studies showing an insignificant effect of atrial fibrillation on survival, although others imply a deleterious effect on prognosis, particularly in patients with New York Heart Association class IV heart failure.[40,41] A recent analysis of approximately 1500 patients in the Veterans Administration Vasodilator/Heart Failure Trials (V-HeFT 1 and 2), which included patients with mild to moderate congestive heart failure, showed that neither mortality nor morbidity was increased by the presence of atrial fibrillation (Table 3).[28] It should be emphasized that the clinical features and subsequent course among patients included in these trials are not the same as those in class IV heart failure described in another large study, in which it appeared that atrial fibrillation did increase overall mortality and the risk of sudden death.[41]

Impact on Morbidity

The Risk of Stroke

Atrial fibrillation is clearly a major risk factor for stroke, and its effect appears to be independent of associated cardiovascular abnormalities.[6,7,12,42-45] What is less clear and of relevance to our understanding of the randomized trials of coumarin and aspirin in nonrheumatic atrial fibrillation is the multifactorial, pathophysiological mechanisms that could predispose to stroke (Fig 7).[46] The majority of strokes in the anterior circulation in a recent series of 154 patients with atrial fibrillation were considered to be due to cerebral embolism, which is readily explicable on the basis of traditional hypotheses, implicating stasis in the left atrium or left

TABLE 3. Cumulative Mortality and Embolic Events in the Veterans Administration Vasodilator in Heart Failure Trials (V-HeFT) 1 and 2: 2-Year Cumulative Mortality

	Atrial Fibrillation	Sinus Rhythm	P
V-HeFT 1	0.34	0.30	NS
V-HeFT 2	0.20	0.21	NS
	Embolic Events (% patients)		
V-HeFT 1	3	6	NS
V-HeFT 2	4	5	NS

NS = not significant
Data adapted from Reference 28, Table 4.

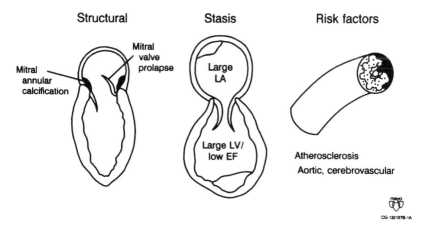

FIGURE 7. *Pathophysiological mechanisms and associations between atrial fibrillation and stroke. LA = left atrium; LV = left ventricle; EF = ejection fraction. Reproduced with permission from* Contemporary Internal Medicine.

ventricle leading to thrombosis and embolism.[47] Less clear-cut, however, is the association between stroke and mitral annular calcification, aortic atherosclerosis, and atrial fibrillation. The beneficial effects of aspirin in some patients[43]; the strong association between atrial fibrillation, hypertension, and stroke[6,7]; and the increase in the attributable risk of stroke from atrial fibrillation with age[45] suggest that in some patients, atrial fibrillation may be a marker of other vascular diseases that predispose to stroke.[46]

Bleeding

In one study of an outpatient population undergoing anticoagulation for a variety of conditions, atrial fibrillation was an independent predictor of bleeding.[48] The mechanisms are speculative (particularly in the face of low risk of bleeding in the randomized trials of nonrheumatic atrial fibrillation)[43] but do raise the issue of atrial fibrillation as a marker of a "friable" cerebrovasculature or the possibility of subclinical infarcts becoming hemorrhagic when the patient is given anticoagulants.

Hemodynamic Effects

The adverse consequences of rapid heart rate and the loss of atrial transport function in elderly patients with impaired left ventricular diastolic function are easily understood.[2] One small series provided evidence that uncontrolled atrial fibrillation can cause reversible left ventricular systolic dysfunction, analogous to the entity of "tachycardia-induced cardiomyopathy"[49] (Fig 8). This is probably a relatively infrequent event, but the proportion of patients in whom atrial fibrillation exacerbates preexisting left ventricular dysfunction is unknown.

Lone Atrial Fibrillation

The entity of "lone" atrial fibrillation refers to atrial fibrillation in the absence of underlying structural heart disease or other overt

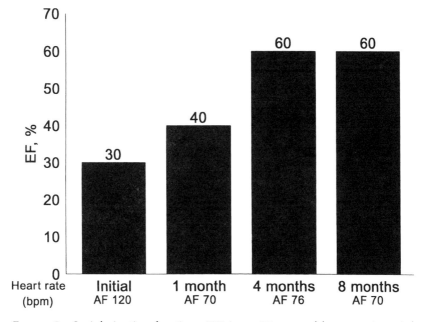

FIGURE 8. *Serial ejection fractions (EF) in an 80-year-old woman in atrial fibrillation, documenting gradual improvement with rate control despite persistence of atrial fibrillation. Reproduced with permission from Reference 49.*

precipitating conditions—thyrotoxicosis, infections, exposure to toxins, etc.[50-54] The role of alcohol is not established, but there is accumulating evidence of its role in the initiation of atrial fibrillation in patients with or without organic heart disease.[55]

The prevalence of lone atrial fibrillation depends to some extent on the definitions used and the zeal with which underlying cardiovascular disease is excluded. Among patients presenting with atrial fibrillation in the Framingham study, 5% were considered to have lone atrial fibrillation, but this increased to 31% at follow-up[50]: of 362 patients <60 years old with a diagnosis of atrial fibrillation in Olmsted County,[51] 2.7% were diagnosed with lone atrial fibrillation, and among 2593 patients >60 years old in Olmsted County, 2.1% received this diagnosis.[56] In another study of an emergency room population, lone atrial fibrillation was diagnosed in 4.7%; in the majority, the arrhythmia was transient.[57] In the CHS, of 277 patients with atrial fibrillation out of a total population of 5201 patients, only 21 (7.6%) had neither clinical nor subclinical disease, and two of these patients had extensive repolarization changes on the electrocardiogram.[9] Clearly, the diagnosis and prevalence of lone atrial fibrillation depend on the vagaries of definitions and the extent and sophistication of techniques aimed at identifying underlying clinical or subclinical cardiac disease.

Early studies suggested a benign prognosis in patients with lone atrial fibrillation,[52-55] but two databases, namely, the Framingham study and Olmsted County, provide us with the most useful follow-up data of lone atrial fibrillation, since too few patients with this clinical entity were included in the randomized trials of anticoagulants, platelet-inhibitor agents, and placebo in nonrheumatic atrial fibrillation, and in any event, the follow-up in these trials was relatively short.[43] At first glance, the three large studies of lone atrial fibrillation suggest a different natural history. In the Framingham study, the risk of stroke was increased approximately 4.5-fold, but in the Olmsted County population <60 years old, neither mortality nor stroke risk was increased in comparison with an age- and sex-matched population. Crucial to resolving these apparently contradictory results is an appreciation of the different definitions of atrial fibrillation in the two studies and the different baseline characteristics of the populations under analysis (Table 3).

In the Framingham study, 56% of patients were >70 years old, and 32% had a history of treated or controlled hypertension. Moreover, it should be emphasized that both age and hypertension are powerful risk factors for stroke among patients with nonrheumatic atrial fibrillation.[45,50,58,59] Not only were the Olmsted County patients at less risk on the basis of age, but patients with a history of hypertension were excluded.[51] Both studies used acceptable definitions of lone atrial fibrillation (based on an absence of overt heart disease), but the outcome was substantially different, in accordance with what one would expect in view of variations in baseline characteristics and the risk of stroke in the two patient populations.[58,59]

Preliminary data in Olmsted County patients >60 years old but without hypertension have been reported.[56] This population falls into an intermediate-risk category on the basis of increased age but an absence of hypertension. In this study, neither survival nor the rate of stroke differed in comparison with age- and sex-matched controls, but the incidence of combined transient ischemic attacks and strokes was increased. It is likely that the inclusion of larger numbers of patients might well have documented an increased risk of stroke in addition to transient ischemic attacks.

Fig 9 illustrates another aspect of the different natural histories of younger and older patients in the Olmsted County population with "lone" atrial fibrillation. [51,56] Among patients <60 years old, only 9% developed chronic atrial fibrillation during the course of the study; atrial fibrillation was recurrent in 70%. In contrast, among older patients (>60 years old), atrial fibrillation was chronic in 58% at the time of diagnosis and in 67% at the time of last follow-up. The latter patients, therefore, are more analogous to the Framingham patients, who by definition had established atrial fibrillation on entry. Nonetheless, there are no clear data as yet to document a greater risk of stroke or mortality in chronic, as opposed to paroxysmal, recurrent atrial fibrillation, although one would intuitively expect the former to be the case[12] (Fig 9).

The results from these three studies of lone atrial fibrillation are entirely consistent with the impact of age, hypertension, and perhaps left atrial dilation and the chronicity or otherwise of atrial fibrillation on the risk of stroke and the development of cardiovascular disease.[58,59] These concepts underlie a logical (although unproven) approach to the estimation of the risks and benefits of anticoagulants and platelet inhibitors in the individual patients.

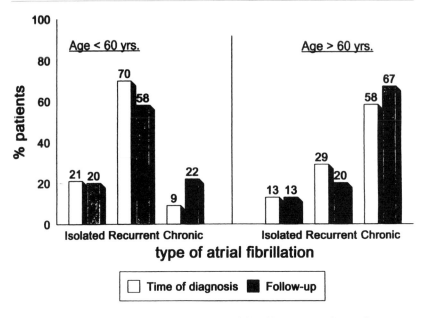

FIGURE 9. *Clinical course of "lone" atrial fibrillation in Olmsted County. Data adapted from References 48 and 53.*

Natural History of Atrial Flutter

The epidemiology of atrial flutter, in contrast to that of atrial fibrillation, is characterized by a paucity of data. In two large databases, the Framingham study and the Veterans Administration studies of heart failure, patients were labeled as having atrial fibrillation if the electrocardiogram documented either flutter or fibrillation.[1,6,12,28] Whether the data from these studies can be subgrouped according to the nature of the inital arrhythmia is uncertain, but such information has not been presented to date.

Anecdotal reports and accumulating clinical evidence imply that atrial fibrillation and flutter frequently coexist in the same patient.[60] In a recent study using 24-hour ambulatory electrocardiographic monitoring of 96 patients (half of whom were in the perioperative period after surgery), alternation of flutter and fibrillation during the 24-hour period was documented in 35% of postoperative patients and in 15% of nonsurgical patients.[60] Further supportive evidence is provided by analysis of patients with recurrent, paroxysmal supraventricular tachycardia and/or atrial fibrillation who were undergoing pharmacological studies.[61] Of the patients with documented atrial fibrillation, 12% of recurrent arrhythmias were observed to be regular, presumably atrial flutter or paroxysmal supraventricular tachycardia. Conversely, among patients with paroxysmal supraventricular tachycardia, 6.5% of occurrences were irregular (presumably, atrial fibrillation).

The bulk of evidence suggests that atrial flutter is very uncommon in patients without underlying heart or lung disease, but the independence of this arrhythmia is unknown, at least in adults as opposed to children or in patients who have had prior surgical repair of congenital heart disease. Two studies suggest that the risk of embolism in patients with atrial flutter in comparison with atrial fibrillation is low, particularly among perioperative patients and in patients undergoing cardioversion.[60,62]

In summary, the independence of atrial flutter from atrial fibrillation or their coexistence is unclear, but a frequent association is well documented. A close relationship and a common origin between the two arrhythmias is very plausible, and it is likely that chronic atrial fibrillation is the final common pathway of patients presenting with both paroxysmal atrial fibrillation and paroxysmal atrial flutter. Insufficient evidence currently exists to draw any conclusions about the independent impact of atrial flutter on survival, prognosis, and the risk of stroke, with the possible exception of patients undergoing cardioversion. Intuitively, one would expect that the preservation of atrial contraction during atrial flutter would reduce the risk of stasis and thromboembolism, and preliminary echocardiographic and clinical data tend to substantiate this.[63] In this study, which used biplane transesophageal echocardiography, thrombus formation in the left atrial appendage was associated with a low peak emptying velocity at that site, and among patients with atrial flutter, left atrial appendage peak emptying velocity was significantly higher than in patients with atrial fibrillation.[63] Both the prevalence of thrombus formation and spontaneous echo contrast were similar for patients with atrial flutter and sinus rhythm but substantially higher among patients with atrial fibrillation.[63] Nonetheless, the evidence available does not answer the critical question regarding the role of anticoagulants and platelet inhibitors in patients with atrial flutter as opposed to those with persistent atrial fibrillation.

Conclusions

The epidemiology of atrial fibrillation provides a critical perspective on the magnitude of the problems from a demographic and socioeconomic standpoint, in addition to a clearer picture of subsets of patients who are not only at increased likelihood of developing the arrhythmia but also at a greater risk for morbid events once the diagnosis has been made. The association of atrial fibrillation as a direct cause as opposed to a marker of cardiovascular risk requires further study. The outcome of these investigations could shed light on the efficacy or otherwise of different therapeutic approaches using anticoagulant and antiplatelet agents.

The optimum therapy for atrial fibrillation remains a subject of controversy and is addressed elsewhere in this monograph. Nonetheless, the existence of the controversy and the debate over therapy focus attention on the importance of prevention and on further studies aimed at the evaluation of the role of traditional as opposed to new risk factors in the development of atrial fibrillation. Whether those risk factors that predisposed to the development of atrial fibrillation 30 years ago apply to the current population to a similar degree is a crucial issue; fortunately, this is the subject of current investigation in several large studies.

Atrial fibrillation is an old arrhythmia familiar to physicians since the turn of the century. It is now a subject of intense investigation for those interested in these electrophysiological mechanisms, their role in the pathogenesis of heart failure, and the issues of rate control as opposed to the complexities involved in the maintenance of sinus rhythm. Several randomized trials are addressing the issues of the risks and benefits of anticoagulant and platelet-inhibitor therapy as modalities for reducing the risks of stroke in an expanding elderly population at increased risk of bleeding. Atrial fibrillation, a well-established entity, has provoked an understandable resurgence of interest into the implications of its pathophysiology, epidemiology, and therapy.

References

1. Kannel WB, Wolf PA. Epidemiology of atrial fibrillation. In: *Atrial Fibrillation: Mechanisms and Management.* Falk RH, Podrid PJ, eds. New York, NY: Raven Press, Ltd; 1992.

2. Pai SM, Torres V. Atrial fibrillation: new management strategies. *Curr Probl Cardiol.* 1993;18:233–300.
3. Kannel WB, Abbott RD, Savage DD, McNamara PM. Epidemiologic features of atrial fibrillation: the Framingham Study. *N Engl J Med.* 1982;306:1018–1022.
4. Murgatroyd FD, Camm AJ. Atrial arrhythmias. *Lancet.* 1993;341:1317–1322.
5. Bialy D, Leahman MH, Shumacher DN, et al. Hospitalization for arrhythmias in the United States: importance of atrial fibrillation. *J Am Coll Cardiol.* 1992;19:41. Abstract.
6. Wolf PA, Abbott RD, Kannel WB. Atrial fibrillation: a major contributor to stroke in the elderly. *Arch Intern Med.* 1987;147:1561–1564.
7. Wolf PA, Dawber TR, Thomas HE, et al. Epidemiologic assessment of chronic atrial fibrillation and risk of stroke: the Framingham Study. *Neurology.* 1978;28:973–977.
8. Vaidya PN, Bhoseley PN, Rao DB, et al. Tachyarrhythmias in old age. *J Am Geriatr Soc.* 1976;24:412–414.
9. Furberg KD, Psaty BM, Manolio TA, et al. Prevalence of atrial fibrillation in elderly subjects: the Cardiovascular Heath Study. In press.
10. Page RL, Wilkinson WE, Clair WK, et al. Asymptomatic arrhythmias in patients with symptomatic paroxysmal atrial fibrillation and paroxysmal supraventricular tachycardia. *Circulation.* In press.
11. Sgarbossa EB, Pinski SL, Maloney JD, et al. Chronic atrial fibrillation and stroke in paced patients with sick sinus syndromes: relevance of clinical characteristics and pacing modality. In press.
12. Kannel WB, Abbott RD, Savage DD, et al. Coronary heart disease and atrial fibrillation: the Framingham Study. *Am Heart J.* 1983;106:389–396.
13. Onundarson PT, Thorgeirsson G, Jonmudsson E, et al. Chronic atrial fibrillation: epidemiologic features and 14 year follow-up: a case control study. *Eur Heart J* 1987;8:521–527.
14. Ostrander LD, Brandt RL, Kjeilsberg MO, et al. Electrocardiographic findings among the adult population of a total natural community, Tecumseh, Michigan. *Circulation.* 1965;31:888.
15. Flegel KM, Shipley MJ, Rose G. Risk of stroke in non-rheumatic atrial fibrillation. *Lancet* 1987;1:526.
16. Kitchin AH, Milne JS. Longitudinal survey of ischemic heart disease in randomly selected sample of older population. *Br Heart J.* 1977;39:889.
17. Lake FR, Cullen KJ, de Klerk NH, et al. Atrial fibrillation and mortality in an elderly population. *Aust N Z J Med* 1989;19:321.
18. Van Gelder IC, Crijns HJ, Van Gilst WH, et al. Prediction of uneventful cardioversion and maintenance of sinus rhythm from direct-current electrical cardioversion of chronic atrial fibrillation and flutter. *Am J Cardiol.* 1991;68:41–46.
19. Murgatroyd FD, Curzen NP, Aldergather J, et al. Clinical features and drug therapy in patients with paroxysmal atrial fibrillation: results from the CRAFT multi-center registry. *J Am Coll Cardiol.* 1993;21:380. Abstract.
20. Murphy JG, Gersh BJ, McGoon MD, et al. Long-term outcome after surgical repair of isolated atrial septal defect: follow-up 27–32 years. *N Engl J Med.* 1990;323:1645–1650.

21. Benjamin EJ, Plehn JF, D'Agostino RB, et al. Mitral annular calcification and the risk of stroke in an elderly cohort. *N Engl J Med.* 1992;327:374–379.
22. Fried LP, Borhani NO, Enwright P, et al. The Cardiovascular Health Study: design and rationale. *Ann Epidemiol.* 1991;1:263–276.
23. Newman AB, Siscovick D, Manolio TA, et al. The ankle-arm index as a marker of atherosclerosis in the Cardiovascular Health Study. *Circulation.* 1993;88:837–845.
24. Lie JT, Falk RH. Pathology of atrial fibrillation: insights from autopsy studies. In: *Atrial Fibrillation: Mechanisms and Management.* Falk RH, Podrid PJ, eds. New York, NY: Raven Press, Ltd; 1992.
25. Goldberg RJ, Seeley D, Becker RC, et al. Impact of atrial fibrillation on the in-hospital and long-term survival of patients with acute myocardial infarction: a community-wide perspective. *Am Heart J.* 1990;119:996.
26. Cameron A, Schwartz MJ, Kronmal RA. Prevalence and signficance of atrial fibrillation in coronary artery disease (CASS Registry). *Am J Cardiol.* 1988;61:714.
27. Pai RG, Rawles JM. The QT interval in atrial fibrillation. *Br Heart J.* 1989;61:510–513.
28. Carson PE, Johnson GR, Dunkman WB, et al. The influence of atrial fibrillation on prognosis in mild to moderate heart failure: the V-HeFT studies. *Circulation.* 1993;87(suppl VI):VI-102–VI-110.
29. Convert G, Delaye J, Biron A, Gonin A: Etude pronostique des myocardiopathies primitives non obstructives. *Arch Mal Coeur.* 1980;73:227–237.
30. Keogh AM, Baron DW, Hickie JB. Prognostic guides in patients with idiopathic or ischemic dilated cardiomyopathy assessed for cardiac transplantation. *Am J Cardiol.* 1990;65:903–908.
31. Fuster V, Gersh BJ, Guiliani ER, et al. The natural history of idiopathic dilated cardiomyopathy. *Am J Cardiol.* 1981;47:525–531.
32. Diaz RA, Obasohan A, Oakley CM. Prediction of outcome in dilated cardiomyopathy. *Br Heart J.* 1987;58:393–399.
33. Likoff MJ, Chandler SL, Kay KR: Clinical determinants of mortality in chronic congestive heart failure secondary to idiopathic dilated or to ischemic cardiomyopathy. *Am J Cardiol.* 1987;59:634–638.
34. Kelly TL, Cremo R, Nielson C, Shabetai R. Prediction of outcome in late-stage cardiomyopathy. *Am Heart J.* 1990;119:1111–1121.
35. Juilliere Y, Danchin N, Briancon S, et al. Dilated cardiomyopathy: long-term follow-up and predictors of survival. *Int J Cardiol.* 1988;21:269–277.
36. Koide T, Kato A, Takabatake Y, et al. Variable prognosis in congestive cardiomyopathy: role of left ventricular functions, alcoholism, and pulmonary thrombosis. *Jpn Heart J.* 1980;21:451–463.
37. Delius W, Sebening H, Weghmann N, et al. Klinik und Verlauf der congestive Cardiomyopathie ungeklärter Ätiologie. *Dtsch Med Wochenschr.* 1976;101:635–647.
38. Unverferth DV, Magorien RD, Moeschberger ML. Factors influencing the one-year mortality of dilated cardiomyopathy. *Am J Cardiol.* 1990;65:903–908.

39. Romeo F, Pelliccia F, Cianfrocca C, Cristofani R. Predictors of sudden death in idiopathic dilated cardiomyopathy. *Am J Cardiol.* 1989;63:138–140.
40. Hoffman T, Meinertz T, Kasper W, et al. Mode of death in idiopathic dilated cardiomyopathy: a multivariate analysis of prognostic determinants. *Am Heart J.* 1988;116:1455–1463.
41. Middlekauff HR, Stevenson WG, Stevenson LW. Prognostic significance of atrial fibrillation in advanced heart failure. *Circulation.* 1991;84:40–48.
42. Godtfredsen J. Atrial fibrillation: course and prognosis: a follow-up study of 1212 cases. In: Kulbertus HE, Olsson JB, Schlepper M, eds. *Atrial Fibrillation.* Mölndal, Sweden: AB Hassle; 1982:134–145.
43. Cairns JA, Connelly SJ. Nonrheumatic atrial fibrillation: risk of stroke and antithrombotic therapy. *Circulation.* 1991;84:469–481.
44. Peterson P, Godtfredsen J. Embolic complications in paroxysmal atrial fibrillation. *Stroke.* 1986;17:622–626.
45. Wolf PA, Abbott RD, Kannel WB. Atrial fibrillation as an idependent risk factor for stroke: the Framingham study. *Stroke.* 1991;22:983–988.
46. Chesebro JH, Fuster V, Halpein JL. Atrial fibrillation: risk marker for stroke. *N Engl J Med.* 1990;323:1556–1558. Editorial.
47. Bogousslavsky J, VanMelle G, Rigli F, et al. Pathogenesis of anterior circulation stroke in patients with non-valvular atrial fibrillation: Lausanne stroke registry. *Neurology.* 1991;40:1046–1050.
48. Landefeld CS, Goldman L. Major bleeding in outpatients treated with warfarin: incidence and prediction by factors known at the start of our patient therapy. *Am J Med.* 1989;87:144.
49. Grogan M, Smith HC, Gersh BJ, et al. Left ventricular dysfunction due to atrial fibrillation in patients initially believed to have idiopathic dilated cardiomyopathy. *Am J Cardiol.* 1992;69:1570–1573.
50. Brand FN, Abbott RD, Kannel WB, et al. Characteristics and prognosis of lone atrial fibrillation: 30-year follow-up in the Framingham study. *JAMA.* 1985;254:3449–3453.
51. Kopecky SL, Gersh BJ, McGoon MD, et al. The natural history of lone atrial fibrillation: a population-based study over three decades. *N Engl J Med.* 1987;317:669–674.
52. Parkinson J, Campbell M. Paroxysmal auricular fibrillation: record of 200 patients. *Q J Med.* 1930;23:67–100.
53. Selzer A. Atrial fibrillation revisited. *N Engl J Med.* 1982;306:1044–1045.
54. Philips E, Levine SA. Auricular fibrillation without other evidence of heart disease. *Am J Med.* 1949;7:478–489.
55. Leather RA, Kerr CR. Atrial fibrillation in the absence of overt cardiac disease. In: *Atrial Fibrillation: Mechanisms and Management.* Falk RH, Podrid PJ, eds. New York, NY: Raven Press, Ltd; 1992.
56. Kopecky SL, Gersh BJ, McGoon MD, et al. Lone atrial fibrillation in the elderly: a marker for cardiovascular risk. In press.
57. Davidson E, Weinberger I, Rotenberg Z, et al. Atrial fibrillation: cause and time of onset. *Arch Intern Med.* 1989;149:457–459.
58. The Stroke Prevention in Atrial Fibrillation Investigators. Predictors of

thromboembolism in atrial fibrillation, I: clinical features of patients at risk. *Ann Intern Med.* 1992;116:1–5.

59. The Stroke Prevention in Atrial Fibrillation Investigators. Predictors of thromboembolism in atrial fibrillation, II: echocardiographic features of patients at risk. *Ann Intern Med.* 1992;116:6–12.
60. Tunick PA, Mcelhaney L, Mitchell T, et al. The alternation between atrial flutter and atrial fibrillation. *Chest.* 1992;101:34–36.
61. Clair WK, Wilkenson WE, McCarthy EA, et al. Spontaneous occurrence of symptomatic paroxysmal atrial fibrillation and paroxysmal supraventricular tachycardia in untreated patients. *Circulation.* 1993;87: 1114–1122.
62. Arnold AZ, Mick MJ, Masureck RP, et al. Role of prophylatic anticoagulation for direct current cardioversion in patients with atrial fibrillation or atrial flutter. *J Am Coll Cardiol.* 1992;19:851–855.
63. Santiago, DW, Warshofsky, M, LiMandri, G, et al. Left atrial appendage function and thrombus formation in atrial flutter. *Circulation* 1993;88(2):I-19. Abstract.

Chapter 1

Editorial Comments

Edward L.C. Pritchett, MD

From the point of view of a clinician who treats patients with atrial fibrillation, this disorder requires attention for two reasons that have been shown to be amenable to medical therapy: (1) atrial fibrillation causes symptoms that can be relieved with antiarrhythmic drug therapy, and (2) atrial fibrillation increases the risk of stroke, but this risk can be reduced with anticoagulation therapy. Other medical consequences, such as an increased risk of cardiovascular death, occur in patients with atrial fibrillation, but it has not been shown that these events can be altered with medical therapy.

Epidemiological research has shown that atrial fibrillation is one of the most common arrhythmias, perhaps the most common, today. This type of research has identified patients with atrial fibrillation by reviewing screening electrocardiograms recorded in specified subject groups, as was done in the Framingham Heart Study.[1] In a widely known report from this study published in 1982, the electrocardiograms of study subjects were "sampled" for a few seconds every 2 years at the time of scheduled follow-up visits for a total follow-up period of 22 years.[1] If atrial fibrillation was present on electrocardiograms recorded on two of these biennial examinations, then atrial fibrillation was considered to be present in that patient. The cumulative 22-year incidence of atrial fibrillation was 21.5 per thousand in men and 17.1 per thousand in women. This type of screening almost certainly identified patients who were permanently in atrial fibrilla-

From DiMarco JP, Prystowsky EN (eds): *Atrial Arrhythmias: State of the Art.* Armonk, NY, Futura Publishing Company, Inc., © 1995.

Dr. Pritchett's research is supported in part by grant RO1-HL40392 from the National Heart, Lung and Blood Institute, Bethesda, MD; by grant MO1 RR00030 from the National Center for Research Resources, National Institutes of Health, Bethesda, MD; and by contract N01-ES-35357 from the National Institute of Environmental Health Sciences, Research Triangle Park, NC.

tion or had "chronic" atrial fibrillation, as these authors used the term. This study found that the incidence of chronic atrial fibrillation increased with age but was not influenced by gender. Patients with chronic atrial fibrillation had an increased risk of cardiovascular mortality and total mortality. Other observations from the Framingham Heart Study established an increased risk of stroke in these same patients.[2,3] Several recent randomized clinical trials have shown convincingly that the risk of stroke can be reduced by anticoagulation therapy with warfarin or aspirin.[4–7]

From the point of view of clinicians who treat patients with atrial fibrillation, the type of patient reported in the Framingham Heart Study is relatively uncomplicated compared with those patients who have sinus rhythm that is punctuated with periods of atrial fibrillation. Such patients are often said to have "paroxysmal," "intermittent," or "transient" atrial fibrillation. There is less epidemiological information about this group of patients compared with those who are permanently in atrial fibrillation. The Framingham Heart Study included some information about this form of atrial fibrillation in a report on coronary artery disease and atrial fibrillation that was published in 1983.[8] In that report, they compared the 2-year incidence of chronic atrial fibrillation (as defined above) with the 2-year incidence of atrial fibrillation identified by electrocardiogram recorded in the area's only hospital. The investigators found that the incidence of this transient atrial fibrillation was about equal to the incidence of chronic atrial fibrillation. The incidence increased with age in both types and was slightly greater in men than in women (Fig 1). The overall 2-year incidence was approximately two per thousand subjects for both chronic and transient atrial fibrillation. This estimate, now more than 10 years old, has never been confirmed. The lack of more estimates of the incidence of transient atrial fibrillation is an important gap in epidemiological data on atrial fibrillation because patients with this type of atrial fibrillation are likely to require substantial amounts of health care resources, including the use of class I and class III antiarrhythmic drugs, which are usually initiated in the hospital, and they require additional hospitalizations for acute care when atrial fibrillation recurs.

There is not much additional epidemiological information about the paroxysmal, transient, or intermittent type of atrial fibrillation, except that the Stroke Prevention in Atrial Fibrillation (SPAF) study found that in control patients (taking no anticoagulants), the point estimate of the risk of stroke for intermittent compared with permanent was 0.9; that is, the risk of stroke was about equal in the two types of atrial fibrillation.[9] The 95% confidence interval (0.5, 1.6) for this estimate of the risk, however, was quite broad. If the true relative risk of stroke were only 0.5 in the patients with intermittent atrial fibrillation, then these patients could be greatly reassured. Similarly, if the true relative risk of stroke were 1.6, then these patients should receive particularly aggressive anti-coagulation. Since patients with transient atrial fibrillation are in arrhythmia only part of the time, it is feasible that the incidence of stroke is lower compared with patients who have permanent atrial fibrillation. Alternatively, the risk of stroke may be higher in patients with transient atrial fibrillation because the transition from atrial fibrillation to sinus rhythm is a time of high risk of stroke, and they have more of these transitions.[10] Thus, an important missing bit of epidemiological information is a more precise estimate of stroke risk in patients with intermittent atrial fibrillation.

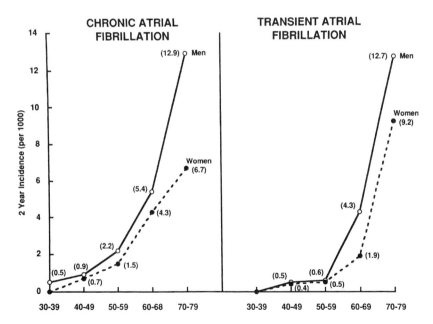

FIGURE 1. *Cumulative 2-year incidence of "chronic" and "transient" atrial fibrillation reported in the Framingham Heart Study. The incidence for both types increased with age and was slightly higher in men compared with women. From Kannel et al[8]; reprinted with permission of the author and the publisher.*

In patients who have paroxysmal atrial fibrillation, little is known about how the successive occurrences of atrial fibrillation in individual patients are related or what baseline factors influence the occurrence of atrial fibrillation. This information is not really epidemiology of the same type as studied in the Framingham Heart Study. The phrase "behavior" of paroxysmal atrial fibrillation was used by Greer et al[11] to define the chain of clinical events formed by the serial occurrences of atrial fibrillation in an individual patient. Greer et al reported that in many patients, the successive occurrences of paroxysmal atrial fibrillation were random events; that is, they were independent, were identically distributed, and followed an exponential probability distribution (Fig 2). In a few patients, apparent nonrandomness was found (Figs 3 and 4). Understanding this behavior is important for planning controlled clinical trials of antiarrhythmic drugs in which the behavior of untreated patients must be predicted. Few studies of behavior have been published, and more are needed.

An important feature of arrhythmia behavior is the frequency with which symptomatic arrhythmias occur. Recent studies reported by Klein et al[12] have looked at factors that increase the frequency with which paroxysmal atrial fibrillation and paroxysmal supraventricular tachycardia occur. Frequency of occurrence was estimated by the time to first recurrence in an untreated observation period. The most important factor was age; advancing age was associated with a significantly shorter time to recurrence. Neither gender nor associated cardiovascular disease influenced time to recurrence when adjustment was made for the effect of age.

Another feature of patients with arrhythmias that is not strictly epidemiological is the occurrence of asymptomatic arrythmias. Page et al[13] recently studied the occurrence of asymptomatic atrial fibrillation in a group of patients known to have symptomatic atrial fibrillation. The ratio of the rate at which asymptomatic arrhythmia events occurred compared with symptomatic events was 12.1; that is, asymptomatic atrial fibrillation was far more common than symptomatic atrial fibrillation in this group of patients. The incidence of asymptomatic atrial fibrillation in the general population and its impact on the risk of stroke are additional important gaps in our understanding of the epidemiology of atrial fibrillation.

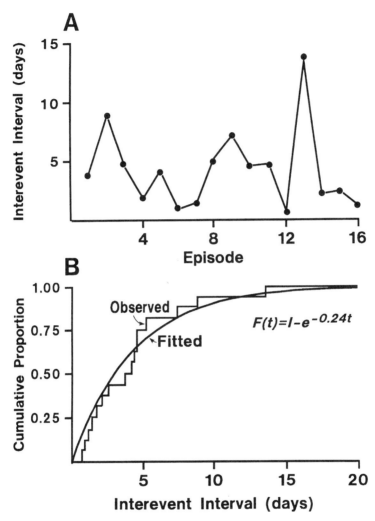

A

B

$$F(t)=1-e^{-0.24t}$$

FIGURE 2. *Time intervals between successive occurrences of sympto-matic atrial fibrillation in a single patient (A). In this patient, the interevent intervals appeared to be independent, to be identically distributed, and to follow an exponential probability distribution. The observed data (B, step function) fit a calculated exponential probability distribution (smooth curve). From Greer et al[11]; reprinted with permission of the author and the publisher.*

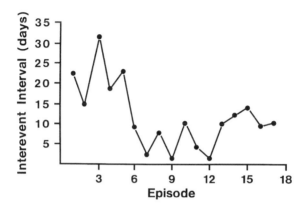

FIGURE 3. *Successive time intervals between episodes of symptomatic paroxysmal atrial fibrillation. In this patient, interevent intervals appeared to be nonrandom; all of the last 12 intervals were shorter than all of the first 5 intervals. From Greer et al[11]; reprinted with permission of the author and the publisher.*

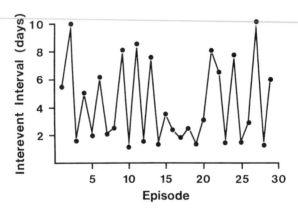

FIGURE 4. *Successive time intervals between episodes of symptomatic paroxysmal atrial fibrillation. Interevent intervals appeared to be nonrandom; long periods alternated with short ones. From Greer et al ; reprinted with permission of the author and the publisher.*

References

1. Kannel WB, Abbott RD, Savage DD, et al. Epidemiologic features of chronic atrial fibrillation: the Framingham Study. *N Engl J Med.* 1982; 306:1018–1022.
2. Wolf PA, Abbott RD, Kannel WB. Atrial fibrillation: a major contributor to stroke in the elderly: the Framingham Study. *Arch Intern Med.* 1987;147:1561–1564.
3. Wolf PA, Kannel WB, McGee DL, et al. Duration of atrial fibrillation and imminence of stroke: the Framingham Study. *Stroke.* 1983;14:664–667.
4. Stroke Prevention in Atrial Fibrillation Investigators. Stroke Prevention in Atrial Fibrillation Study: final results. *Circulation.* 1991;84:527–539.
5. Boston Area Anticoagulation Trial for Atrial Fibrillation Investigators. Effect of low-dose warfarin on the risk of stroke in patients with nonrheumatic atrial fibrillation. *N Engl J Med.* 1990;323:1505–1511.
6. Petersen P, Boysen G, Godtfredsen J, et al. Placebo-controlled, randomised trial of warfarin and aspirin for prevention of thromboembolic complications in chronic atrial fibrillation: the Copenhagen AFASAK Study. *Lancet.* 1989;1:175–179.
7. Connolly SJ, Laupacis A, Gent M, et al. Canadian atrial fibrillation anticoagulation (CAFA) study. *J Am Coll Cardiol.* 1991;18:349–355.
8. Kannel WB, Abbott RD, Savage DD, et al. Coronary heart disease and atrial fibrillation: the Framingham Study. *Am Heart J.* 1983;106:389–396.
9. Stroke Prevention in Atrial Fibrillation Investigators. Predictors of thromboembolism in atrial fibrillation, I: clinical features of patients at risk. *Ann Intern Med.* 1992;116:1–5.
10. Bjerkelund CJ, Orning OM. The efficacy of anticoagulant therapy in preventing embolism related to D.C. electrical conversion of atrial fibrillation. *Am J Cardiol.* 1969;23:208–216.
11. Greer GS, Wilkinson WE, McCarthy EA, et al. Random and nonrandom behavior of symptomatic paroxysmal atrial fibrillation. *Am J Cardiol.* 1989;64:339–342.
12. Klein GJ, Guiraudon GM, Sharma AD, et al. Demonstration of macroreentry and feasibility of operative therapy in the common type of atrial flutter. *Am J Cardiol.* 1986;57:587–591.
13. Page RL, Wilkinson WE, McCarthy EA, et al. Frequency of asymptomatic paroxysmal supraventricular tachycardia in patients followed by trans-telephonic electrocardiogram monitor. *J Am Coll Cardiol.* 1992; 19:64A. Abstract.

Chapter 2

Role of the Autonomic Nervous System in Atrial Arrhythmias

Menashe B. Waxman, MD; Douglas Cameron, MD; and Robert W. Wald, MD

Introduction

In 1913, the participation of the autonomic nervous system in human tachycardias was first documented when Cohn and Fraser[1] published two cases of paroxysmal supraventricular tachycardia that were terminated by carotid sinus pressure. Although the ability of vagal stimulation to terminate paroxysms of rapid regular heart action in humans had been reported in separate papers by Bensen[2] and by Priesendorff[3] in 1880, Cohn and Fraser provided the first electrocardiographic proof of the nature of the tachycardia and its termination. Cohn and Fraser's work is of further historic interest because the electrocardiogram during normal sinus rhythm revealed a pattern of Wolff-Parkinson-White conduction, a condition that was not described until 1930, a full 17 years later.[4] Of additional interest, one of Cohn and Fraser's patients was able to regularly terminate the tachycardia by a deep inspiration. The perceptiveness of Cohn and Fraser is understood by the fact that the mechanism of respiration-induced termination of supraventricular tachycardia was not elucidated until 1980, when it was shown that a deep breath greatly increases blood pressure and activates vagal tone via baroreceptors.[5]

General Considerations

While this chapter is concerned with the relationship between the autonomic nervous system and supraventricular tachycardias,[6]

From DiMarco JP, Prystowsky EN (eds): *Atrial Arrhythmias: State of the Art.* Armonk, NY, Futura Publishing Company, Inc., © 1995.

Supported in part by grants in-aid from the Heart and Stroke Foundation of Ontario.

information has been drawn from and comparisons will be made to ventricular arrhythmias where relevant.[7–15]

Afferent and Efferent Innervation of the Heart

A network of afferent and efferent nerve fibers serves autonomic functions throughout the body, including the heart and blood vessels.[16] Baroreceptors[17] and frequently chemoreceptors[18] as well are located in the carotid sinuses, the aortic arch, and other areas of the circulatory system, such as the kidneys, as well as the heart.[19] These receptors send afferent impulses relating to the pressure and chemical milieu to the medullary centers, which in turn regulate the outflow of vagal and sympathetic tone. An increase in afferent impulses from the carotid sinus baroreceptors[17] in response to a blood pressure increase (such as after phenylephrine administration) or in response to direct mechanical deformation (carotid sinus massage)[20] results in a reflex increase in vagal tone and a reciprocal decrease in sympathetic tone. Along with afferent impulses from one source, the vasomotor center's function is affected by competing or additive signals from other regions such as the lungs, heart, extrathoracic organs, and other parts of the central nervous system itself.[21]

We have limited information about the transduction of mechanical or chemical signals into nerve impulses, central integration and processing of the afferent signals, and the means by which this information is converted into physiologically meaningful efferent signals. Also, the efferent neural anatomy and the delivery of neurotransmitters to the end organ is incompletely understood.[21] While this lack of knowledge may be inconsequential in certain settings, it becomes paramount when the anatomy and function of the entire system or any part of it (such as the target organ) are altered by age, disease, surgery, or drugs. Tachycardias disturb cardiac function and hence alter autonomic nervous system behavior.[6,11,12,22] Supraventricular tachycardias, by virtue of their autonomic responsiveness, offer a particularly good opportunity to study the interaction between the autonomic nervous system and clinical tachycardias.[5,11,12,22–24]

In general, there is a reciprocal pattern of vagal and sympathetic activity. For example, stimulation of the baroreceptors by an elevation of blood pressure results in a reduction of sympathetic activity and a reciprocal rise in vagal activity. Conversely, when baroreceptor activation diminishes or ceases during hypotension, sympathetic activity is increased while vagal activity is reduced. There are, however, instances in which both cardiac vagal and sympathetic activity are activated together. One example is the result of chemoreceptor stimulation by perfusion of the carotid sinus with sodium cyanide or CO_2-rich solution.[25]

Physiological and Pharmacological Methods of Manipulating Vagal and Sympathetic Tone

Perturbations of autonomic tone result in complex direct and reflex responses in cardiovascular function, which can enhance or diminish the actual effect of the intervention (Tables 1 and 2). Of these, heart rate, blood pressure, and ventricular volume appear to be of greatest significance. Since alterations of vagal tone are the most commonly used maneuvers in the study of supraventricular tachycardias, the complexity of the effects of vagal maneuvers and of their interpretation will be illustrated at several levels.

TABLE 1. Effects of Common Vagal Interventions During Normal Sinus Rhythm

Maneuver	Sympathetic Tone	Heart Rate	Blood Pressure	End-Diastolic Volume	Contractility	Vagal Tone
Carotid sinus massage	↓	↓	↓	↑	↓	↑
Valsalva, phase 2	↑	↑	↓	↓	↑	↓
Valsalva, phase 4	↑	↓	↑	↑	↑	↑
Supine position	↓	↓	↑	↑	↓	↑
Phenylephrine	↓	↓	↑	↑	−↑	↑
Edrophonium	↓	↓	−	↑	↓	↑
Atropine	↓↑	↑	↑↓	↓	↑	↓

TABLE 2. Effects of Common Adrenergic Interventions During Normal Sinus Rhythm

Maneuver	Sympathetic Tone	Heart Rate	Blood Pressure	End-Diastolic Volume	Contractility	Vagal Tone
Exercise	↑	↑	↑	−↑	↑	↓
Valsalva, phase 2	↑	↑	↓	↓	↑	↓
Valsalva, phase 3	↑	↑	↓	↓	↑	↓
Valsalva, phase 4	↑	↑	↑	↑	↑	↑
Upright position	↑	↑	↑	↓	↑	↓
Amyl nitrite/ nitroprusside	↑	↑	↓	↓	↑	↓
Norepinephrine	↓	↑	↑	↓↑	↑	↑
Epinephrine	↑↓	↑	↑	↓↑	↑	↓↑
Isoproterenol	↑↓	↑	↓↑	↓	↑	↓

General

Clinically and experimentally, the effects of vagal tone on the heart are measured by changes in sinus rate or atrioventricular (AV) nodal conduction time.[11,12,20,26,27] While efferent vagus nerve stimulation affects the refractory period of the atrial myocardium,[28] we lack a noninvasive marker of this effect. Thus, we infer autonomic effects on the atrial myocardium by observing rate and AV conduction changes. It remains to be established whether, and to what degree, the response of the sinus node and the AV node to alterations in autonomic tone correlates with changes in atrial myocardium.

Physiology of the Carotid Sinus Baroreceptors

Activation of efferent vagal tone in humans involves mainly blood pressure elevation by phenylephrine or the Valsalva maneuver or mechanical stimulation of the carotid baroreceptors by carotid sinus massage or by negative pressure around the carotid sinuses.[17,27] Arterial blood pressure is sensed by baroreceptors distributed in the carotid sinuses and the aortic arch. The nerve of Hering, a branch of the ninth cranial nerve, emanates from the sinus and courses up to the vasomotor center of the medulla, while the vagus nerve carries afferent impulses from the aortic arch baroreceptors. Baroreceptor activation reflexly increases vagal tone and decreases sympathetic tone, resulting in additive effects on the depression of the sinus node and AV conduction.[20] Both carotid sinus massage and phenylephrine activate baroreceptors and slow the heart rate, but the former reduces the blood pressure because of decreased sympathetic tone, while the vasoconstrictor effect of phenylephrine raises and maintains an elevated blood pressure.

Baroreceptor activation can be graded by varying the extent and duration of carotid sinus massage or the dose of administered phenylephrine. This reflects the fact that afferent traffic in the nerve of Hering is proportional to the blood pressure increase or intensity of carotid sinus massage.[17] The quantitative aspects of carotid sinus massage allow one to seek a sufficient but avoid an excessive increase in vagal tone. Depending on the means of baroreceptor stimulation, the accompanying blood pressure elevation or reduction can exert arrhythmogenic or antiarrhythmic effects, respectively.[11,12,14] Likewise, heart rate slowing can exert a powerful effect on arrhythmias.[11,12,14] This has to be considered whenever vagal tone is modified by baroreceptor stimulation. A reduction in perfusion pressure, such as occurs following amyl nitrate inhalation or nitroprusside administration, reduces baroreceptor firing and leads to vagal tone withdrawal and sympathetic tone increase.[29]

Differential Effects of Right- and Left-Sided Carotid Sinus Massage

Right- and left-sided carotid sinus massage can have qualitatively and quantitatively different effects on sinus node slowing, AV conduction, and blood pressure experimentally[30] and clinically.[31] The basis for these differences has not been elucidated. Depending on the site of origin of a particular supraventricular tachycardia, the effects created by carotid sinus massage may be lateralized. The effectiveness of carotid sinus massage may be enhanced by the concomitant use of other techniques to increase vagal tone,[20] as described in the following sections.

Edrophonium

The anticholinesterase edrophonium (5 to 10 mg IV) increases the concentration of acetylcholine by inhibiting its hydrolysis at the neuroeffector junction, thereby simulating an increased vagal tone.[32] The drug has nicotinic and muscarinic side effects (lacrimation, salivation, abdominal cramps, nausea, sweating, muscle twitching) in addition to the desired slowing of the heart rate and of AV nodal conduction within 30 to 40 seconds of its administration. Carotid sinus massage, if used as an additional agent, should be performed at this time. In contrast to carotid sinus massage, the administration of edrophonium does not noticeably alter blood pressure. However, edrophonium has other widespread effects, including but not limited to autonomic ganglionic stimulation and bronchoconstriction, which may interact with its cardiac effects.[20,32]

The Valsalva Maneuver

The Valsalva maneuver activates autonomic reflexes in a complex fashion.[27,33] At the onset of the strain, the blood pressure and vagal tone rise transiently (phase 1). This is followed by reduced venous return, cardiac dimensions, blood pressure, and pulse pressure, while sympathetic tone increases (phase 2). On release of the strain, there is a marked transient fall in blood pressure (phase 3), which is rapidly followed by an increase in venous return, cardiac dimensions, and blood pressure, and the latter activates vagal tone (phase 4). Thus, vagal tone is activated as a result of high sympathetic tone and an elevated blood pressure after release of the strain. The slower onset and offset of sympathetic tone compared with vagal tone is crucial to the development of the overshoot in blood pressure and the resultant reflex increase in vagal tone. The increase in vagal tone during phase 4 may terminate paroxysmal supraventricular tachycardia (Fig 1).[23] When used to augment the effect of the Valsalva maneuver, carotid sinus massage should be applied 5

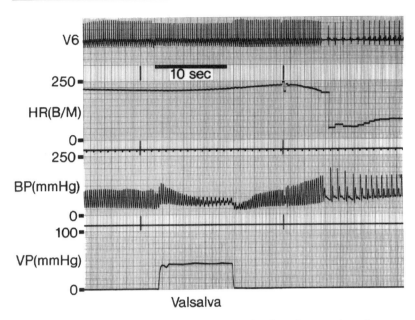

FIGURE 1. *Simultaneous recording of ECG lead V₆, beat-to-beat heart rate in beats per minute [HR(B/M)], blood pressure (BP), and Valsalva pressure (VP) during an episode of paroxysmal supraventricular tachycardia. Following a 10-second Valsalva strain of 40 mm Hg, the blood pressure rises above control; this is accompanied by slowing and termination of the tachycardia (MB Waxman, unpublished observations).*

to 10 seconds after the release of a strong Valsalva maneuver, at a time when the blood pressure is considerably above control.[20]

Phenylephrine

Phenylephrine, an α-adrenergic agonist, elevates the blood pressure and reflexly increases vagal tone.[17] An initial bolus of 50 µg should be doubled sequentially until the desired end point, but not exceeding 1 mg or a systolic blood pressure above 180 mm Hg. One to 3 minutes must be allowed between injections for the blood pressure to normalize. If the desired end point is not achieved by administration of phenylephrine alone, eg, termination of paroxysmal supraventricular tachycardia,[20,23] carotid sinus massage may be applied 30 to 60 seconds after an intravenous bolus of phenylephrine, at a time when the blood pressure has increased substantially above control. Phenylephrine is ill-advised if the resting systolic blood pressure exceeds 160 mm Hg and should not be used in patients with suspected intracranial vascular malformations, ischemic heart disease, or heart failure. Also, it should be used with great care in persons > 60 years old.[20] One must anticipate that if a tachycardia breaks or slows significantly in response to phenylephrine, the blood pressure may rise very significantly.

Head-Dependent Position

The relatively simple maneuver of head-dependent tilting results in an increase in venous return, which affects the blood pressure only minimally during normal sinus rhythm but has a marked pressor effect during supraventricular tachycardia. This maneuver increases vagal tone, and this may terminate the tachycardia (Fig 2).[5] Carotid sinus massage may be applied after the subject is placed in a head-dependent body position to further enhance vagal tone.

Atropine

Atropine antagonizes the effects of vagal tone by competitive muscarinic receptor blockade. However, interpretation of the action of atropine is complex because (1) it causes significant hypotension when administered in the upright position,[34] possibly as a result of its ganglionic blocking properties[35]; (2) it accelerates the sinus rate[20]; and (3) it blocks presynaptic muscarinic receptors on postganglionic sympathetic nerve terminals,[36] thus removing an inhibitory influence on the release of norepinephrine.

Effects of Heart Disease on Activation of Autonomic Tone and the Interaction Between Autonomic Tone and Cardiac Response

In heart disease, baroreceptor function and the ability to enhance vagal tone through baroreceptor stimulation are significantly attenuated.[17] Sympathetic responsiveness is also greatly diminished in

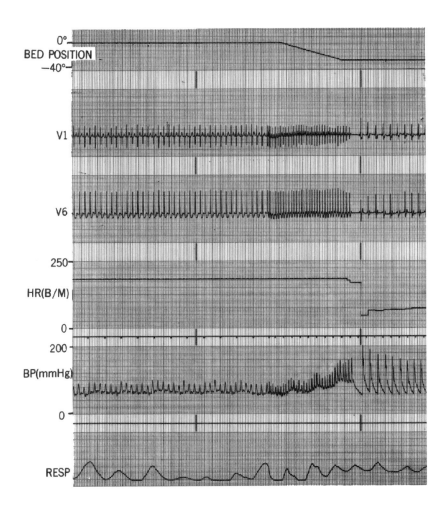

FIGURE 2. *Simultaneous recording of bed position, ECG leads V_1 and V_6, beat-to-beat heart rate in beats per minute [HR(B/M)], blood pressure (BP), and respiratory activity (RESP) during paroxysmal supraventricular tachycardia. Turning the bed to a dependent position ($-40°$) raised the blood pressure, and the tachycardia slowed and terminated. Time markers indicate 1 second. Reproduced with permission from Reference 5.*

heart failure, as evidenced by the failure of the Valsalva maneuver to generate a postrelease overshoot in blood pressure.[27,33] The inability to mount a sympathetic response has the additional effect of preventing enhancement of vagal tone by the Valsalva maneuver.[37]

Even a modest tachycardia may cause a major fall in cardiac output and blood pressure in the face of ventricular dysfunction.[38] When coronary perfusion is limited, the reduction in ventricular compliance during tachycardia is exaggerated, causing a further reduction in cardiac output and blood pressure[39] and, therefore, an even larger increase in sympathetic tone. Disease states characterized by impaired diastolic function are particularly vulnerable to reduced diastolic filling periods and the loss or inappropriate timing of atrial systole. Moreover, the diseased heart exhibits minimal hemodynamic improvement in response to sympathetic tone because of cardiac denervation[40] and reduced responsiveness to autonomic tone and other stimuli.[41] The failure of hemodynamic compensation maintains high sympathetic tone, and this may accelerate or transform the tachycardia. For similar reasons, vagal tone remains depressed, and this also contributes to a failure to restrain sympathetic tone.

Interaction Between Vagal and Sympathetic Systems

At the level of the neuroeffector junction and beyond, the parasympathetic and sympathetic systems interact in four ways: (1) vagal stimulation inhibits the release of norepinephrine at sympathetic nerve terminals[42]; (2) sympathetic stimulation releases neuropeptide Y, which in turn interferes with the actions of vagal stimulation, possibly by inhibiting the release of acethycholine[43]; (3) α-adrenergic stimulation with phenylephrine attenuates the bradycardia induced by direct vagus nerve stimulation[44]; and (4) acetylcholine antagonizes the intracellular production of cyclic AMP by catecholamines in ventricular tissue.[45]

Discrepancy Between Neural Sympathetic Stimulation and Circulating Catecholamines

Exogenously administered catecholamines, especially isoproterenol, are often used to simulate the effects of enhanced sympathetic neural stimulation, yet there may be important differences between these methods of adrenergic stimulation. First, exogenous catecholamines have different electrophysiological actions from neural sympathetic stimulation on the dispersion of refractoriness in the ventricles as well as the ventricular fibrillation threshold.[46,47] These differences have been ascribed to the more "uniform" distribution of the blood supply compared with that of the sympathetic nerves. Second, experiments have shown a discrepancy between circulating levels of catecholamines and left ventricular contractility during exercise and during an infusion of catecholamines.[48] When augmentation of left ventricular contractility was used as an end point, activation of neural sympathetic tone by moderate exercise doubled the left ventricular dP/dt in conscious dogs at the same time as the plasma norepinephrine and epinephrine levels doubled. By contrast, when norepinephrine and epinephrine were infused, sufficient quantities had to be given to raise their level 10-fold or more to achieve a 50% rise in left ventricular dP/dt. Thus, the levels of circulating catecholamines do not reflect the concentration of norepinephrine within the synaptic clefts.[48] Similar reasons may contribute, in part, to the difference between the action of exogenously administered isoproterenol and neural sympathetic tone.

Nonautonomic Effects of the Maneuvers Used to Alter Vagal and Sympathetic Tone: Heart Rate and Cardiac Volume

Heart Rate

The evidence for an independent role of background heart rate on the susceptibility to supraventricular arrhythmias is limited and applies mainly to atrial fibrillation. This evidence is largely clinical and suggests that atrial fibrillation and flutter in humans may be more likely to occur in the setting of bradycardia. Pacing may inhibit the development of atrial fibrillation that is dependent on[49] or independent of vagal tone.[50] The susceptibility to atrial fibrillation in the setting of bradycardia may be similar to the enhanced susceptibility of the ventricular myocardium to arrhythmias in the setting of bradycardia. Rate slowing increases the temporal dispersion of excitability and can depress conduction by allowing diastolic depolarization, either or both of which factors may permit or facilitate reentrant arrhythmias.[51]

The difficulty of assigning susceptibility to atrial fibrillation to a particular factor such as heart rate is illustrated in a model of experimental atrial fibrillation in the dog in which atrial fibrillation was induced by epicardial application of methylcholine chloride. When the sinus node region was destroyed or depressed by injection of alcohol or concentrated sodium pentobarbital into the sinoatrial nodal artery, preexisting atrial fibrillation ceased spontaneously and became much more difficult to reinduce, and its duration became much shorter. When the atria were paced, the ability to induce atrial fibrillation was restored toward control. Not only did bradycardia not predispose these animals to atrial fibrillation, but either the presence of the sinus node or, more likely, a background of regular atrial depolarization proved to be vital to cholinergically induced atrial fibrillation.[52]

Cardiac Volume or Filling Pressure

It has long been assumed that cardiac chamber dilatation and high intracavitary pressures increase the heart's susceptibility to arrhythmias. There is, however, only a limited body of evidence regarding this relationship that successfully factors out the contribution of myocardial disease, which frequently coexists with cardiac dilatation. For example, the ventricular arrhythmias that develop during the combination of the inhalational anesthetic cyclopropane with catecholamines are extremely sensitive to aortic blood pressure.[53] In humans it has been shown that an abrupt reduction in ventricular volume by the Valsalva maneuver may terminate certain forms of ventricular tachycardia independent of autonomic blockade.[9]

Three recent reports of atrial flutter illustrate how autonomic maneuvers influence the electrophysiological properties of the atria by a mechanism independent of changes in autonomic tone.[54-56] In a report of a patient with atrial flutter and high-degree AV block, the flutter cycle abruptly lengthened immediately after a QRS complex, implying a close relationship to ventricular systole. This relationship is probably mechanically mediated by a transient increase in atrial pressure, which must follow ventricular systole, since the fluttering atria contract against closed AV valves.[54] In a second study, the Valsalva strain phase, passive upright tilting, and the expiratory phase of respiration shortened the cycle length of atrial flutter in humans, and this is unaffected by combined β-adrenergic receptor and muscarinic receptor blockade.[55] The changes in cycle length were ascribed to a decrease in cardiac volume that occurs in response to these interventions (Fig 3). In a third report involving atrial flutter in humans and dogs, the occurrence of 1:1 AV conduction slowed the flutter rate by a mechanism related to a rise in atrial pressure.[56] Other investigators have shown that atrial stretch can affect the rate of atrial flutter[57] or the refractory period of the atria[58] in humans.

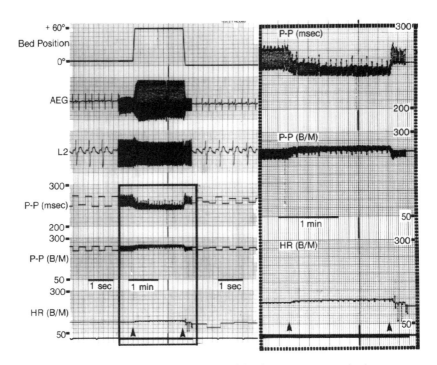

FIGURE 3. *Simultaneous recording of bed position, atrial electrogram (AEG), electrocardiogram lead 2 (L2), flutter cycle interval [P-P(msec)], beat-to-beat flutter rate [P-P(B/M)], and beat-to-beat heart rate in beats-per-minute [HR(B/M)]. The bed is rotated from 0° to +60° at the first arrow-head, and the flutter cycle begins to shorten immediately, the maximum reduction being 15 msec. The changes in cycle length reverse when the bed is returned to 0° (second arrowhead). Since the A-V conduction ratio remains constant (2:1), the ventricular rate increases slightly at +60°. The right panel is an enlargement of the lower tracings contained within the rectangle. There is beat-to-beat alternans in the flutter cycle interval. The longest flutter cycle intervals occur at intervals of about 5 seconds and coincide with the inspiratory phase of respiration. Each prolongation of the flutter cycle interval is accompanied by a small reduction in the heart rate (see enlargement). Reproduced with permission from Reference 55.*

Thus, it is important to appreciate that the Valsalva maneuver and other maneuvers that alter autonomic functions[6,11,14,33] have additional effects that may alter the electrophysiological properties of cardiac tissues.

Diagnostic Considerations

Altering autonomic tone, especially vagal tone, is useful in diagnosing conduction disturbances and is particularly valuable in assessing tachycardias (Table 3).[20] The results of such maneuvers in the diagnosis of tachycardias, including supraventricular tachycardias, have been published.[6,11,12,20] In addition, adenosine is proving to be an alternative or adjunct to manipulations of autonomic tone in tachycardia diagnosis.[59]

Initiation of Tachycardias

Atrial Fibrillation

Vagal Tone

The administration or application of acetylcholine or methylcholine to the atria or vagal efferent stimulation can reproducibly

TABLE 3. Effects of Increased Vagal Tone on Common Tachycardias

Tachycardia	Response to Increased Vagal Tone
Sinus tachycardia	Gradual slowing and reacceleration
Atrial flutter	Transient AV block
	Occasional reversion to atrial fibrillation
Atrial fibrillation	Transient AV block
Paroxysmal supraventricular tachycardia, (with or without accessory AV bypass tract)	Slowing and termination
Ventricular tachycardia (with AV dissociation or VA association)	Selective slowing of the atrial rate, no change in ventricular rate
	Occasional reversion to sinus rhythm

AV = atrioventricular; VA = ventriculoatrial.

induce atrial fibrillation.[60] Also, rapid electrical pacing of the atria in the presence of vagal stimulation can induce prolonged episodes of atrial fibrillation, whereas rapid atrial pacing without concomitant vagal stimulation produces very short-lived episodes of atrial fibrillation.[61] In connection to this atrial flutter can be transformed to atrial fibrillation in dogs by vagus nerve stimulation[62] or occasionally in humans by increased vagal tone.[20]

Coumel[63] described a type of paroxysmal atrial fibrillation in humans that they attribute to increased vagal tone with the following characteristics: (1) repeated attacks last minutes to hours; (2) attacks typically start at night, during rest, or after meals; (3) the arrhythmia is preceded by progressive mild bradycardia, and the onset of atrial fibrillation is preceded by further sinus rate slowing; (4) analysis of heart rate variability reveals oscillations consistent with increased vagal tone; (5) the arrhythmia is often heralded by atrial bigeminy before the onset of atrial flutter, which is subsequently replaced by atrial fibrillation; (6) exercise or emotional stress does not trigger atrial fibrillation; (7) in the presence of premonitory symptoms (premature beats), atrial fibrillation can be prevented by exercise: (8) atrial fibrillation can be induced by vagotonic maneuvers (Fig 4), but these maneuvers fail to induce the arrhythmia during atrial pacing; (9) sinus node function is normal; (10) the arrhythmia remains episodic; and (11) chronic atrial pacing has been found to be highly effective in preventing recurrences of atrial fibrillation in a limited number of cases.

The mechanism of induction of atrial fibrillation by cholinergic stimulation is not fully understood, although several factors are likely to contribute: the shortening of atrial myocardial refractory period and the nonuniformity of this shortening,[28,64] the production of intra-atrial conduction delays,[65] and the accompanying bradycardia, which increases susceptibility to reentry (see section on heart rate).[51] In addition, cholinergic stimulation or the administration of acetylcholine exerts a powerful negative inotropic effect on atrial tissue,[66] which may raise intra-atrial pressure and lead to atrial distension. Atrial distension may alter the electrophysiological properties of cells[54–58] and predispose to arrhythmias (see section on cardiac volume or filling pressure).[51,67] In view of the nocturnal occurrence of so-called vagally induced atrial fibrillation, it is interesting to note that obstructive sleep apnea, a condition that causes transient increases in vagal tone, can also cause atrial fibrillation.[68]

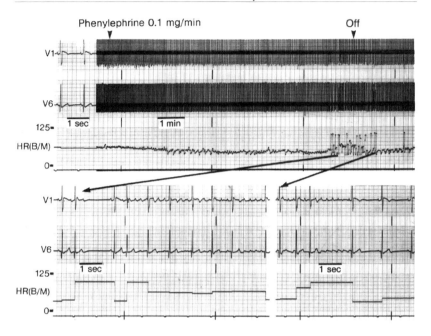

FIGURE 4. *Simultaneous recording of ECG leads V_1 and V_6 and beat-to-beat heart rate in beats per minute [HR(B/M)] in a patient with paroxysmal atrial fibrillation. An infusion of phenylephrine 0.1mg per minute increases vagal tone, slows the heart rate, and induces a short run of atrial fibrillation (see blowup in bottom panel) (MB Waxman, unpublished observations).*

Adrenergic Tone

Coumel[63] also described a different group of patients with adrenergically induced atrial fibrillation with the following clinical characteristics: (1) the heart rate trend suggests enhanced sympathetic tone preceding the paroxysms; (2) episodes occur primarily during the day, during exercise, or with emotional stress; (3) the arrhythmia begins at a specific heart rate (often 90 beats per minute) that is reached gradually; and (4) analysis of heart rate variability confirms the predominance of sympathetically mediated oscillations.

While adrenergic influences are most frequently proarrhythmic, a recent study showed that adrenergic stimulation with isoproterenol had a protective effect against repetitive atrial responses. In 3 of 11 patients with supraventricular tachycardias, isoproterenol reduced the stimulus-latency period, the atrial refractory period, and the intra-atrial and interatrial conduction times. In these 3 patients, the ability to induce repetitive atrial responses or atrial flutter or both was abolished during isoproterenol infusion.[69]

In a recent assessment of the prevalence of Coumel's "vagotonic" and "adrenergic" patterns of atrial fibrillation in 38 patients with paroxysmal atrial fibrillation, a point score of symptoms suggested that the onset of atrial fibrillation is more commonly associated with factors causing increased vagal tone than adrenergic tone.[70] Baroreflex testing with phenylephrine in 28 of these patients[17] revealed no relationship between the vagal score and baroreflex sensitivity. This suggests that "vagal" paroxysmal atrial fibrillation is not due to increased vagal efferent traffic or enhanced sinus node responsiveness to vagal tone. The authors concluded that the abnormality may reside in the atrial myocardium itself.

Paroxysmal Supraventricular Tachycardia

Paroxysmal supraventricular tachycardia is usually initiated by premature atrial beats occurring spontaneously or administered artificially.[5,20,23,24] Among 23 patients who suffered from paroxysmal supraventricular tachycardia, the arrhythmia could be induced without programmed stimulation at least once in 5 of the patients (22%) by exercise or isoproterenol.[11] In each case, exercise or isoproterenol evoked a premature atrial beat, which started the tachycardia. At times, even in the presence of well-timed beats, it may be impossible to induce sustained or nonsustained paroxysms of supraventricular tachycardia without an appropriate adjustment in autonomic tone.

In some instances, paroxysmal supraventricular tachycardia can paradoxically be initiated by vagotonic maneuvers, the very interventions that classically terminate them.[23] One such setting is that of a concealed accessory AV bypass tract. In this case, carotid sinus massage slows AV node conduction sufficiently to allow a retrograde impulse from the ventricles to find the atria excitable and induces a paroxysm of supraventricular tachycardia (Fig 5). In such cases, carotid sinus massage, applied to terminate an ongoing episode of tachycardia, may leave sufficient AV nodal slowing in its

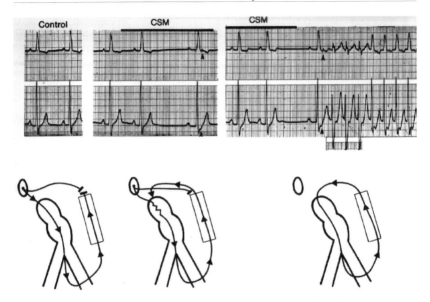

FIGURE 5. *Simultaneous recording of ECG lead 1 and lead 2 in a patient with a concealed left-sided accessory AV pathway. In the middle panel, carotid sinus massage (CSM) slows the rate, prolongs the PR interval, and induces an atrial echo beat (see arrowhead). In the right panel, another application of carotid sinus massage prolongs the PR interval, induces an atrial echo beat, and initiates a paroxysm of supraventricular tachycardia. The tachycardia exhibits tachycardia-dependent left anterior hemiblock during the first three beats. The accompanying diagrams indicate the mechanisms underlying the initiation of the echo beats and of the tachycardia (MB Waxman, unpublished observations).*

wake to cause the immediate reinitiation of the tachycardia. This mechanism of tachycardia initiation, while not widely reported, may not be a particularly exotic one and, in addition to being responsible for many putative "failures" of carotid sinus massage termination of paroxysmal supraventricular tachycardia, may be responsible for some and perhaps most cases of the "incessant" variety of paroxysmal supraventricular tachycardia.

Numerous studies have reported the usefulness of adrenergic stimulation with isoproterenol or of the upright posture, as well as of muscarinic receptor blockade with atropine as a means of facilitating the induction of paroxysmal supraventricular tachycardia during electrophysiological testing, as follows.

1. Isoproterenol commonly facilitates the induction of paroxysmal supraventricular tachycardia by programmed stimulation.[71,72] While in the majority of studies, isoproterenol facilitates the induction of paroxysmal supraventricular tachycardia in a broad spectrum of patients, in one study the ability to so induce the tachycardia depended on an antecedent history of spontaneous exercise-induced episodes.[73] The electrophysiological basis for these observations includes a variety of effects, including speeding of conduction and shortening of the refractory properties within the AV node and/or accessory bypass tracts, particularly in the retrograde direction.[72] These changes may induce or facilitate the induction of paroxysmal supraventricular tachycardia in a variety of ways.

2. Upright tilting has also been used to facilitate the induction of paroxysmal supraventricular tachycardia.[11,74] Upright tilting enhances anterograde slow pathway and retrograde fast pathway (V-A) conduction in patients with reentrant AV nodal supraventricular tachycardia.[74]

3. Atropine was shown to permit the induction of reentrant paroxysmal supraventricular tachycardia in patients with[75] and without[76] spontaneous tachycardias. The facilitation of tachycardia induction was due to facilitation of retrograde conduction in the fast pathway.[75]

Tachycardia Termination

Termination of Paroxysmal Supraventricular Tachycardia by Increased Vagal Tone

Vagal stimulation depresses AV node conduction[26] and interrupts paroxysmal supraventricular tachycardias.[5,20,23,24] In 68 patients with paroxysmal supraventricular tachycardia, the extent of vagal stimulation needed to terminate the tachycardia could be measured when methods such as the Valsalva maneuver (Fig 6) or drugs like edrophonium or phenylephrine were used.[23] The level of vagal tone needed to terminate the tachycardia is decreased or augmented when background sympathetic tone is reduced or elevated, respectively. Tachycardia termination by increased vagal tone was preceded by slowing due to depression of AV nodal conduction by a maximum of 40 to 220 milliseconds (mean, 79.7 ± 3.8 milliseconds).[23] If vagal stimulation is not sufficiently powerful to terminate the tachycardia, the transient slowing in the tachycardia rate may cause some confusion between paroxysmal supraventricular tachycardia and sinus tachycardia.

In addition to physician-applied or -directed interventions such as

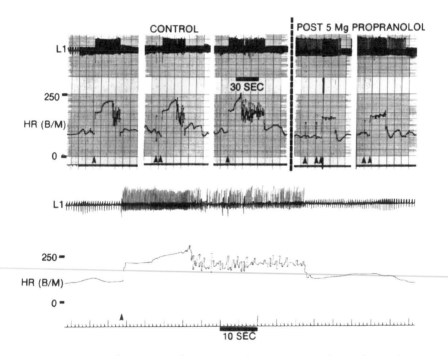

FIGURE 6.   *Transformation of paroxysmal supraventricular tachycardia to atrial fibrillation. Simultaneous recording of ECG lead 1 and beat-to-beat heart rate in beats per minute [HR(B/M)] during five episodes of paroxysmal supraventricular tachycardia induced by premature beats (see arrows). During control, the initial tachycardia rate is 180 to 190 beats per minute, and the compensatory sympathetic reflex first accelerates the tachycardia rate to 225 to 250 beats per minute, then transforms the tachycardia to atrial fibrillation (see irregularity of heart rate display), which ends spontaneously in each case. The enlargement at the bottom represents the third control panel. After propranolol, the initial rate of induced paroxysmal supraventricular tachycardia is slower (160 beats per minute), there is little reflex acceleration, and atrial fibrillation does not develop. Reproduced with permission from Waxman MB et al. Cardiol Clin. 1983.*

carotid sinus massage, Valsalva maneuver, and edrophonium or phenylephrine administration, there are several patient-initiated maneuvers that raise vagal tone and may terminate paroxysmal supraventricular tachycardia. Deep breaths (Fig 7) or rapidly assuming a recumbent or dependent position (Fig 2) during paroxysmal supraventricular tachycardia elevates the blood pressure by augmenting venous return.[5] This stimulates vagal tone through baroreceptors and may terminate the tachycardia (Figs 2 and 7). Muscarinic receptor blockade with atropine does not interfere with the blood pressure rise caused by a deep breath or the dependent body position, but it inhibits termination of the tachycardia (Fig 7).[5] The ability of deep breaths to elevate blood pressure and terminate tachycardias depends

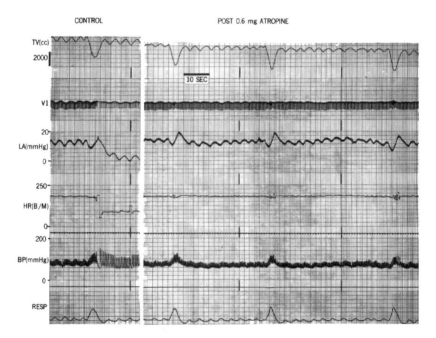

FIGURE 7. *Simultaneous recordings of tidal volume (TV), left atrial pressure (LA), beat-to-beat heart rate in beats per minute [HR(B/M)], arterial blood pressure (BP), and respiration (resp) during two episodes of paroxysmal supraventricular tachycardia. During control (left), a deep inspiration augments the blood pressure and terminates the tachycardia. After atropine (right), deep breaths raise the blood pressure but fail to terminate the tachycardia. Reproduced with permission from Reference 5.*

on body position, tidal volume, and vagal sensitivity of the AV node, and therefore in some cases this maneuver may slow the tachycardia transiently but fail to terminate it.[5]. The mechanism of the marked increase in blood pressure in response to a deep breath or a dependent body position during paroxysmal supraventricular tachycardia may be due in part to significant redistribution and pooling of blood in the venous system. During sinus rhythm and in the face of normal atrial and venous pressure, a deep inspiration may augment venous return by a limited amount because the inferior vena cava collapses as it enters the thorax in response to a markedly negative intrathoracic pressure. By contrast, the elevated right atrial and venous pressure during paroxysmal supraventricular tachycardia may prevent the inferior vena cava from collapsing as it enters the thorax in response to a deep breath. This could account for an augmented increase in venous return, which may be a major component of the blood pressure increase in response to a deep breath.

A comprehensive list of patient- and physician-activated measures for raising vagal tone is presented in Table 4.[11,20]

TABLE 4. Methods of Activating Vagal Tone

Method	Action
Carotid sinus massage	Direct stimulation of baroreceptors
Valsalva maneuver (phase 1, 4)	↑ BP—stimulation of baroreceptors
Coughing	Valsalva maneuver
Sneezing	Valsalva maneuver
Gagging	Valsalva maneuver
Vomiting	Valsalva maneuver
Squatting	↑ BP—stimulation of baroreceptors
Head-dependent position	↑ BP—stimulation of baroreceptors
Cold immersion	↑ BP—stimulation of baroreceptors
Breath holding and facial immersion in water	Diving reflex
Deep breath	↑ BP—stimulation of baroreceptors
Eyeball compression	? Reflex vagal stimulation
Anticholinesterase (edrophonium)	↑ [ACh] at vagal nerve endings
α-Agonists (phenylephrine, methoxamine)	↑ BP—stimulation of baroreceptors
Digitalis Glycosides	Reflex and direct vagal stimulation
Adenosine triphosphate	Cardiac C fibers

↑—increased; BP—blood pressure, ACL—acetylcholine.

Termination of Paroxysmal Supraventricular Tachycardia by an Increase in Sympathetic Tone

When paroxysmal supraventricular tachycardia involves an accessory AV bypass tract, the AV nodal effects of altered autonomic tone slow or speed the tachycardia, which, in turn, may affect other tissues involved in the reentrant circuit, such as the His bundle, bundle branches, ventricles, accessory AV bypass tract, and atria. Therefore, augmentation of either vagal or sympathetic tone may terminate such tachycardias by different mechanisms. One can monitor the beat-to-beat changes that occur in anterograde AV nodal and retrograde bypass tract conduction times during autonomic maneuvers, as well as identifying whether the tachycardia ends with (AV nodal block) or without a retrogade P wave (bypass tract block). This allows one to identify the mechanism of tachycardia termination.[24,77] When a person is placed in a head-dependent position during ongoing paroxysmal supraventricular tachycardia, the blood pressure rises and vagal tone is increased. This slows conduction in an anterograde direction (AV node) while leaving conduction in the retrograde direction (AV bypass tract) unaffected. This slows the tachycardia, and it may terminate. Since the tachycardia ends as a result of AV nodal block, it ends with a retrograde P wave (Fig 8, left). Conversely, tilting a person upright during paroxysmal supraventricular tachycardia reduces the blood pressure and activates sympathetic tone. As a result, conduction time in the anterograde limb (AV node) increases while conduction time in the retrograde direction (AV bypass tract) is generally unchanged. The tachycardia then accelerates, and it may terminate as a result of tachycardia-dependent (phase 3) block in the retrograde limb. In this case, the tachycardia ends without a retrograde P wave (Fig 8, right)

Interactions Between Tachycardia and Autonomic Tone

Effect of Tachycardia on Autonomic Tone

Irrespective of their origin, mechanism, or cause, tachycardias alter cardiovascular function because they affect cardiac filling and stroke volume.[38,78,79] Blood pressure and pulse pressure decline in

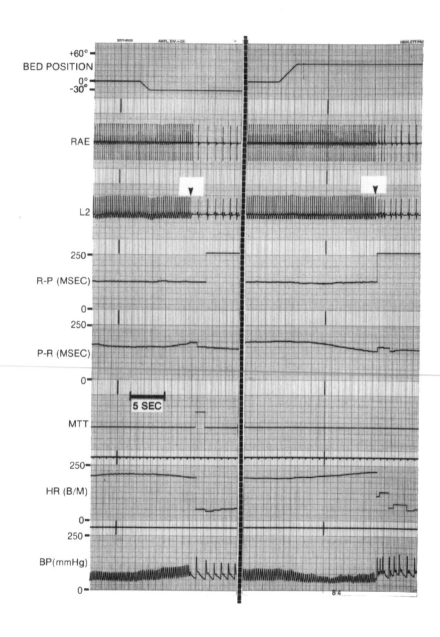

direct relationship to the rate, AV synchrony, and cardiac function.[38,80] This reduces afferent activity to the vasomotor center from the pressure-sensitive fibers in the carotid sinus.[17] In turn, this augments sympathetic efferent tone and reduces vagal efferent tone. Tachycardias generally cause a maximum blood pressure fall at their onset,[22,38] and thus, the maximal stimulus for compensatory sympathetic enhancement and vagal withdrawal occurs at this time.[24] These changes are vital to the restoration of cardiac output and blood pressure. Depending on the location of the arrhythmia, its innervation, and its responsiveness to autonomic tone,[20] these alterations in neural tone can significantly affect the arrhythmia rate. These changes in autonomic tone also determine the blood pressure overshoot after the tachycardia terminates, which in turn activates vagal tone and slows the heart rate transiently.[24]

During a tachycardia, ventricular and atrial mechanoreceptors (C fibers) may be activated as a result of an increase in atrial and ventricular diastolic pressure (Fig 9) interacting with a reduced cardiac volume and an increased sympathetic tone.[19,81] Activation of C fibers leads to a reflex withdrawal of sympathetic tone and an enhancement of vagal tone.[81] Thus, during a tachycardia, the car-

---

FIGURE 8. *Termination of paroxysmal supraventricular tachycardia separately by increased vagal tone and increased sympathetic tone. Simultaneous recording of bed position, right atrial electrogram (RAE), lead 2 (L2), retrograde V-A conduction (R-P), anterograde AV conduction (P-R), mode of tachycardia termination (MTT), beat-to-beat heart rate in beats per minute [HR(B/M)], and blood pressure (BP) in a patient with paroxysmal supraventricular tachycardia that incorporates an AV bypass tract. Left, the patient is turned from 0° to − 30°, thus raising the BP, and the tachycardia slows and ends. Slowing is traceable to P-R interval prolongation (AV node slowing), while the R-P interval (bypass tract conduction) remains constant. The tachycardia breaks due to AV nodal block and so ends with a retrograde P wave; this is denoted by the MTT circuits, which emit a positive pulse. Right, the patient is turned from 0° to +40°, the BP falls, and the tachycardia speeds and breaks. The speeding is related to P-R interval shortening (AV nodal acceleration), while the R-P interval remains constant. The tachycardia terminates secondary to phase 3–dependent block in the bypass tract and so ends without a retrograde P wave, and the MTT circuit does not emit a positive pulse. Reproduced with permission from Waxman MB et al. Cardiol Clin. 1983.*

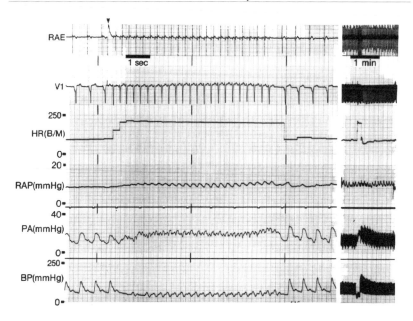

FIGURE 9. *Simultaneous recording of right atrial electrogram (RAE), ECG lead V$_1$, beat-to-beat heart rate in beats per minute [HR(B/M)], right atrial pressure (RAP), pulmonary artery pressure (PA), and systemic arterial blood pressure (BP) from a patient with Wolff-Parkinson-White syndrome. At the arrowhead, a premature atrial beat initiates a run of nonsustained supraventricular tachycardia at a rate of 225 beats per minute. There is considerable hypotension, a small rise in right atrial filling pressure, and a dramatic rise in pulmonary artery pressure, especially the pulmonary artery diastolic pressure. The panel on the right is a compressed record of the same event. Reproduced with permission from Reference 22.*

diac C fibers[81] and extracardiac baroreceptors[17] may act in opposite directions with respect to sympathetic tone. This is perhaps similar to the response to a reduction in venous return by passive upright tilting combined with intravenous isoproterenol that may result in dramatic paradoxic bradycardia in individuals who are susceptible to vasodepressor reactions.[82] Like Sharpey-Schafer and his colleagues[83] in 1958, as well as Oberg and Thoren[84] in 1972, we also concluded that adrenergic stimulation coupled with a reduced cardiac volume leads to an overly powerful cardiac contraction, and this activates cardiac afferent C fibers.[82,85] This in turn leads to a reflex increase in efferent vagal tone and heart rate slowing.[81] In complementary experiments in rats, the inferior vena cava was occluded for 60 seconds during an infusion of isoproterenol. This caused a marked paradoxical bradycardia, which, as in the clinical setting, is mediated by activation of cardiac vagal afferents,[86,87] Although not proven, it is quite likely that tachycardias could provide the necessary ingredients needed to activate cardiac C fibers, namely, a reduced venous return combined with marked sympathetic activation.[22] If activated during paroxysms of tachycardia, these reflexes many aggravate their symptomatic manifestations but may also bring about their spontaneous termination.

During tachycardia, stretch receptors in the atria and possibly in the ventricles cause release of atrial natriuretic factor during tachycardia, a hormone that not only promotes diuresis[88] but also relaxes vascular smooth muscle.[89] Thus, released atrial natriuretic factor can affect the recovery of blood pressure during a tachycardia. The loss of atrial contraction during atrial fibrillation, its diminished efficacy during atrial flutter, or its abnormal timing relative to the cardiac cycle in cases of paroxysmal supraventricular tachycardia may contribute significantly to the hemodynamic and neural effects of a tachycardia.

Effect of Autonomic Tone on Tachycardia Rate Modulation

Paroxysmal Supraventricular Tachycardia

The rate of reentry arrhythmias such as paroxysmal supraventricular tachycardia depends on the properties of conduction velocity and refractoriness of the participating tissues.[51] The AV node is an integral component of these tachycardias,[5,23,24] and vagal tone prolongs refractoriness and slows conduction, while sympathetic tone shortens refractoriness and speeds conduction through this structure.[26] Whenever the properties of the AV node are rate-limiting, changes in vagal and sympathetic tone will slow or speed the tachycardia, respectively. As in the case of sinus rhythm,[17] the rate of paroxysmal supraventricular tachycardia varies inversely with the level of blood pressure.[5] Conversely, stimuli that lower the blood pressure, such as a passive upright tilt, increase the tachycardia rate by raising sympathetic tone and reducing vagal tone.[11,12] To study the separate actions of vagal and sympathetic tone on the tachycardia rate, one can administer vagal and sympathetic agonists and antagonists separately. When a tachycardia involves an accessory AV bypass tract, autonomic tone alters the rate by changing anterograde AV nodal conduction time (PR interval), leaving retrograde conduction (RP interval) unchanged.[24,77] Tachycardias confined to the AV node involve a slow anterograde and a fast retrograde pathway.[90] In these, autonomic maneuvers alter the rate largely, but not exclusively, through the anterograde slow pathway. The location of the retrograde limb during paroxysmal supraventricular tachycardia confined to the AV node is not known,[90] and it is either poorly innervated or minimally responsive to autonomic tone as well as sympathetic and vagal agonists or antagonists. Perhaps this uneven responsiveness of various regions of the AV node is related to a developmental or acquired abnormality responsible for the genesis of dual AV nodal pathways and paroxysmal supraventricular tachycardia.

Atrial Flutter and Fibrillation

Although the ventricular response rate during atrial flutter or fibrillation is influenced by the atrial rate and the intrinsic conduction properties of the AV node and ventricular conducting system, autonomic tone also plays a major role. As in paraoxysmal supraventricular tachycardia, in which sympathetic and vagal tone speed or slow the tachycardia rate, respectively, through their actions on the AV node, the ventricular response during flutter or fibrillation is similarly affected. In this regard, raising the sympathetic tone and observing the resultant increase in the heart rate is a common clinical test of the adequacy of AV blockade by digitalis and/or β-adrenergic blocking drugs in patients with atrial fibrillation or flutter. Passive upright tilting reduces venous return and produces a reflex increase in sympathetic tone.[91] This is illustrated in a patient with atrial flutter and a well-controlled resting ventricular rate who develops 1:1 AV conduction after passive upright tilting. This response is blocked by propranolol, a β-adrenergic receptor antagonist (Fig 10). Adrenergic stimulation (isoproterenol) also facilities anterograde accessory AV pathway conduction during atrial fibrillation.[92]

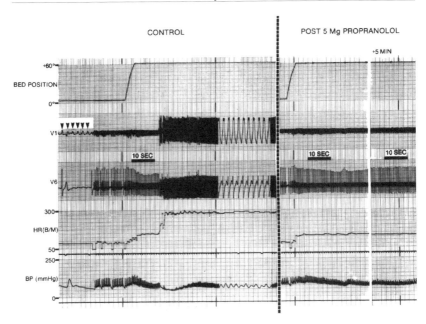

Figure 10. *Simultaneous recording of bed position, ECG lead V_6, beat-to-beat heart rate in beats per minute [HR(B/M)], and blood pressure (BP) in a patient with atrial flutter. The arrowheads denote the atrial activity. After passive upright tilting to +60°, the blood pressure falls, and 1:1 AV conduction develops with rate-dependent right bundle branch block (left). After propranolol, passive upright tilting fails to provoke 1:1 AV conduction. Reproduced with permission from Waxman MB et al. Cardiol Clin. 1983;00:000–000.*

Brief Disturbances in Autonomic Tone May Have Long-Lasting Effects on a Tachycardia

The initial changes in blood pressure and sympathetic tone at the onset of a tachycardia can cause long-lasting changes in autonomic tone.[22] This is illustrated in a patient with paroxysmal supraventricular tachycardia in whom the increased sympathetic tone at the onset of a tachycardia keeps the rate very high (Fig 11). In this patient, paroxysmal supraventricular tachycardia at 200 beats per minute was initiated by a premature atrial beat, and the blood pressure fell markedly (systolic blood pressure, 30 mm Hg).

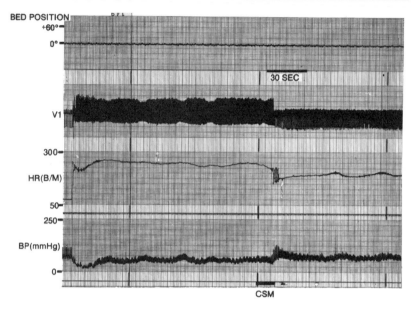

FIGURE 11. *Simultaneous recording of surface ECG lead V_1, beat-to-beat heart rate in beats per minute [HR(B/M)], and blood pressure (BP) from a patient with recurrent paroxysmal supraventricular tachycardia. A single premature atrial starts the tachycardia, and its initial rate is 200 beats per minute. There is considerable hypotension, and the rate rises to 260 beats per minute while the blood pressure recovers modestly. Carotid sinus massage (CSM) causes a dramatic reduction in the rate; this is accompanied by a considerable augmentation in blood pressure. The fall in the heart rate and the increase in the blood pressure persisted indefinitely. Reproduced with permission from Reference 22.*

Sympathetic tone was activated, the tachycardia accelerated to 260 beats per minute, and the blood pressure recovered modestly. However, the very high tachycardia rate prevented the systolic blood pressure from rising above 75 mm Hg, and the persistent hypotension maintained high sympathetic tone. Thus, the high rate and low blood pressure were linked in a positive feedback loop. Carotid sinus massage slowed the tachycardia rate to 200 beats per minute, and although sympathetic tone was probably reduced by the maneuver itself, the blood pressure actually rose. The slowing persisted indefinitely, even though the neural effects of carotid sinus massage lasted for only several seconds. The slowing of the rate allowed the cardiac output and blood pressure to rise and allowed the sympathetic tone to remain lower. As a consequence, the tachycardia rate did not reaccelerate, and in turn, this allowed the blood pressure to stay higher.

Tachycardia Transformation

Transformation of Paroxysmal Supraventricular Tachycardia to Atrial Fibrillation

Individuals suffering from paroxysmal supraventricular tachycardia may also experience episodes of atrial fibrillation. This is particularly well appreciated in patients with Wolff-Parkinson-White syndrome, since the transformation of paroxysmal supraventricular tachycardia to atrial fibrillation may result in a rapid ventricular rate and ventricular fibrillation.[93] The mechanism of this transformation, particularly in patients with Wolff-Parkinson-White syndrome, is thus of more than academic interest. If the transformation from supraventricular tachycardia to atrial fibrillation is in some way connected mechanistically, then one expects that ablating the bypass tract will not only cure the supraventricular tachycardia but also eliminate the transformation to atrial fibrillation. Conversely, if the atrial fibrillation develops by a different mechanism, possibly as a consequence of atrial disease, then interruption of the bypass tract would not be expected to affect the recurrence rate of atrial fibrillation. Surgical ablation of accessory AV bypass tract reduces the likelihood of recurrence of atrial fibrillation in most patients with the Wolff-Parkinson-White syndrome.[94] This supports the concept that atrial fibrillation may develop by a mechanism of transformation from paroxysmal supraventricular tachycardia, possibly as a result of a neural reflex.[11]

As has been stated, the period immediately following the onset of the tachycardia is accompanied by marked hypotension and intense sympathetic compensation to restore the blood pressure. The rise in sympathetic tone inevitably facilitates AV node conduction, and this accelerates that tachycardia rate at the same time as the blood pressure is being restored. It is during this phase of tachycardia acceleration that we have observed the transformation of supraventricular tachycardia to atrial fibrillation. Interventions that reduce the rate of supraventricular tachycardia or reduce the reflex response to the tachycardia inhibit the transformation to atrial fibrillation. Specifically, we studied a group of individuals who exhibited transformation of supraventricular tachycardia to atrial fibrillation before and after the administration of propranolol[11,22] and found that propranolol blocks this transformation (Fig 6).

On the basis of these observations, we hypothesized that the transformation of supraventricular tachycardia to atrial fibrillation is secondary to the large rate increase during the tachycardia. In support of this concept, we have observed that one can induce atrial fibrillation in the same individuals by other maneuvers that activate the adrenergic system and raise the rate of the supraventricular tachycardia.[22] Thus, in cases in which atrial fibrillation does not develop spontaneously, reflex increases in adrenergic tone may induce atrial fibrillation.

Transformation of Atrial Flutter to Fibrillation

Vagotonic maneuvers can occasionally transform atrial flutter to atrial fibrillation.[20] The mechanism of this transformation may be similar to the process whereby increased vagal tone induces atrial fibrillation directly from sinus rhythm. The electrophysiological basis for this observation may be related to the uneven distribution of vagal input to the atria, which increases the dispersion of atrial refractoriness, combined with a marked shortening of atrial refractoriness.[28]

Spontaneous Termination of Supraventricular Tachycardia

The reflex neural effects following the onset of a tachycardia are responsible for spontaneous early termination of paroxysmal supraventricular tachycardia.[24] In 20 patients with paroxysmal supraventricular tachycardia, we found nine individuals in whom the tachycardia consistently terminated spontaneously within a mean of 28 ± 5 seconds after its onset. The mechanism was due to reflex changes in autonomic tone. The onset of the tachycardia causes hypotension, which activates an increase in sympathetic tone. Initially this results in enhanced AV nodal conduction time, and the tachycardia rate increases. At the same time, the increased sympathetic tone restores the blood pressure to or even above control values. The blood pressure elevation then stimulates the baroreceptors, which in turn increase efferent vagal tone; the latter depresses conduction in the AV node, and the tachycardia slows and then terminates (Fig 12).[24] Activation of vagal tone is the essential final mechanism responsible for spontaneous termination of tachycardia. Pretreatment with atropine prevented the spontaneous termination of tachycardia without interfering with the blood pressure recovery.

Cardiac adrenergic responsiveness to the tachycardia was another essential component of spontaneous termination of paroxysmal supraventricular tachycardia, since β-adrenergic receptor blockade inhibits spontaneous reflex termination.[24] β-Adrenergic receptor blocking drugs inhibited spontaneous termination by two mechanisms. In some, propranolol greatly slowed the rate of the induced tachycardia. Therefore, the initial hypotension at the onset of tachycardia was blunted; as a consequence, there was a minimal rise of sympathetic tone, and the tachycardia did not terminate spontaneously (Fig 13, panels 6 and 7). This is analogous to inhibition of spontaneous termination of paroxysmal supraventricular tachycardia after patients are placed in a head-dependent position of $-20°$, thereby reducing background sympathetic tone (Fig 13, panels 4 and 5). Thus, the result following propranolol is almost identical to that seen when patients are at $-20°$ (Fig 13, compare panels 6 and 7 with panels 4 and 5). These observations suggest that an important mechanism by which propranolol blocks spontaneous termination of supraventricular tachycardia is by reducing the initial rate of the tachycardia, thereby decreasing the initial hypotensive stimulus necessary for the augmentation of sympathetic tone. Other studies have found that α-adrenergic activation is central to the recovery of the blood pressure in cases of ventricular tachycardia.[95]

In other cases, β-adrenergic receptor blockade inhibited spontaneous termination of the tachycardia by a second mechanism (Fig 14). In these patients, treatment with propranolol did not significantly reduce the initial rate of the tachycardia, but it slowed the rate of recovery of blood pressure, which in turn led to an insufficient activation of vagal tone.[25] The tachycardia failed to spontaneously terminate in these cases, undoubtedly because of a decreased cardiac contractile response to augmented adrenergic

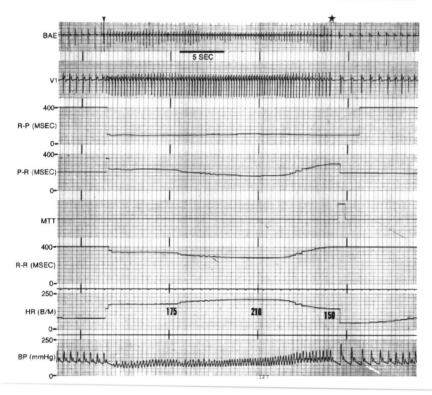

FIGURE 12. *Autonomic reflex response following the onset of tachycardia. Simultaneous recording of bipolar atrial electrogram (BAE) lead V_1, retrograde V-A conduction time (R-P), antegrade AV conduction time (P-R), mode of tachycardia termination (MTT), RR interval beat-to-beat heart rate in beats per minute [HR(B/M)] and blood pressure (PB) in a patient with a concealed left-sided bypass tract. At the arrow, paroxysmal supraventricular tachycardia at a rate of 175 beats per minute is started by a premature atrial stimulus, and the blood pressure falls to 75 mm Hg. Within several seconds, sympathetic tone begins to increase; this accelerates the tachycardia to 210 beats per minute and elevates the blood pressure above control values. This augments vagal tone, which slows the tachycardia to 150 beats per minute, and it then terminates. The changes in rate are all traceable to alterations in AV node conduction time (P-R), while bypass tract conduction time (R-P) remains constant. Since the tachycardia terminates due to block in the AV node, it ends with a P wave (see star), and the MTT circuit exerts a positive pulse to denote this. Reproduced with permission from Reference 24.*

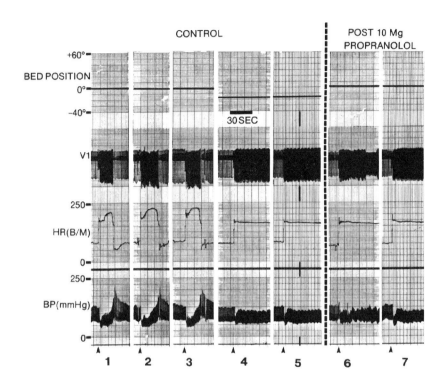

FIGURE 13. *Simultaneous recording of bed position, ECG lead V_1, beat-to-beat heart rate in beats per minute [HR(B/M)], and blood pressure (BP) from a patient with paroxysmal supraventricular tachycardia. During control conditions (panels 1–3), three episodes of tachycardia are initiated at 0°. Each episode causes considerable hypotension, but the blood pressure recovers sufficiently to cause reflex termination of the tachycardia within 30 seconds or less in each case. In panels 4 and 5, two episodes of tachycardia induced after the patient is placed in a head-dependent position of − 20° exhibit a considerably slower rate of 170 beats per minute. The accompanying hypotension is considerably less severe, and the tachycardia no longer terminates spontaneously. In panels 6 and 7, supraventricular tachycardia is initiated after 10 mg of propranolol, and the rate of the tachycardia slows to 170 beats per minute. The hypotension is less pronounced compared with the control record, and the tachycardias do not terminate spontaneously. Reproduced with permission from Reference 24.*

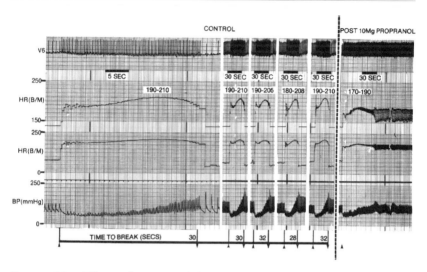

FIGURE 14. *Effects of propranolol on spontaneous termination of paroxysmal supraventricular tachycardia. Simultaneous recordings of lead V$_6$, beat-to-beat heart rate in beats per minute [HR(B/M)] on two scales, and blood pressure (BP) during six episodes of tachycardia. The upgoing arrows denote the premature stimuli that start the tachycardias, and the downgoing arrows signal the moment of spontaneous termination. The numbers at the bottom denote the times at which spontaneous termination occurs. Each episode of tachycardia is accompanied by a large fall in blood pressure, which quickly begins to recover. As pressure recovery is taking place, the tachycardia accelerates, and each panel contains the initial and maximum rates. In all five episodes during control conditions, the tachycardia slows and terminates when the blood pressure exceeds initial values. After propranolol during a sixth episode of tachycardia, the recovery of blood pressure is greatly slowed, and thus, the episode does not end. Marked RR interval alternans is seen once the pressure recovers. Reproduced with permission from Reference 24.*

tone.[96] Thus, propranolol inhibits spontaneous reflex termination of paroxysmal supraventricular tachycardia by reducing the initial afferent stimulus needed to activate sympathetic tone (secondary to tachycardia slowing) and by reducing the effectiveness of the efferent increase in sympathetic tone.

The reflex neural mechanism responsible for early spontaneous termination of paroxysmal supraventricular tachycardia is summarized in Fig 15. The hypotensive stimulus following the onset of tachycardia reduces vagal tone and augments β-adrenergic tone. These effects cause the heart rate and blood pressure to rise. When the blood pressure exceeds pretachycardia levels, the baroreceptors are stimulated; this leads to increased vagal tone and reduced β-adrenergic tone. If the rise in vagal tone is sufficient, the tachycardia slows and terminates. Peripheral α-adrenergic tone also rises,

MECHANISM OF SPONTANEOUS TERMINATION OF PSVT

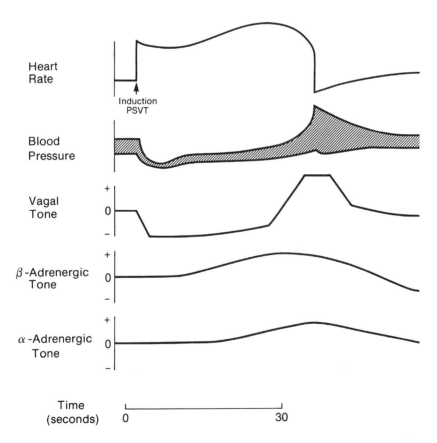

FIGURE 15. *Summary of the reflex neural mechanism responsible for early spontaneous termination of paroxysmal supraventricular tachycardia (PSVT). Reproduced with permission from Reference 24.*

but this aspect was not examined in this study.[24] One can draw an analogy between the mechanism of spontaneous termination of supraventricular tachycardia[24] and the reflex changes that follow a Valsalva maneuver.[27] The blood pressure recovery following Valsalva maneuver resembles the blood pressure recovery in cases of paroxysmal supraventricular tachycardia with spontaneous termination. If the tachycardia fails to terminate spontaneously, the arrhythmia stabilizes and may continue indefinitely until its equilibrium is disturbed. A Valsalva maneuver can cause such a disturbance. By inhibiting the return of blood to the heart, the Valsalva maneuver activates powerful sympathetic reflexes that in turn cause an overshoot in the blood pressure after release of the strain phase, and this can terminate the tachycardia (see Fig 1).[23]

Conclusions

It is obvious that autonomic tone may be instrumental in initiating, accelerating, transforming, and ultimately terminating certain supraventricular tachycardias. The mechanisms of interaction between the autonomic nervous system and supraventricular tachycardias vary with different arrhythmias, age, and cardiac function. In addressing these mechanisms of action, one must consider that the effects of the autonomic nervous system on cardiac arrhythmias are mediated through alterations in heart rate, blood pressure, contractility, and cardiac dimensions as well as the direct electrophysiological effects of neurotransmitters.

References

1. Cohn AE, Fraser FR. Paroxysmal tachycardia and the effect of stimulation of the vagus nerves by pressure. *Heart* 1913–1914;5:93–108.
2. Bensen. Ein Fall Innervationsstörung des Herzens. *Berl Klin Wochenschr.* 1880;17:248–249.
3. Preisendorff P. Ueber reflektorische Vagusneurose. *Dtsch Archiv F Klin Med.* 1880;17:387–388.
4. Wolff L, Parkinson J, White PD. Bundle-branch block with short P-R interval in healthy young people prone to paroxysmal tachycardia. *Am Heart J.* 1930;5:684–704.

5. Waxman MB, Bonet JF, Finley JP, Wald RW. Effects of respiration and posture in paroxysmal supraventricular tachycardia. *Circulation.* 1980;62:1011–1120.

6. Waxman M, Wald RW, Cameron DA. The effects of autonomic tone on supraventricular tachycardias. In: Zipes DP, Jalife J, eds. *Cardiac Electrophysiology: From Cell to Beside.* 2nd ed. Philadelphia, Pa: WB Saunders Co., 1993.

7. Waxman MB, Downar E, Berman ND, Felderhoff CH. Phenylephrine (neosynephrine) terminated ventricular tachycardia. *Circulation.* 1974;50:656–664.

8. Waxman MB, Wald RW. Termination of ventricular tachycardia by an increase in cardiac vagal drive. *Circulation.* 1977;56:385–391.

9. Waxman MB, Wald W, Finley JP, Bonet JF, Downar E, Sharma AD: Valsalva termination of ventricular tachycardia. *Circulation.* 1980;62:843–851.

10. Waxman MB, Staniloff H, Wald RW: Respiratory and vagal modulation of ventricular tachycardia. *J Electrocardiol.* 1981;14:83–90.

11. Waxman MB, Cameron DA, Wald RW. Interactions between the autonomic nervous system and tachycardias in man. In: Zipes DP, ed. *Cardiology Clinics, Arrhythmias, II.* Philadelphia, Pa: WB Saunders Co; 1983:143–185.

12. Waxman MB, Wald RW. The effects of autonomic tone on tachycardias. In: Surawicz B, Reddy CP, Prystowsky EN, eds. *Tachycardias.* Boston, Mass: Martinus Nijhof; 1984:67–102.

13. Waxman M, Sharma AD, Lascault GR, Cameron DA, Wald RW. The protective effect of vagus nerve stimulation on catecholamine-halothane induced ventricular fibrillation in dogs. *Can J Physiol Pharmacol.* 1989;67:801–809.

14. Waxman MB, Cameron DA, Wald RW. The effects of vagal tone on ventricular tachyarrhythmias. In: Levy M, Schwartz P, eds. *Vagal Control of the Heart.* Mt Kisco, NY: Futura Publishing Co; 1993.

15. Corr PB, Yamada KA, Witkowski FX. Mechanisms controlling cardiac autonomic function and their relation to arrhythmogenesis. In: Fozzard HA, Haber E, Jennings RB, Katz AM, Morgan HE, eds. *The Heart and Cardiovascular System.* New York, NY: Raven Press; 1986:1343–1403.

16. Randall WC, Ardell JL. Nervous control of the heart: anatomy and pathophysiology. In: Zipes DP, Jalife J, eds. *Cardiac Electrophysiology: From Cell to Bedside.* Philadelphia, Pa: WB Saunders Co; 1990:291–299.

17. Eckberg DL, Sleight P. *Human Baroreflexes in Health and Disease.* Oxford, UK: Oxford University Press; 1992.

18. Coleridge JCG, Coleridge HM. Chemoreflex regulation of the heart. In: Berne RM, Sperelakis N, Geiger SR, eds. *Handbook of Physiology, sec 2, The Cardiovascular System.* Bethesda, Md: American Physiological Society; 1979; 1: chap 18.

19. Hainsworth R. Reflexes from the heart. *Physiol Rev* 1991;71:617–658.

20. Waxman MB, Cameron DA, Wald RW, Lascault GR. The use of autonomic maneuvers for diagnosis and treatment of cardiac arrhythmias.

In: Wagner GS, Waugh RA, Ramo BW, eds. *Cardiac Arrhythmias.* New York, NY: Churchill Livingstone: 1983:57–108.

21. Abboud FM, Thames MD. Interaction of cardiovascular reflexes in circulatory control. In: Shepherd JT, Abboud FM, eds. *Handbook of Physiology: Periperal Circulation and Organ Blood Flow, sec 2, The Cardiovascular System.* Bethesda, Md: American Physiological Society; 1983: 675–753.

22. Waxman MB, Cameron DA. The reflex effects of tachycardias on autonomic tone. *Ann N Y Acad Sci.* 1990;601;378–393.

23. Waxman MB, Wald RW, Sharma AD, et al. Vagal techniques for termination of paroxysmal supraventricular tachycardia. *Am J Cardiol.* 1980;46:655–664.

24. Waxman MB, Sharma AD, Cameron DA, et al. Reflex mechanisms responsible for early spontaneous termination of paroxysmal supraventricular tachycardia. *Am J Cardiol.* 1982;49:259–272.

25. Koizumi K, Terui N, Kollai M. Neural control of the heart: significance of double innervation reexamined. *J Auton Nerv Syst.* 1983;7:279–294.

26. Levy MN, Zieske H. Autonomic control of cardiac pacemaker activity and atrioventricular transmission. *J Appl Physiol* 1969;27:465–470.

27. Eckberg DL. Parasympathetic cardiovascular control in human disease: a critical review of methods and results. *Am J Physiol* 1980;239:H581–H593.

28. Allessi R, Nusynowitz M, Abildskov JA, et al. Nonuniform distribution of vagal effects on the atrial refractory period. *Am J Physiol* 1958;194:406–410.

29. Vatner SF, Pagani M, Rutherford JD, Millard RW, Manders TW. Effects of nitroglycerine on cardiac function and regional blood flow distribution in conscious dogs. *Am J Physiol* 1978;234:H242–H244.

30. Wang SC, Borison HL. Decussation of the pathways in the carotid sinus cardiovasvular reflex: an example of the principle of convergence. *Am J Physiol* 1947;150:722–728.

31. Brown KA, Maloney JD, Smith HC, Hartzler GO, Ilstrup DM. Carotid sinus reflex in patients undergoing coronary angiography: relationship of degree and location of coronary artery disease to response to carotid sinus massage. *Circulation* 1980;62:697–703.

32. Day MD. Anticholinesterase agents. In: *Autonomic Pharmacology.* Edinburgh, Scotland. Churchill and Livingstone; 1979:53–64.

33. Sharpey-Schafer EP. Effect of respiratory acts on the circulation. In: Hamilton WF, Dow P, eds. *Handbook of Physiology.* Washington, DC: Am Physiological Society; 1965; 3:1875–1886.

34. Kalser MH, Frye CW, Gordon AS. Postural hypotension induced by atropine sulphate. *Circulation.* 1954;10:413–422.

35. Brown AM. Cardiac sympathetic adrenergic pathways in which synaptic transmission is blocked by atropine sulphate. *J Physiol (Lond).* 1967;191;271–288.

36. Langer SZ. Presynaptic regulation of the release of catecholamines. *Pharmacol Rev.* 1981;32:337–361.

37. Elisberg EI. Heart rate response to the Valsalva maneuver as a test of circulatory integrity. *JAMA.* 1963;186:200–205.

38. Lima JAC, Weiss JL, Guzman PA, Weisfeldt ML, Reid PR, Traill A: Incomplete filling and incoordinate contraction as mechanisms of hypotension during ventricular tachycardia in man. *Circulation.* 1983;68:928–938.
39. Fifer MA, Bourdillon PD, Lorell BH. Altered left ventricular diastolic properties during pacing induced angina in patients with aortic stenosis. *Circulation.* 1986;74:675–683.
40. Chidsey CA, Braunwald E. Sympathetic activity and neurotransmitter depletion in congestive heart failure. *Pharmacol Rev.* 1966;18:685–700.
41. Bristow MR, Ginsburg R, Umans V, Fowler M, Minobe W, Rasmussen R, Zera P, Menlove R, Shah P, Jamieson S, Stinson EB: β_1-β_2-Adrenergic-receptor subpopulations in nonfailing and failing human ventricular myocardium: coupling of both receptor subtypes to muscle contraction and selective β_1-receptor down-regulation in heart failure. *Circ Res.* 1986;59:297–309.
42. Levy MN, Blattberg B. Effect of vagal stimulation on the overflow of norepinephrine into the coronary sinus during cardiac sympathetic nerve stimulation in the dog. *Circ Res.* 1976;38:81–85.
43. Potter EK. Presynaptic inhibition of cardiac vagal postganglionic nerves by neuropeptide Y. *Neurosci Lett.* 1987;83:101–106.
44. McGratten PA, Brown JH, Brown OM. Parasympathetic effects on in vivo rat heart can be regulated through an α_1-adrenergic receptor. *Circ Res.* 1987;60:465–471.
45. Brown JH. Cholinergic inhibition of catecholamine-stimulable cyclic AMP accumulation in murine atria. *J Cyclic Nucleotide Res.* 1979;5:423–433.
46. Han J, Moe GK: Non uniform recovery of excitability in ventricular muscle. *Circ Res.* 1964;14:44–60.
47. Han J, Darcia de Jalon PD, Moe GK. Adrenergic effects on ventricular vulnerability. *Circ Res.* 1964;14:516–524.
48. Vatner SF. Sympathetic mechanisms regulating myocardial contractility in conscious animals. In: Fozzard HA, Haber E, Jennings RB, Katz AM, Morgan HE, eds. *Heart and Cardiovascular System.* 2nd ed. New York, NY: Raven Press Ltd; 1992; chap 67.
49. Coumel P, Friocourt P, Mugica J, Attuel P, Leclercq JF. Long-term prevention of vagal atrial arrhythmias by atrial pacing at 90/minute:experience with 6 cases. *PACE Pacing Clin Electrophysiol.* 1983;6:552–560.
50. Brandt J, Anderson H, Faraeus T, Schuller H. Natural history of sinus node disease treated with atrial pacing in 213 patients: implications for selection of stimulation mode. *J Am Coll Cardiol.* 1992;20:633–639.
51. Moe GK. Evidence for reentry as a mechanism of cardiac arrhythmias. *Rev Physiol Biochem Pharmacol* 1975;72:56–81.
52. Nadeau RA, Roberge FA, Billette J. Role of the sinus node in the mechanism of cholinergic atrial fibrillation. *Circ Res.* 1970;27:129–138.
53. Dresel PE, Sutter MC. Factors modifying cyclopropane-epinephrine cardiac arrhythmias. *Circ Res.* 1961;9:1284–1290.
54. Waxman MB, Kirsh JA, Cameron DA, Wald RW. The mechanism of flutter interval alternans. *PACE Pacing Clin Electrophysiol.* 1990;13:138–143.

55. Waxman MB, Yao L, Cameron DA, Kirsh JA. Effect of posture, the Valsalva maneuver and respiration on atrial flutter rate: an effect mediated through cardiac volume. *J Am Coll Cardiol.* 1991;17:1545–1552.
56. Waxman MB, Kirsh JA, Cameron DA, Asta JA, Yao L. Slowing of the atrial flutter rate during 1:1 atrioventricular conduction in humans and dogs: an effect mediated through atrial pressure and volume. *J Cardiovasc Electrophysiol.* 1992;3:101–114.
57. Lammers WJEP, Ravelli F, Disertori M, Antolini R, Furlanello F, Allessie MA. Variations in human atrial flutter cycle length induced by ventricular beats: evidence of a reentrant circuit with a partially excitable gap. *J Cardiovasc Electrophysiol.* 1991;2:375–387.
58. Klein LS, Miles WM, Zipes DP. Effect of atrioventricular interval during pacing or reciprocating tachycardia on atrial size, pressure, and refractory period: contraction-excitation feedback in human atrium. *Circulation.* 1990;82:60–68.
59. Rankin AC, Goldroyd KG, Chong E, Cobbe SM. Value and limitations of adenosine in the diagnosis of narrow and broad complex tachycardias. *Br J Heart J.* 1989;62:195–203.
60. Burn JH, Vaughan Williams EM, Walker JM. Effects of acetylcholine in heart-lung preparations including the production of auricular fibrillation. *J Physiol.* 1955;128:277–293.
61. Wang J, Bourne GW, Wang Z, Villemaire C, Talajic M, Nattel S.Comparative mechanism of antiarrhythmic drug action in experimental atrial fibrillation: importance of use-dependent effects of refractoriness. *Circulation.* 1993;88:1030–1044.
62. Page PL, Hassanalizadeli H, Cardinal R. Transitions among atrial fibrillation, atrial flutter, and sinus rhythm during procainamide infusion and vagal stimulation in dogs with sterile pericarditis. *Can J Physiol Pharmacol.* 1991;69:15–24.
63. Coumel P. Neural aspects of paroxysmal atrial fibrillation. In: Falk RH, Prodrid PJ, eds. *Atrial Fibrillation: Mechanisms and Management.* New York, NY: Raven Press; chap 7.
64. Allessie MA, Lammers WJ, Bonke IM, Hollen J. Intra-atrial reentry as a mechanism for atrial flutter induced by acetylcholine and rapid pacing in the dog. *Circulation.* 1984;70:123–135.
65. Spear JF, Kronhaus KD, Moore EN, Klein RP. The effect of brief vagal stimulation on the isolated rabbit sinus node. *Circ Res.* 1979;44:75–88.
66. Burgen ASV, Terroux KG. On the negative inotropic effect in cat's auricle. *J Physiol (Lond).* 1953;120:449–464.
67. Boyden PA, Hoffman BF. The effects on atrial electrophysiology and structure of surgically induced right atrial enlargement in dog. *Circ Res.* 1981;49:1319–1331.
68. Guilleminault C, Connolly SJ, Winkle RA. Cardiac arrhythmias and conduction disturbances during sleep in 400 patients with sleep apnea syndrome. *Am J Cardiol.* 1983;52:490.
69. Nguyen NX, Yang P-T, Huycke EC, Keung EC, Deedwania P, Sund RJ. Effects of beta-adrenergic stimulation on atrial latency and atrial vulnerability in patients with paroxysmal supraventricular tachycardia. Am J Cardiol. 1988;61:1031–1036.

70. Murgatroyd FD, Camm AJ. Sinus rhythm, the autonomic nervous system and quality of life. In: Kingma JH, van Hemel NM, Lie KL. *Atrial Fibrillation, A Treatable Disease?* Netherlands: Klewer Academic Publishers; 1992:195–210.

71. Waxman MP, Cupps CI. Spontaneous termination of paroxysmal supraventricular tachycardia following disappearance of bundle branch block ipsilateral to a concealed atrioventricular accessory pathway: the role of autonomic tone in tachycardia diagnosis. *PACE Pacing Clin Electrophysiol.* 1986;9:26–35.

72. Brownstein SL, Hopson RC, Martins JV, Aschoff AM, Olshansky B, Constantin L, Kienzel MG. Usefulness of isoproterenol in facilitating atrial ventricular nodal re-entry tachyardia during electrophysiologic testing. *Am J Cardiol.* 1988;61:1037–1041.

73. Brembilla-Perrot B, Terrier de la Chaise A, Pichene MF, Aliot E, Cherrier F, Pernot C. Isoprenaline as an aid to the induction of catecholamine dependent supraventricular tachycardias during programmed stimulation. *Br Heart J* 1989;61:348–355.

74. Mann DE, Raiter MJ. Effects of upright posture on atrial ventricular nodal re-entry and dual atrial ventricular nodal pathways. *Am J Cardiol.* 1988;62:408–412.

75. Wu D, Denes P, Bauernfeind R, Dhingra RC, Wyndham C, Rosen KM. Effects of atropine on production and maintenance of atrial ventricular nodal re-entrant tachycardia. *Circulation.* 1979;59:779–788.

76. Akhtar M, Damato AN, Batsford OUP, Caracta AR, Ruskin JN, Weisfogel GM, Lau SH: Induction of atrial ventricular nodal re-entrant tachycardia after atropine: report of five cases. *Am J Cardiol.* 1975;36:286–291.

77. Waxman MB, Wald RW McGillivray R, Cameron DA, Sharma AD, Huerta F. Continuous on-line beat to beat analysis of AV conduction. *PACE Pacing Clin Electrophysiol.* 1981;4:262–273.

78. Freeman GL, Little WC, O'Rourke RA. Influence of heart rate on left ventricular performance in conscious dogs. *Circ Res.* 1987;61:455–464.

79. Schlepper M, Weppner HG, Merle H. Hemodynamic effects of supraventricular tachycardias and their alteration by electrically and verapamil induced termination. *Cardiovasc Res.* 1978;12:28–33.

80. Linderer T, Chatterjee K, Parmley WW, Sievers RE, Glantz SA, Tyberg JV. Influence of atrial systole on the Frank-Starling relation and the end-diastolic pressure-diameter relation of the left ventricle. *Circulation.* 1983;67:1045–1053.

81. Thoren P. Role of cardiac vagal C-fibers in cardiovascular control. *Rev Physiol Biochem Pharmacol.* 1979;86:1–94.

82. Waxman MB, Yao L, Cameron DA, Wald RW, Roseman J. Isoproterenol induction of vasodepressor-type reaction in vasodepressor-prone persons. *Am J Cardiol.* 1989;63:58–65.

83. Sharpe-Schafer EP, Hayter CJ, Barlow ED. Mechanism of acute hypotension from fear or nausea. *Br Med J.* 1958;2:878–880.

84. Oberg B, Thoren P. Increased activity in left ventricular receptors during hemorrhage or occlusion of caval veins in the cat: a possible cause of vasovagal reaction. *Acta Physiol Scand.* 1972;85:164–173.

85. Waxman MB, Cameron DA, Wald RW. The role of ventricular afferents in the vasovagal reaction. *J Am Coll Cardiol.* 1993;21:1138–1141.
86. Waxman MB, Asta JA, Cameron DA. Vasodepressor reaction induced by inferior vena cava occlusion and isoproterenol. *Can J Physiol Pharmacol.* 1992;70:872–881.
87. Waxman MB, Asta JA, Cameron DA. Localization of the reflex pathway responsible for the vasodepressor reactor induced by inferior vena cava occlusion and isoproterenol. *Can J Physiol Pharmacol.* 1992;70:882–889.
88. Tikkanen I, Metsarinne K, Fyhrquist F. Atrial natriuretic peptide in paroxysmal supraventricular tachycardia. *Lancet.* 1985;2:40–41.
89. Maack T, Kleinert HD. Renal and cardiovascular effects of atrial natriuretic factor. *Biochem Pharmacol.* 1987;35:2057–2064.
90. Wu D. Dual atrioventricular nodal pathways: a reappraisal. *PACE Pacing Clin Electrophysiol.* 1982;5:72–89.
91. Burke D, Sundlof G, Wallin BG. Postural effects on muscle nerve sympathetic activity in man. *J Physiol.* 1977;272:399–414.
92. Szabo TS, Klein GJ, Sharma AD, Yee R, Milstein S. Usefulness of isoproterenol during atrial fibrillation in evaluation of asymptomatic Wolff-Parkinson-White pattern. *Am J Cardiol.* 1989;63:187–192.
93. Klein GJ, Bashore TM, Sellers TD, Pritchett ELC, Smith WM, Gallagher JJ. Ventricular fibrillation in the Wolff-Parkinson-White syndrome. *N Engl J Med.* 1979;301:1080–1085.
94. Chen PS, Pressley JC, Tang ASL, Packer DL, Gallagher JJ, Prystowski EN. New observations on atrial fibrillation before and after surgical treatment in patients with the Wolff-Parkinson-White syndrome. *J Am Coll Cardiol.* 1992;19:974–981.
95. Ellenbogen KA, Smith ML, Thames MD, Mohanty PK. Changes in regional adrenergic tone during sustained ventricular tachycardia associated with coronary artery disease or idiopathic dilated cardiomyopathy. *Am J Cardiol.* 1990;65:1334–1338.
96. Feldman T, Carroll JD, Munkenbeck F, Alibali P, Feldman M, Coggins DL, Gray KR, Bump T. Hemodynamic recovery during simulated ventricular tachycardia: role of adrenergic receptor activation. *Am Heart J* 1983;115:576–587.

Chapter 2

Editorial Comments

Douglas P. Zipes, MD

Waxman[1], et al, in their fine review on the role of the autonomic nervous system (ANS) in atrial arrhythmias, provides a brief discussion on the physiology of autonomic innervation and a superb summary on how sympathetic and vagal discharge can initiate and terminate supraventricular tachycardias, modulate their rate, and transform one tachycardia into another. The report is an excellent discourse on clinical cardiac electrophysiology and, parenthetically, illustrates how an astute clinician scientist can make important physiological observations in patients.

In this editorial commentary, I would like to enlarge the scope of Waxman's presentation and discuss the role of the ANS and arrhythmogenesis in more general terms. My goal is to provide the clinician with a broader, "user-friendly" framework to illustrate how the ANS can affect arrhythmia development. I structure the discussion about what I descriptively call the four Ps of neurocardiology, explaining how the ANS can *precipitate, promote, prevent,* and *predict* the development of cardiac arrhythmias.

Before I embark on this discussion, it is important to caution that the effects of ANS stimulation can be mediated by multiple processes, including a direct action of the ANS on cardiac excitable properties such as conduction, refractoriness, and automaticity[2] and indirect effects on myocardial and coronary blood flow, myocardial metabolism, platelet adhesiveness, development of oxygen free radicals, and so forth.[3-5] Often the precise mechanisms by which the ANS acts can only be conjectured for many clinically occurring arrhythmias.

This study was supported in part by the Herman C. Krannert Fund, Indianapolis: Grants HL-42370 and HL-07182 from the National Heart, Lung and Blood Institute, National Institutes of Health, Bethesda, Maryland; and the American Heart Association, Indiana Affiliate, Indianapolis, Indiana.

From DiMarco JP, Prystowsky EN (eds): *Atrial Arrhythmias: State of the Art.* Armonk, NY, Futura Publishing Company, Inc., © 1995.

Precipitate

This term is used to indicate that the ANS interacts with an apparently normal heart to cause the development of a cardiac arrhythmia. Thus, the substrate (heart) is presumably normal and the trigger is the ANS discharge. Whether the heart is truly totally normal in some of these examples can be questioned,[6] but at least no evidence of structural heart disease can be found with conventional tests in most examples. The ANS may be qualitatively or quantitatively abnormal.

Examples in this category include precipitation of idiopathic atrial[7] and ventricular fibrillation[8,9] and other arrhythmias in patients with normal hearts, hypersensitive carotid syndrome, and vasodepressor syncope.[10] In many of these examples, behavioral or psychological factors such as depression, bereavement,[11] fear, or anger[12] and physical activity known to increase sympathetic discharge while decreasing vagal "tone" can be linked to the precipitating event.

Initiation of atrial fibrillation by autonomic stimulation serves as a good model to illustrate the influence of autonomic modulation. In tachyarrhythmias initiated and maintained by reentry, shortening of the effective refractory period, particularly if it occurs heterogeneously, can precipitate fibrillation.[13] Vagal stimulation causes such heterogeneous shortening of refractoriness in the atria and can incite atrial fibrillation in a completely normal animal, such as the dog. The atrial fibrillation will be sustained for as long as the vagal stimulation continues.[14] This may be the mechanism responsible for atrial fibrillation that occurs during sleep, when vagal "tone" is heightened.[7] The effects of sympathetic stimulation on atrial refractoriness are more complex, since β-adrenegic receptor stimulation shortens refractoriness, whereas α-adrenergic receptor stimulation appears to prolong it.

Interestingly, in a canine model attempting to replicate the maze surgical procedure by radiofrequency ablation, we have found that vagal denervation of the atrium occurs routinely as a consequence of the ablation lesions.[15] It is possible that part of the success of the surgical maze procedure can be attributed to vagal denervation of the atrium. Naturally, mechanisms other than neural, such as atrial stretch, may also be important in heterogeneously altering atrial refractoriness and precipitating atrial fibrillation.[16,17]

Promote

In this category, the ANS interacts with a structurally abnormal heart to cause the development of cardiac arrhythmias. Thus, the substrate is abnormal and is triggered by the ANS, which may be normal or abnormal.

Many arrhythmias exist in this category, probably the most common one including the examples of supraventricular tachycardias Waxman et al noted.[1] In these examples, the abnormal cardiac substrate may be the presence of an accessory pathway, dual atrioventricular nodal inputs, or a dilated atrium. The ANS can also interact with an abnormal ventricular substrate and cause ventricular tachyarrhythmias such as those found in the long-QT syndrome[18] and possibly in left ventricular hypertrophy.[19] The increased incidence of sudden cardiac death, myocardial infarction, and stroke in the morning upon arising[20] may be related to sympathetic discharge interacting with partially obstructed coronary or cerebral arteries. It is well known that the ANS can also directly influence the development of cardiac arrhythmias caused by ischemia and infarction and is in turn modulated by these events, since ischemia and infarction can cause autonomic dysfunction.[21]

Prevent

Alterations in the ANS can preclude the development of cardiac arrhythmias in situations in which the cardiac substrate is either abnormal or normal. This can occur by blockade of the promoting role played by the ANS as well as by a direct action. If, for example, discharge of the ANS is required to cause the onset of the arrhythmia, ANS blockade will prevent the arrhythmia. Conversely, direct ANS discharge can also prevent the development of some arrhythmias.

Examples of prevention of clinically occurring arrhythmias by ANS modulation abound. β-Adrenergic receptor blockade can prevent a host of supraventricular and some ventricular tachyarrhythmias. β-Blockade reduces sudden and total mortality in patients after myocardial infarction. Vagal stimulation appears to prevent some ventricular arrhythmias,[22] particularly those associated with ischemia.[23] α-Adrenergic receptor blockade can prevent reperfusion ventricular arrhythmias in animals[24] and in experimental[25,26] and possibly clinical ventricular arrhythmias[27] associated with the long-QT-interval syndrome. The efficacy of sympathetic neural interruption and β-adrenergic receptor blockade for this syndrome is well established.[18] Autonomic modulation can even come from the pericardium, and experimental examples exist of pericardial prevention of ventricular fibrillation during coronary occlusion-reperfusion and sympathetic stimulation.[28]

Predict

Finally, the ANS can be used to identify individuals at increased risk for developing a cardiac event such as a cardiac arrhythmia by finding the presence of reduced heart rate variability[29,30] or reduced baroreceptor sensitivity.[31]

In summary, the four Ps of neurocardiology provide an easy-to-remember descriptive classification of how the ANS can modulate the development of cardiac arrhythmias. Studies such as those presented by Waxman et al[1] as well as future work will no doubt expose the mechanisms of these interactions, and this will facilitate the choice of very specific ANS interventions in patients with cardiac arrhythmias.

References

1. Waxman MB, Cameron D, Wald RW. The role of the autonomic nervous system in atrial arrhythmias. In: DiMarco JP, Prystowsky EN (eds.) *Atrial Arrhythmias: State of the Art.* Armonk, NY. Futura Publishing Co. 1995.
2. Inoue H, Zipes DP. Changes in atrial and ventricular refractoriness and in atrioventricular nodal conduction produced by combinations of vagal and sympathetic stimulation that result in a constant spontaneous sinus cycle length. *Circ Res.* 1987;60:942–951.
3. Pappano A. Parasympathetic control of cardiac electrical activity. In: Zipes DP, Jalife J, eds. *Cardiac Electrophysiology. From Cell to Bedside.* Baltimore, Md: WB Saunders; 1990
4. Corr PB, Yamada KA, Witkowski FX. Mechanisms controlling cardiac autonomic tone function and their relation to arrhythmogenesis. In:

Fozzard HA, ed. *The Heart and Cardiovascular System.* New York, N.Y., Raven Press, 1986.

5. Randall WC, Ardell JL. Nervous control of the heart: anatomy and pathophysiology. In: Zipes DP, Jalife J, eds. *Cardiac Electrophysiology. From Cell to Bedside.* Baltimore, Md: WB Saunders; 1990:291–299.

6. Mitrani R, Klein LS, Miles WM, Burt RW, Wellman HN, Zipes DP. Regional cardiac sympathetic denervation in patients with ventricular tachycardia in the absence of coronary artery disease. *J Am Coll Cardiol.* 1993;23:1344–1353.

7. Coumel P. Neural aspects of paroxysmal atrial fibrillation. In: Falk RH, Podrid PJ, eds. *Atrial Fibrillation: Mechanisms and Management.* New York, NY: Raven Press; 1992:109–125.

8. Lown B, Temte JV, Reich P, et al. Basis for recurring ventricular fibrillation in the absence of coronary heart disease and its management. *N Engl J Med.* 1976:623–629.

9. Belhassen B, Viskin S. Idiopathic ventricular tachycardia and fibrillation. *J Cardiovasc Electrophysiol.* 1993;4:356–368.

10. Kapoor WN. Evaluation and management of the patient with syncope. *JAMA.* 1992;268:2553–2560.

11. Engel GL. Sudden and rapid death during psychological stress: folk lore or folk wisdom? *Ann Intern Med.* 1971;74:771.

12. Verrier RL, Dickerson LW, Nearing BD. Behavioral states and sudden cardiac death. *PACE Pacing Clin Electrophysiol.* 1992;15:1387–1393.

13. Allessie MA. Reentrant mechanisms in atrial flutter and fibrillation. In: Zipes DP, Jalife J, eds. *Cardiac Electrophysiology. From Cell to Bedside.* Baltimore, Md: WB Saunders; 1994.

14. Zipes DP, Mihalick MJ, Robbins GT. Effects of selective vagal and stellate ganglion stimulation on atrial refractoriness. *Cardiovasc Res.* 1974; 8:647–655.

15. Elvan A, Pride HP, Zipes DP. Replication of the "maze" procedure by radiofrequency catheter ablation reduces the ability to induce atrial fibrillation. *PACE Pacing Clin Electrophysiol.* In press. Abstract.

16. Kaseda S, Zipes DP. Contraction-excitation feedback in the atria: a cause of changes in refractoriness. *J Am Coll Cardiol.* 1988;11:1327–1336.

17. Klein LS, Miles WM, Zipes DP. Effect of the atrioventricular interval during pacing or reciprocating tachycardia on atrial size, pressure and refractory period: contraction-excitation feedback in human atrium. *Circulation.* 1990;82:60–68.

18. Schwartz PJ, Locati E, Priori SG, et al. The long QT syndrome. In: Zipes DP, Jalife J, eds. *Cardiac Electrophysiology. From Cell to Bedside.* Baltimore, Md: WB Saunders; 1994. In press.

19. Ben-David J, Zipes DP, Ayers GM, et al. Canine left ventricular hypertrophy predisposes to ventricular tachycardia induction by phase-2 early afterdepolarizations following BAY K 8644 administration. *J Am Coll Cardiol.* 1992;20:1576–1584.

20. Muller JE, Stone PH, Turi ZG, et al. Circadian variation in the frequency of onset of acute myocardial infarction. *N Engl J Med.* 1985;313: 315.
21. Zipes DP. Influence of myocardial ischemia and infarction on autonomic innervation of the heart. *Circulation* 1990;82:1095–1105.
22. Waxman MB, Sharma AD, Asta J, et al. The protective effect of vagus nerve stimulation on catecholamine-halothane-induced ventricular fibrillation in dogs. *Can J Physiol Pharmacol.* 1988;67:801–809.
23. Hull SS, Vanoli E, Adamson PB, et al. Exercise training confers anticipatory protection from sudden death during acute myocardial ischemia. *Circulation.* 1994;89:548–552.
24. Sheridan BJ, Penkoske PA, Sobel BE, Corr PB. Alpha adrenergic contributions to dysrhythmias during myocardial ischemia and reperfusion in cats. *J Clin Invest.* 1980:65:161–171.
25. Kaseda S, Zipes DP. Effects of alpha adrenoceptor stimulation and blockade on early afterdepolarizations and triggered activity induced by cesium in canine cardiac Purkinje fibers. *J Cardiovasc Electrophysiol.* 1990;1:31–40.
26. Ben-David J, Zipes DP. Alpha adrenoceptor stimulation and blockade modulates cesium-induced early afterdepolarizations and ventricular tachyarrhythmias in dogs. *Circulation.* 1990;82:225–233.
27. Zipes DP. The long QT syndrome: a Rosetta stone for sympathetic related arrhythmias. *Circulation.* 1991;84:1414–1419. Editorial.
28. Miyazaki T, Zipes DP. Pericardial prostaglandin biosynthesis prevents the increased incidence of reperfusion-induced ventricular fibrillation produced by efferent sympathetic stimulation in dogs. *Circulation.* 1990;82:1008–1019.
29. Kleiger RE, Miller JP, Bigger JT Jr, et al. Decreased heart rate variability and its association with increased mortality after acute myocardial infarction. *Am J Cardiol.* 1987;59:256–262.
30. Bigger JT Jr, Fleiss JL, Steinman RC, et al. Frequency domain measures of heart period variability and mortality after myocardial infarction. *Circulation.* 1992;85:164–171.
31. LaRovere MT, Specchia G, Mortara A, et al. Baroreflex sensitivity, clinical correlates, and cardiovascular mortality among patients with a first myocardial infarction. *Circulation.* 1988;78:816–824.

Chapter 3

Tachycardia-Induced Tachycardia: A Mechanism of Initiation of Atrial Fibrillation

Eric N. Prystowsky, MD

Arrhythmias can occur as the result of one tachycardia degenerating into another tachycardia, a phenomenon I refer to as tachycardia-induced tachycardia. Several different arrhythmias can degenerate into atrial fibrillation, atrial flutter possibly being the most common. In this situation, there is usually an intrinsic atrial abnormality. More intriguing is the initiation of atrial fibrillation as a result of a nonatrial tachycardia; for example, degeneration of atrioventricular (AV) reentry into atrial fibrillation (Fig 1). This situation is particularly pernicious in patients in whom a rapid preexcited ventricular response over the accessory pathway leads to another type of tachycardia-induced tachycardia: atrial fibrillation producing ventricular fibrillation (Fig 2).[1-6] Other examples of nonatrial tachycardias initiating atrial fibrillation are AV node reentry (Fig 3)[7] and ventricular tachycardia (Figs 4 and 5).

Potential factors affecting conversion of sustained nonatrial tachycardias to atrial fibrillation include tachycardia cycle length, electrophysiological characteristics of accessory pathways, intrinsic atrial vulnerability, and contraction-excitation feedback. These issues, as well as the problem of sudden cardiac death in patients with Wolff-Parkinson-White (WPW) syndrome, are the subject of this chapter.

From DiMarco JP, Prystowsky EN (eds): *Atrial Arrhythmias: State of the Art.* Armonk, NY, Futura Publishing Company, Inc., © 1995.

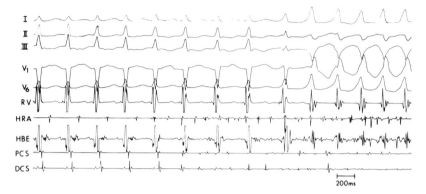

FIGURE 1. *Atrioventricular (AV) reentry degenerating into atrial fibrillation. Simultaneous tracings are ECG leads I, II, III, V_1, and V_6 and intracardiac electrograms from the right ventricle (RV), high right atrium (HRA), His bundle area (HBE), proximal coronary sinus (PCS), and distal coronary sinus (DCS). The left portion of the figure demonstrates AV reentry using a left free wall accessory pathway. Note that the fifth atrial electrogram recorded on the HRA is premature, and shortly thereafter atrial fibrillation is present. The end of the tracing shows wide QRS complexes due to conduction over the left free wall accessory pathway. Note that degeneration of AV reentry into atrial fibrillation appears to occur first in the HRA recording.*

Tachycardia Cycle Length

Many investigators have demonstrated that AV reentry can degenerate into atrial fibrillation.[8–11] Surgical ablation of the accessory pathway precludes AV reentry and also prevents recurrences of atrial fibrillation in almost all of these patients.[10,11] This could be due to factors related to the accessory pathway itself, as discussed subsequently, or to electrophysiological changes in the atrium resulting from AV reentry. Wyndham et al[12] evaluated the effects of atrial paced cycle length on atrial vulnerability in patients without WPW syndrome. Repetitive atrial responses were commonly initiated during the shorter paced cycle length.[12] Thus, one might predict that atrial fibrillation would occur more commonly in patients with faster AV reentrant rates.

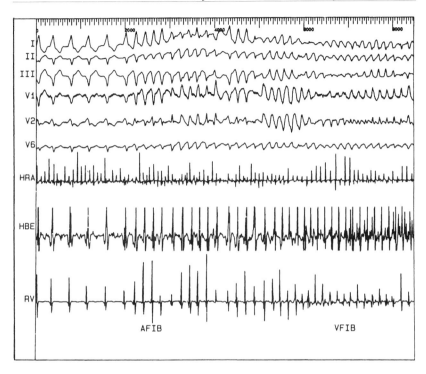

FIGURE 2. *Atrial fibrillation (AFIB) with a rapid preexcited ventricular response that degenerates into ventricular fibrillation (VFIB). Other abbreviations as in Fig 1. Reproduced with permission from Reference 6.*

Sharma et al[11] compared characteristics of 19 patients with WPW syndrome with and without a history of atrial fibrillation. In patients with atrial fibrillation, the cycle length of AV reentry was 307 ± 61 msec compared with 333 ± 34 msec for those without atrial fibrillation. Although the trend was toward a shorter cycle length in patients with atrial fibrillation, this difference was not statistically significant. Chen and associates[10] evaluated electrophysiological characteristics of 342 patients who underwent surgical treatment for WPW syndrome, 166 of whom had a history of atrial fibrillation. The cycle length of AV reentry was 304 ± 42 msec compared with 321 ± 54 msec ($P<.005$) in patients with and without a history of atrial fibrillation, respectively. Spontaneous conversion of AV reentry to atrial fibrillation at electrophysiological study occurred more frequently in patients with (29 of 146, 20%) than without (9 of 116, 5%) a history

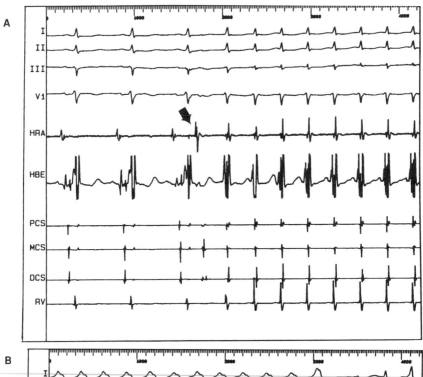

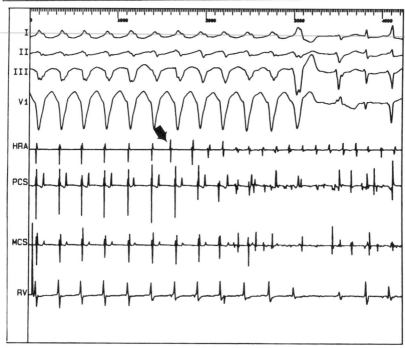

FIGURE 3. *Atrioventricular (AV) node reentry producing atrial fibrillation. A, Premature atrial complex (PAC) (arrow) produces a sudden increase in AV node conduction and initiation of AV node reentry. This PAC blocks over the fast conduction pathway, and anterograde conduction occurs over the slow conduction pathway; subsequent retrograde conduction is over a fast conducting pathway. B, This patient also had AV node reentry with left bundle branch block aberrancy. During this episode of tachycardia, there was degeneration into atrial fibrillation following a PAC from the HRA (arrow). MCS = mid coronary sinus electrogram; other abbreviations as in Fig 1.*

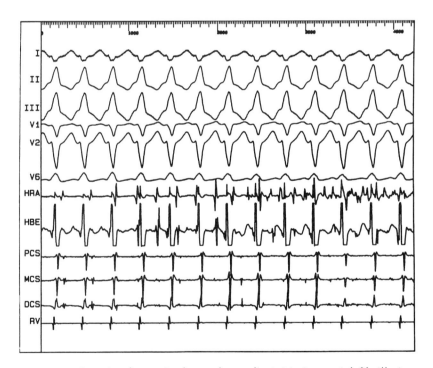

FIGURE 4. *Sustained ventricular tachycardia initiating atrial fibrillation. This patient had normal ventricular function with a right ventricular outflow tract tachycardia. There was 1:1 ventriculoatrial conduction during tachycardia. As clearly demonstrated on the high right atrial (HRA) electrogram, atrial fibrillation occurred during sustained ventricular tachycardia. Other abbreviations as in Figs 1 and 3.*

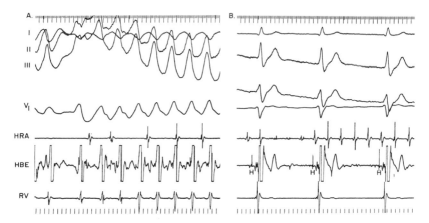

FIGURE 5. *Induction of atrial fibrillation during sustained monomorphic ventricular tachycardia in a patient with ventriculoatrial block. A, This patient had ventriculoatrial block at all paced cycle lengths. During sustained ventricular tachycardia, atrial extrasystoles were noted. B, Atrial fibrillation occurred during ventricular tachycardia and is clearly noted after ventricular tachycardia terminated. Of note, this patient would present to the emergency room with symptoms of tachycardia that caused presyncope. By the time he arrived at the emergency room he always felt better, and atrial fibrillation was the documented arrhythmia. At electrophysiological study, he consistently had atrial fibrillation as a consequence of sustained ventricular tachycardia. Abbreviations as in Fig 1.*

of atrial fibrillation. Further, when atrial fibrillation resulted from AV reentry, the cycle length of AV reentry that degenerated into atrial fibrillation was significantly shorter (289 ± 26 vs 316 ± 51 msec, P<.005). In certain subgroups of patients, however, there was no significant difference between the cycle length of tachycardia in patients with and without atrial fibrillation.

Data from these two studies[10,11] suggest that faster rates of AV reentry appear to predispose to the development of atrial fibrillation. The differences in tachycardia rate in patients with and without atrial fibrillation in these studies is not that striking and may be related to the referral bias at both institutions. Regardless, in our experience it is extremely uncommon to observe degeneration of AV reentry into atrial fibrillation at electrophysiological study in patients with relatively slow AV reentry, eg, 150 beats per minute. Electrophysiological changes in the atria that occur during AV reentry may also be caused by hemodynamic factors, as discussed below.

Tachycardia-induced tachycardia is also a mechanism to produce atrial fibrillation in patients with AV node reentry.[7] In patients with documentation of both arrhythmias, the rate of AV node reentry is typically relatively rapid (Fig 3). AV node reentry is a relatively common arrhythmia that is frequently studied in the electrophysiology laboratory. Regardless, few data have been reported on the occurrence of atrial fibrillation in patients with AV node reentry. Further, transition of AV node reentry into atrial fibrillation at electrophysiological study has been a relatively rare observation in our experience. This could be due, in part, to differences in tachycardia rate between AV and AV node reentries. For example, Wathen et al[13] reported a mean cycle length of 390 ± 75 msec for AV node reentry. In contrast, the cycle length of AV node reentry was 338 ± 70[14] and 328 ± 53 msec[15] in other studies.

If we assume, for the sake of discussion, that differences in tachycardia cycle length are not that dissimilar in patients referred for AV and AV node reentries, then alternative factors should be considered to explain the apparently increased frequency of atrial fibrillation in patients with WPW syndrome. Two possible factors are (1) contributions of the accessory pathway per se to initiation and maintenance of atrial fibrillation and (2) differences in ventriculoatrial intervals during tachycardia. Alternatively, the difference in frequency of spontaneous atrial fibrillation between AV and AV node reentries may be more apparent than real. For example, atrial fibrillation in WPW syndrome may lead to a rapid preexcited ventricular response with symptoms such as syncope or presyncope, and the altered hemodynamics may favor maintenance of atrial fibrillation. These patients would probably be referred for further evaluation. In contrast, if AV node reentry degenerated into atrial fibrillation, the ventricular rate would probably be slower, with fewer hemodynamic consequences and a greater possibility of spontaneous termination.

Accessory Pathway Characteristics

Several investigators have noted that the anterograde effective refractory period of the accessory pathway is shorter in patients with than without atrial fibrillation.[10,16,17] In one study, anterograde accessory pathway effective refractory period was shorter (279 ± 26 msec) in the atrial fibrillation group than in the control group (304 ± 75 msec) (P=.03).[16] In this same study, 19% of episodes of atrial fibrillation started at a site closest to the accessory pathway.[16] In another investigation, electrophysiological characteristics of the accessory pathway were compared in patients with WPW syndrome with or without a history of spontaneous atrial fibrillation.[17] The anterograde effective refractory period of the accessory pathway was shorter in patients with a history of atrial fibrillation (252 ± 34 vs 297 ± 67 msec, P<.01). Chen et al[10] also observed a significantly shorter anterograde effective refractory period in patients with WPW syndrome and a history of atrial fibrillation. Of note, these authors[10] presented follow-up data on three patients who had surgical ablation of accessory pathways with only anterograde conduction. These individuals presented with atrial fibrillation and a rapid preexcited ventricular response. Atrial fibrillation did not recur in any patient after successful ablation of the accessory pathway. These authors[10] postulated that the structural and functional heterogeneity of the accessory pathways in these three patients might have been responsible for the initiation, maintenance, or both of atrial fibrillation. Reentry in this instance could be a consequence of anisotropic discontinuous propagation.[18] Preliminary data from Jackman et al[19] suggest that accessory pathway networks may generate arrhythmias mimicking atrial flutter and fibrillation.

In summary, a rather consistent finding in patients with WPW and atrial fibrillation has been a shorter anterograde accessory pathway effective refractory period compared with patients without a history of atrial fibrillation. Spontaneous atrial fibrillation occurs less frequently in patients with concealed accessory pathways.[10,17] These data, bolstered by the observations of Chen et al[10] and Jackman et al[19] in a few select patients, support the hypothesis that anterograde accessory pathway function may play a role in the initiation or maintenance of atrial fibrillation in some patients with WPW syndrome. Conversely, a short anterograde accessory pathway effective refractory period might merely lead to a faster preexcited ventricular response during atrial fibrillation, with a greater likelihood that the patient would be referred for further workup.

Intrinsic Atrial Vulnerability

Electrophysiological evaluation of patients with WPW syndrome involves placement of catheters in the high right atrium,

His bundle area, right ventricle, and coronary sinus. Thus, throughout the study, simultaneous atrial electrograms are recorded from the high right atrium, base of the left atrium, and interatrial septum near the His bundle. Of note, the catheter recording site in the high right atrium may be in proximity to the trabeculations near the crista terminalis. In atrial pectinate muscle bundles from the atrial appendage taken at surgery, Spach et al[18] demonstrated microreentry based on anistropy in very small muscle bundles. Spontaneous degeneration of AV reentry into atrial fibrillation at electrophysiological study is commonly noted first on the high right atrial tracing[16] (Fig 1). The paucity of recording sites precludes identification of the earliest area of atrial disorganization before the onset of atrial fibrillation in patients with AV reentry. However, it appears reasonable to speculate that the unique electrophysiological-anatomic characteristics of the right atrium provide a welcome milieu for the development of atrial fibrillation.

Several investigators have implicated atrial vulnerability as a cause for atrial fibrillation in patients with WPW syndrome and AV reentry.[9,16,17,20] Sung et al[9] reported on seven patients with spontaneous conversion between AV reentry and atrial flutter-fibrillation at electrophysiological study. In all patients, repetitive atrial responses could be initiated by single premature atrial stimuli, and the right atrium appeared to be more vulnerable than the left atrium. In five patients, paroxysms of atrial flutter-fibrillation were initiated with single atrial premature stimuli. In another study of patients with WPW syndrome, Della Bella et al[17] initiated atrial fibrillation with a single atrial extrastimulus introduced during sinus rhythm in 5 of 31 patients with versus 1 of 26 without a history of spontaneous atrial fibrillation. Gaita et al[20] also demonstrated greater atrial vulnerability in patients with WPW syndrome who had a history of atrial fibrillation. Their atrial stimulation protocol included introduction of single and double extrastimuli during two atrial paced cycle lengths and incremental atrial pacing to a rate of 250 beats per minute. Sustained atrial fibrillation was initiated in 15 of 23 patients with a history of spontaneous atrial fibrillation but in only 7 of 54 symptomatic patients without atrial fibrillation.

Conflicting data exist regarding the importance of electrophysiological characteristics of the right atrium in patients with WPW syndrome and atrial fibrillation. Fujimura et al[16] evaluated electrophysiological characteristics of the right atrium in 79 patients in whom atrial fibrillation lasting ≥30 seconds occurred during electrophysiological study without attempts to induce it with rapid atrial pacing. The results were compared with data from 53 patients without a history of spontaneous atrial fibrillation in whom atrial fibrillation could not be intentionally induced with rapid atrial pacing. The P-A interval was 54 ± 14 msec in the atrial fibrillation group compared with 42 ± 12 msec (P<.0001) in the control group. The functional refractory period of the right atrium was shorter in patients with atrial fibrillation (226 ± 38 vs 240 ± 30 msec, P=.049). The effective refractory period of the right atrium was shorter in the atrial fibrillation group but did not reach statistical significance (194 ± 37 vs 208 ± 31 msec, P=.057). In contrast, Della Bella et al[17] noted no significant differences in P-A interval or atrial effective refractory period between patients with WPW syndrome with and without a history of spontaneous atrial fibrillation.

Contraction-Excitation Feedback

It is well known that supraventricular tachycardia can cause alterations in hemodynamics.[21] The peripheral circulatory effects of supraventricular tachycardia can often be easily recognized by changes in blood pressure, but intra-atrial and intraventricular pressure and volume changes also may occur. In the era of surgical ablation of accessory pathways, it was common to observe, in open-chest surgery in humans, sudden dilatation of the atria after onset of AV reentry. Changes in mechanical stress can alter cardiac membrane potential, a phenomenon referred to as contraction-excitation feedback[22]. It is possible that such electrophysiological changes, especially if they are inhomogeneous throughout the atria, could lead to disorganization and the development of atrial fibrillation.

Klein et al[23] investigated the effects of variable AV intervals on right atrial (RA) pressure and refractoriness and echocardiographic left atrial size in patients with and without supraventricular tachycardia. During pacing at a cycle length of 400 msec, minimal values for all three parameters were at an AV interval of 120 msec, and maximal value was at an AV interval of 0 msec. The maximal changes for all 10 patients in RA effective refractory period, RA peak pressure, and left atrial size were 22.5 ± 3 msec, 10.4 ± 1.8 mm Hg, and 0.55 ± 0.05 cm, respectively. In addition, there was a weak correlation of RA effectory refractory period with left atrial size and RA peak pressure.

Calkins et al[24] investigated the effects of changes in AV relationship on human RA refractoriness with and without autonomic blockade. Right atrial refractoriness was determined at AV intervals of 0, 120, and 160 msec. Continuous RA pacing was used during refractory period determination. The peak RA pressures were 16 ± 4 and 7 ± 4 mm Hg at AV intervals of 0 and 160 msec, respectively. The corresponding RA effective refractory periods were 196 ± 19 and 195 ± 20 msec. Autonomic blockade with intravenous atropine (0.04 mg/k) and propranolol (0.2 mg/kg) did not alter the results. Consistent with the observations of Klein et al,[23] the peak RA pressure occurred at an AV interval of 0 msec. In contrast, Calkins et al[24] noted no prolongation of RA refractoriness with increased RA pressure. Some of these differences may be related to methodology between studies.

A subsequent study by Calkins et al [25] evaluated changes in RA refractoriness due to acute increases in RA pressure. Acute increases in RA pressure were produced by shortening of the AV relationship during the final two beats of RA drive train. The authors[25] noted a shortening of RA effective refractory period from 208 ± 19 to 199 ± 21 msec (P<.001), with a corresponding increase in RA peak pressure from 7 ± 3 to 15 ± 5 mm Hg (P<.001). Thus, acute increases in RA pressure shortened, not lengthened, RA refractoriness. Autonomic blockade yielded similar results.

It is clear from the studies of Klein et al[23] and Calkins et al[24,25] that contraction-excitation feedback can occur in the human right atrium under appropriate conditions. Importantly, the discrepant results among these studies range from no change in RA refractoriness to lengthening and shortening of RA refractoriness at similar AV relationships. Thus, other than the observation that changes in RA pressure can be associated with changes in RA refractoriness, minimal conclusions can be drawn regarding what occurs during AV or AV node reentry. Contraction-excitation feedback alterations of RA refractoriness could explain the development of atrial fibrillation in the patient with ventricular tachycardia and no ventriculoatrial conduction (Fig 5).

Summary of Observations

Tachycardia-induced tachycardia can yield atrial fibrillation by a variety of potential mechanisms. In patients with atrial tachycardia or atrial flutter that initiates atrial fibrillation, the most important factor may be diseased atrial myocardium. In patients with ventricular tachycardia without ventriculoatrial conduction, contraction-excitation feedback may play a major role in the pathogenesis of atrial fibrillation. In my experience, however, initiation of atrial fibrillation during ventricular tachycardia at electrophysiological study is exceedingly uncommon, regardless of ventriculoatrial conduction properties. Since the most marked increases in RA pressure occur during simultaneous atrial and ventricular activation, one might anticipate a high frequency of atrial fibrillation in association with AV node reentry. However, degeneration of AV node reentry into atrial fibrillation rarely occurs at electrophysiological study. These observations do not support electrophysiological changes due to contraction-excitation feedback as a major cause of atrial fibrillation during tachycardia-induced tachycardia.

In patients with WPW syndrome, various lines of evidence suggest that atrial vulnerability, rate of AV reentry, and short anterograde accessory pathway refractoriness may all contribute to the development of atrial fibrillation during AV reentry. It is quite likely that degeneration of AV reentry into atrial fibrillation is multifactorial. My bias is that rapid tachycardia rates are very important to the development of atrial fibrillation but certainly not the sole factor.

It is tempting to implicate the accessory pathway in at least the maintenance of atrial fibrillation, especially if one discounts referral bias for the apparently increased frequency of atrial fibrillation in AV reentry compared with AV node reentry. In our experience, patients sent for evaluation of AV and AV node reentries have similar tachycardia cycle lengths and usually no structural heart disease. After catheter or surgical ablation of accessory pathways, approximately 95% of patients with a history of spontaneous atrial fibrillation never experience this arrhythmia again. Initiation of atrial fibrillation during AV reentry at electrophysiological study typically occurs at a distance from the accessory pathway, suggesting that disorganization within the accessory pathway per se is usually not the cause of atrial fibrillation. Regardless, anterograde conduction in the accessory pathway network after initiation of atrial fibrillation may be important for maintenance of this arrhythmia. This may explain why sustained atrial fibrillation is more common in patients with overt preexcitation than in patients with retrograde conduction only in the accessory pathways or AV node reentry.

Asymptomatic Patients With Ventricular Preexcitation

The occurrence of atrial fibrillation with a rapid preexcited ventricular response initiating ventricular fibrillation in patients with WPW syndrome has produced a conundrum—whether to screen asymptomatic patients to uncover those potentially at high risk for sudden cardiac death.[1,6,26,27] Patients resuscitated from ventricular fibrillation consistently have a rapid preexcited ventricular response during induced atrial fibrillation at electrophysiological study.[2,3] Thus, it has been suggested that asymptomatic individuals with ventricular preexcitation undergo electrophysiological evaluation to identify those with a preexcited ventricular response of <250 msec during atrial fibrillation. Presumably, patients at high risk could undergo prophylactic therapy, including radiofrequency endocardial catheter ablation of the accessory pathway.

The nobility of mass screening for possible high-risk individuals notwithstanding, few data are available to substantiate this approach. The incidence of ventricular preexcitation is 0.1% to 0.3% of the general population, yet the incidence of sudden death in asymptomatic individuals is exceedingly low.[1] Whereas the overwhelming majority of patients with WPW syndrome have otherwise normal cardiac structure, normal hearts are rarely reported in autopsy studies of sudden cardiac death.[26] Further, the prevalence of a rapid preexcited ventricular response with atrial fibrillation in asymptomatic individuals is approximately 17%, markedly limiting the specificity of this observation.[1]

In summary, ventricular fibrillation as the first symptom in a patient with ventricular preexcitation is rare, although a substantial number of patients would be identified as high risk by use of a preexcited RR interval < 250 msec during atrial fibrillation induced at electrophysiological study. Pharmacological and nonpharmacological treatments for these patients have risks, and the overwhelming majority of individuals will have a negative risk/benefit ratio. For these reasons, I do not recommend mass screening of asymptomatic patients with ventricular preexcitation to determine those at potential high risk. Some individuals, however, for example, airline pilots or competitive athletes, may be candidates for screening.

References

1. Prystowsky EN, Klein GJ. *Cardiac Arrhythmias: An Integrated Approach for the Clinician.* New York, NY: McGraw-Hill; 1994.
2. Klein GJ, Bashore TM, Sellers TD, Pritchett EL, Smith WM, Gallagher JJ. Ventricular fibrillation in the Wolff-Parkinson-White syndrome. *N Engl J Med.* 1979;301:1080–1085.
3. Fananapazir L, Packer DL, German LD, Greer GS, Gallagher JJ, Pressley JC, Prystowsky EN. Procainamide infusion test: inability to identify patients with Wolff-Parkinson-White syndrome who are potentially at risk of sudden death. *Circulation.* 1988;77:1291–1296.
4. Ahlinder S, Granath A, Holmer S, Mascher G. Wolff-Parkinson-White-syndrom med paroxysmalt atrieflimmer overgaende i ventrikelflimmer. *Nord Med.* 1963;70:50.
5. Dreifus LS, Haiat R, Watanabe T, et al. Ventricular fibrillation: a possible mechanism of sudden death in patients with Wolff-Parkinson-White syndrome. *Circulation.* 1971;43:520.
6. Prystowsky EN, Knilans TK, Evans JJ. Diagnostic evaluation and treatment strategies for patients at risk for serious cardiac arrhythmias, II: ventricular tachyarrhythmias and Wolff-Parkinson-White syndrome. *Mod Concepts Cardiovasc Dis.* 1991;60:55.
7. Hurwitz JL, German LD, Packer DL, Wharton JM, McCarthy EA, Wilkinson WE, Prystowsky EN, Pritchett ELC. Occurrence of atrial fibrillation in patients with paroxysmal supraventricular tachycardia due to atrioventricular nodal entry. *PACE Pacing Clin Electrophysiol.* 1990, 13:705–710.
8. Campbell RWF, Smith RA, Gallagher JJ, Pritchett ELC, Wallace AG. Atrial fibrillation in the preexcitation syndrome. *Am J Cardiol.* 1977;40:515–520.
9. Sung RJ, Castellanos A, Mallon SM, Bloom MG, Gelband H, Myerburg RJ. Mechanisms of spontaneous alteration between reciprocating tachycardia and atrial flutter-fibrillation in the Wolff-Parkinson-White syndrome. *Circulation.* 1977;56:409–416.
10. Chen PS, Pressley JC, Tang ASL, Packer DL, Gallagher JJ, Prystowsky EN. New observations on atrial fibrillation before and after surgical treatment in patients with the Wolff-Parkinson-White syndrome. *J Am Coll Cardiol.* 1992;19:974–981.
11. Sharma AD, Klein GJ, Guiraudon GM, Milstein S. Atrial fibrillation in patients with Wolff-Parkinson-White syndrome: incidence after surgical ablation of the accessory pathway. *Circulation.* 1985;72:161–169.
12. Wyndham CRC, Amat-y-Leon F, Wu D, Denes P, Dhingra R, Simpson R, Rosen KM. Effects of cycle length on atrial vulnerability. *Circulation.* 1977;55:260–267.
13. Wathen M, Natale A, Wolfe K, Yee R, Newman D, Klein G. An anatomically guided approach to atrioventricular node slow pathway ablation. *Am J Cardiol.* 1992;70:886–889.
14. Jackman WM, Beckman KJ, McClelland JH, Wang X, Friday KJ, Roman CA, Moulton KP, Twidale N, Hazlitt HA, Prior MI, Oren J,

Overholt ED, Lazzara R. Treatment of supraventricular tachycardia due to atrioventricular nodal reentry by radiofrequency catheter ablation of slow-pathway conduction. *N Engl J Med.* 1992;327:313–318.

15. Jazayeri MR, Hempe SL, Sra JS, Dhala AA, Blanck Z, Deshpande SS, Avitall B, Krum DP, Gilbert CJ, Akhtar M. Selective transcather ablation of the fast and slow pathways using radiofrequency energy in patients with atrioventricular nodal reentrant tachycardia. *Circulation.* 1992;85:1318–1328.

16. Fujimura O, Klein GJ, Yee R, Sharma AD. Mode of onset of atrial fibrillation in the Wolff-Parkinson-White syndrome: how important is the accessory pathway? *J Am Coll Cardiol.* 1990:15:1082–1086.

17. Della Bella P, Brugada P, Talajic M, Lemery R, Torner P, Lezaun R, Dugernier T, Wellens HJJ. Atrial fibrillation in patients with an accessory pathway: importance of the conduction properties of the accessory pathway. *J Am Coll Cardiol.* 1991;17:1352–1356.

18. Spach MS, Dolber PC, Heidlage JF. Influence of the passive anisotropic properties on directional differences in propagation following modification of the sodium conductance in human atrial muscle: a model of reentry on anisotropic discontinuous propagation. *Circ Res.* 1988; 62:811–832.

19. Jackman W, Wah JYL, Friday K, Khan A, Sakurai M, Lazzara R. Tachycardias originating in accessory pathway networks mimicking atrial flutter and fibrillation. *J Am Coll Cardiol* 1986;7:6A.

20. Gaita F, Giustetto C, Riccardi R, Mazza A, Mangiardi L, Rosettani E, Brusca A. Relation between spontaneous atrial fibrillation and atrial vulnerability in patients with Wolff-Parkinson-White pattern. *PACE Pacing Clin Electrophysiol.* 1990;13:1249–1253.

21. McIntosh HD, Kong Y, Morris JJ Jr. Hemodynamic effects of supraventricular arrhythmias. *Am J Med* 1964;37:712–727.

22. Lab MJ. Contraction-excitation feedback in myocardium. *Circ Res.* 1982;50:757–766.

23. Klein LS, Miles WM, Zipes DP. Effect of atrioventricular interval during pacing or reciprocating tachycardia on atrial size, pressure, and refractory period: contraction-excitation feedback in human atrium. *Circulation.* 1990;82:60–68.

24. Calkins H, El-Atassi R, Leon A, Kalbfleisch S, Borganelli M, Langberg J, Morady F. Effect of the atrioventricular relationship on atrial refractoriness in humans. *PACE Pacing Clin Electrophysiol.* 1992;15:771–778.

25. Calkins H, El-Atassi R, Kalbfleisch S, Langberg J, Morady F. Effects of an acute increase in atrial pressure on atrial refractoriness in humans. *PACE Pacing Clin Electrophysiol.* 1092;15:1674–1680.

26. Prystowsky EN, Fananapazier L, Packer DL, Thompson KA, German LD. Wolff-Parkinson-White syndrome and sudden cardiac death. *Cardiology.* 1987;74(suppl 2):67–71.

27. Klein GJ, Prystowsky EN, Yee R, Sharma AD, Laupacis A. Asymptomatic Wolff-Parkinson-White: should we intervene? *Circulation.* 1989;80:1902–1905.

Chapter 4

Nonvalvular Atrial Fibrillation:
A Risk Marker for Stroke of Cardiac and Vascular Origin

James H. Chesebro, MD; Jonathan L. Halperin, MD; Valentin Fuster, MD, PhD

Nonvalvular atrial fibrillation has a mean age of onset of 64 years; affects 2% to 5% of the general population, which includes more than 1 million Americans; is associated with a fivefold increase in the risk of ischemic stroke and a 5% to 7% yearly risk of stroke, which increases with age; occurs in up to 35% of patients with nonvalvular atrial fibrillation during their lifetime; and is the single most important characteristic associated with stroke in women > 70 years old.[1–5]

Pathogenesis and Risk

Antithrombotic therapy for thromboembolism should be based on pathogenesis and risk.[6] Therapy to prevent thrombus in cardiac chambers should be predominantly antifibrin; this could be heparin to an activated partial thromboplastin time to 1.5 to 2.5 × control in acute cases or warfarin to an international normalized ratio (INR) of 2.0 to 3.0 in chronic cases. Aspirin does not prevent thrombus in cardiac chambers.[7] Conversely, therapy to prevent arterial thrombus should be antiplatelet, such as aspirin or warfarin, to a higher INR of 2.8 to 4.5. Low doses of antithrombin

From DiMarco JP, Prystowsky EN (eds): *Atrial Arrhythmias: State of the Art.* Armonk, NY, Futura Publishing Company, Inc., © 1995.

therapy decrease fibrinogen/fibrin deposition, but higher doses at a very sharp cutoff in dose ranging are necessary to inhibit platelet deposition, which comprises the bulk of an arterial thrombus.[8]

Thus, the mechanism of stroke, the choice of antithrombotic prophylaxis, and the response to therapy are closely related. High- and low-risk clinical subgroups help identify patients who should be treated, and particular risk factors may help identify a rational choice of antithrombotic therapy. For example, risks associated with enlarged cardiac chambers (left ventricular enlargement and dysfunction or left atrial enlargement; heart failure, which indicates enlargement of these chambers; or hypertension, which may lead to these enlargements) suggest the need for antifibrin therapy. However, the absence of any of these risk factors and age > 60 years in patients with nonvalvular atrial fibrillation suggest a higher vascular risk for stroke and are associated with a high responsiveness for prevention of stroke with aspirin alone.[9]

Independent clinical risk factors for stroke and thromboembolism were derived from the placebo group of the Stroke Prevention in Atrial Fibrillation (SPAF) study (Table 1) and include hypertension, heart failure within the past 100 days, and prior thromboembolism.[9]

The echocardiographic predictors of stroke and thromboembolism in patients with nonvalvular atrial fibrillation are summarized in Table 2.[10] Only 3% of patients had no clinical risk factors

TABLE 1. Clinical Risk Factors (Hypertension, Heart Failure, Prior Thromboembolism) For Stroke in Patients With Nonvalvular Atrial Fibrillation

Thromboembolic Risk	Risk of Stroke, %/yr
0 risk factors	2.5 (nondiabetic, 1.4)*
1 risk factor	7.2
≥2 risk factors	17.6

*Age was an independent risk factor only in this group, which is in keeping with the increased risk of atherosclerotic vascular disease with age.

Data derived from Reference 9.

TABLE 2. Independent Echocardiographic Predictors of Stroke and Thromboembolism in 539 Patients From Placebo Group of Stroke Prevention in Atrial Fibrillation Study

Echocardiographic Status	Risk of Stroke/, Thromboembolism %/yr
Normal echocardiogram	1.5
Moderate or severe LV dysfunction (global or any regional hypokinesis)	16.1
Left atrial dimension (two-dimensional surface area)	
If 2.5 cm/m^2	8.7
If 2.0 to 2.5 cm/m^2	5.0
If abnormal LV and LA	20.0

Data derived from Reference 10.
LV = left ventricle; LA = left atrium

and moderate LV dysfunction with a risk of stroke of 4.5% per year. After patients were stratified for clinical risk factors, only 17% of the 539 patients in the SPAF placebo group were reclassified to a higher-risk category by means of the echocardiogram. The echocardiogram reclassified 38% of low-risk patients to a higher-risk category.

Part two of the SPAF study hypothesized that patients without clinical risk factors for stroke would be responsive to aspirin, and indeed they were, since these patients on aspirin (325 mg/d of enteric coated aspirin) had a stroke risk of 0.5% per year, which included men of any age and women <75 years old (women >75 years old had more heart failure and larger cardiac chambers).[11] This clinical observation of increased vascular risk for stroke at age >60 years is consistent with the examination of vascular risk in patients > 60 years old with lone atrial fibrillation,[12] examination of the carotid arteries by Doppler ultrasound,[13,14] autopsy examination of carotid and vertebral arteries in patients with atrial fibrillation and stroke,[15,16] recent concepts concerning thromboembolism in atherosclerotic coronary disease,[17,18] and recent autopsy evidence concerning the prevalence of ulcerated plaques in the aortic arch in patients with cerebral infarction.[19]

Increased Vascular Risk of Stroke at Age >60 Years

From a population-based case-controlled study in patients >60 years old with lone atrial fibrillation (no cardiopulmonary disease, no hypertension even under treatment, and no diabetes) but with atrial fibrillation, the presence of atrial fibrillation does not increase the risk of mortality, myocardial infarction or nonfatal stroke but does slightly increase the risk of transient cerebral ischemia.[12] However, the total vascular risk, including fatal and nonfatal stroke, transient cerebral ischemia, and fatal and nonfatal myocardial infarction, is high overall and totals 4.6% per year. This high risk of vascular events implies that this group of patients may benefit from prophylactic aspirin therapy. In addition, since two thirds of these patients developed chronic atrial fibrillation after their initial presentation with atrial fibrillation, even this group as a whole should not be considered for cardioversion merely on the basis of trying to prevent stroke but rather mainly on the basis of hemodynamics or inability to adequately control the ventricular rate response if atrial fibrillation should result.

Although duplex ultrasound imaging of carotid arteries in patients with atrial fibrillation and stroke shows a low prevalence (10% to 25%) of ipsilateral carotid stenosis,[13,14] small plaques in the carotid arteries are found in almost all patients >65 years old[15,16] and may account for the increased risk of stroke in older individuals. Recent concepts concerning the pathophysiology of thromboembolism in atherosclerotic coronary arteries indicate that lesions that precede a thromboembolic event are not severe stenoses (≤50% stenosis in more than half of patients and ≤75% stenosis in 75% to 90% of patients). The ulcerated or disrupted plaque is derived from these minor obstructive lesions, which are plaques with a lipid pool covered by a thin fibrous cap prone to rupture. Disruption results in immediate formation of a platelet-rich mural thrombus that may grow to occlusion or embolize distally[17,18] (Fig 1).

The aorta is 2 to 4 times more likely to show evidence of severe atherosclerosis than cervical arteries that supply the brain.[20] The prevalence of ulcerated plaques in the aortic arch in patients with

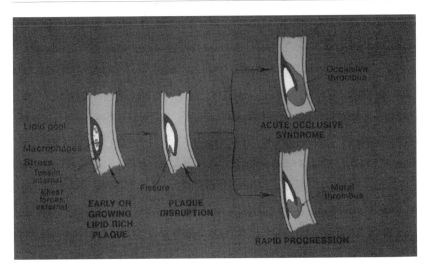

FIGURE 1. *Diagram of plaque disruption of typical fatty plaque with lipid pool in coronary artery. Note macrophages in wall and fibrous cap causing thinning and dissolution of collagen lattice within fibrous cap. Plaque disruption most often occurs at the margin of attachment of the fibrous cap and leads to immediate thrombus formation, which may partially obstruct the artery and cause unstable angina, embolize distally, or occlude the artery and cause myocardial infarction. Reproduced with permission from References 17 and 18.*

stroke is very high in individuals >60 years old. Ulcerated plaques were present in 26% of 239 patients with cerebrovascular disease, were present in 28% of 183 patients with cerebral infarcts, and were especially prevalent in patients with no known cause of cerebral infarction (61% of these 28 patients).[19] In addition, there were strong correlations between the presence of ulcerated plaques in the aortic arch and increasing age >60 years and heart weight (reflects mainly the presence of hypertension). In patients with cerebral infarction, no patient <60 years old had ulcerated plaques in the aortic arch, but with each decade over 60 years, the prevalence of ulcerated plaques in the aortic arch increased, and they were present in 21%, 31%, 34%, and 50% of groups by decade over 60 years, respectively.[19]

Conclusions

Thus, it appears that atrial fibrillation is truly a risk marker for stroke that has both cardiac and vascular origins of pathogenesis. With knowledge of mixed pathogeneses, it is not surprising that patients with nonvalvular atrial fibrillation may have a significant reduction in stroke in response to warfarin and to aspirin and that patients without clinical risk factors (hypertension even under treatment, heart failure, and prior stroke or thromboembolism) are very responsive to aspirin and have a stroke risk on aspirin of only 0.5% per year.[21]

References

1. Halperin JL, Hart RG. Atrial fibrillation and stroke: new ideas, persisting dilemmas. *Stroke.* 1988;19:937–941.
2. Boysen G, Nyboe J, Appleyard M, et al. Stroke incidence and risk factors for stroke in Copenhagen, Denmark. *Stroke.* 1988;19:1345–1353.
3. Cerebral Embolism Task Force. Cardiogenic brain embolism: the second report of the Cerebral Embolism Task Force. *Arch Neurol.* 1989;46:727–743.
4. Wolf PA, Abbott RD, Kannel WB. Atrial fibrillation: a major contributor to stroke in the elderly: the Framingham Study. *Arch Intern Med.* 1987;147:1561–1564.
5. Wolf PA, Abbott RD, Kannel WB. Atrial fibrillation as an independent risk factor for stroke: the Framingham Study. *Stroke.* 1991;22:983–988.
6. Stein B, Fuster V, Halperin JL, Chesebro JH. Antithrombotic therapy in cardiac disease: an emerging approach based on pathogenesis and risk. *Circulation.* 1989;80:1501–1513.
7. Kupper AJF, Verheugt FWA, Peels CH, et al. Effect of low dose acetylsalicylic acid on the frequency and hematologic activity of left ventricular thrombus in anterior wall acute myocardial infarction. *Am J Cardiol.* 1989;63:917–920.
8. Heras M, Chesebro JH, Webster MWI, et al. Hirudin, heparin, and placebo during deep arterial injury in the pig: the in vivo role of thrombin in platelet-mediated thrombosis. *Circulation.* 1990;82:1476–1484.
9. The Stroke Prevention in Atrial Fibrillation Investigators. Predictors of thromboembolism in atrial fibrillation, I: clinical features of patients at risk. *Ann Intern Med.* 1992;116:1–5.
10. The Stroke Prevention in Atrial Fibrillation Investigators. Predictors of thromboembolism in atrial fibrillation, II: echocardiographic features of patients at risk. *Ann Intern Med.* 1992;116:6–12.
11. Stroke Prevention in Atrial Fibrillation Investigators. Warfarin com-

pared to aspirin for prevention of thromboembolism in atrial fibrillation: results of the Stroke Prevention in Atrial Fibrillation II Study. Submitted to *JAMA*.

12. Kopecky SL, Gersh BJ, McGoon MD, et al. Lone atrial fibrillation in the elderly: a population-based long-term study. *Circulation*. 1989;80(suppl II):II-409. Abstract.
13. Tegeler CH, Stroke Prevention in Atrial Fibrillation Study: Carotid Stenosis Study Group. Carotid stenosis in atrial fibrillation. *Neurology*. 1989;38(suppl 1):159. Abstract.
14. Weinberger J, Rothlauf E, Materese E, Halperin J. Noninvasive evaluation of the extracranial carotid arteries in patients with cerebrovascular events and atrial fibrillations. *Arch Intern Med*. 1988;148:1785–1788.
15. Britton M, Gustafson C. Nonrheumatic atrial fibrillation as a risk factor for stroke. *Stroke*. 1985;16:1561–1564.
16. Jorgensen L, Torvik A. Ischemic cerebrovascular diseases in an autopsy series. *J Neurol Sci*. 1966;3:490–509.
17. Fuster V, Badimon L, Badimon JJ, Chesebro JH. The pathogenesis of coronary artery disease and the acute coronary syndromes, I. *N Engl J Med*. 1992;326:242–250.
18. Fuster V, Badimon L, Badimon JJ, Chesebro JH. The pathogenesis of coronary artery disease and the acute coronary syndromes, II. *N Engl J Med*. 1992;326:310–318.
19. Amarenco P, Duyckaerts C, Tzourio C, et al. The prevalence of ulcerated plaques in the aortic arch in patients with stroke. *N Engl J Med*. 1992;326:221–225.
20. Fisher CM, Gore I, Okabe N, White PD. Atherosclerosis of the carotid and vertebral arteries: extracranial and intracranial. *J Neuropathol Exp Neurol*. 1965;24:455–476.
21. Chesebro JH, Fuster V, Halperin J. Atrial fibrillation: risk marker for stroke. *N Engl J Med*. 1990;323:1556–1558.

Chapter 5

Atrial Tachycardias in Pediatric Patients

D. Woodrow Benson, Jr, MD, PhD

Atrial tachycardias affect relatively few pediatric patients, and affected patients should be evaluated to determine whether they have associated heart disease. For example, atrial tachycardias account for only 14% of supraventricular tachycardias in pediatric patients without other heart disease,[1] while among pediatric patients with atrial tachycardias, only 6% have ostensibly normal hearts.[2] Additionally, after certain types of congenital heart disease surgery, atrial tachycardias may occur in up to 40% of late survivors followed for 10 years or more.[3-6] While these tachycardias may manifest some of the ECG features of atrioventricular (AV) reentrant tachycardias, they differ by the lack of interdependence of the atria and ventricles for the continuation of tachycardia. Thus, they may occur with various AV relationships, whereas AV reentrant tachycardias (with rare exceptions) occur only with a 1:1 AV relationship. This variability of the AV relationship serves as an important diagnostic clue in identifying these tachycardias. This is important because the terminology for specific types of atrial tachycardia was coined before the development of clinical electrophysiology, and the definitions are usually based on ECG features.

ECG Features and Definition

Despite the many advances in clinical electrophysiology in the past two decades, only some aspects of atrial tachycardias are understood. The distinction between specific atrial tachycardias is

From DiMarco JP, Prystowsky EN (eds): *Atrial Arrhythmias: State of the Art.* Armonk, NY, Futura Publishing Company, Inc., © 1995.

sometimes obscure, and some terms are used interchangeably. Five terms have been used to describe these tachycardias: atrial fibrillation, atrial flutter, intra-atrial reentry, automatic (ectopic) atrial tachycardia, and chaotic atrial tachycardia.

Atrial fibrillation is characterized by the marked irregularity in atrial depolarizations. Atrial flutter is defined by the ECG appearance of discrete and regular "flutter waves" with a "sawtooth" appearance. During atrial flutter, variations in the ventricular cycle length (RR interval) are usually integer multiples of the atrial cycle length. Further distinctions have been made. For example, the typical ("classic," or "type I") atrial flutter has an atrial rate of 240 to 360 beats per minute, and flutter waves are usually evident in leads II, III, and aVF. Atypical flutter is characterized by slower atrial rate (250 to 300 beats per minute) and discrete P waves instead of flutter waves. Atypical ("type II") atrial flutter has also been used to designate a faster atrial rate.[7] In pediatric patients, a variety of definitions have been used. For example, atrial flutter has been defined as the presence of flutter waves (in any lead) with an atrial rate of 200 to 500 beats per minute.[2] The mechanistic significance of these electrocardiographic distinctions is not known.

Part of the confusion may stem from the fact that atrial flutter is a special case of intra-atrial reentry. This distinction may be especially important when the tachycardia rate and P-wave features are not characteristic of atrial flutter.[8] When distinct P waves are seen that are indistinguishable from sinus P waves, the rhythm is often referred to as "sinus node reentry." Whether or not this truly represents reentry in the sinus node, microreentry in the region of the sinus node, or macroreentry with an exit site of the circuit close to the sinus node remains undetermined.

Atrial automatic tachycardias appear to arise from localized foci within the atrium rather than reentry. Typically, tachycardia rates fluctuate considerably, but over sustained periods of time, the beat-to-beat rate may be quite monotonous. Heart rate may be within the normal range or only moderately increased. However, rates tend to be inappropriately increased for the clinical situation, particularly at rest. Careful scrutiny of P waves in multiple leads during heart rate changes usually reveals subtle changes in P-wave morphology with transitions between sinus rhythm and tachycardia.[9-11] The PR interval may be normal or only slightly prolonged, but like other atrial tachycardias, 2° block may occur without interrupting tachycardia.

Chaotic or multifocal atrial tachycardia is an unusual form of atrial tachycardia characterized by ECG evidence of multiple (three or more) distinct P-wave morphologies during tachycardia with an isoelectric baseline. Although this is typically seen in adults with advanced chronic obstructive pulmonary disease, an identical arrhythmia is also occasionally seen in young infants with otherwise normal hearts.[12-14] Tachycardia rates vary considerably with irregular PP intervals, even when discrete P waves are present. This rhythm disturbance may mimic the electrographic features of other atrial tachycardias.[15]

Basis

In light of experimental and clinical studies, atrial reentry appears to be the basis of most atrial tachycardias in pediatric patients; this is probably not true for automatic or chaotic tachycardias, in which abnormal automaticity appears to be the basis. A role for triggered automaticity has not been defined for atrial tachycardias in pediatric patients. For the population at large, age and underlying heart disease are strongly associated with atrial tachycardias. For example, typical atrial flutter is usually found in patients ≥50 years old with coronary artery or hypertensive cardiovascular disease or both, whereas the pediatric patient with atrial tachycardia is usually a long-term survivor of "atrial" surgery for congenital heart disease.

The most important aspect of atrial fibrillation in the first two decades of life is its rarity; this is not surprising in light of the known association of atrial fibrillation with age and its increased incidence beyond 60 years of age. Atrial fibrillation has been reported in the fetus, neonate, child, and adolescent, but except for the article by Radford and Izukawa,[16] reports are usually in the form of single case studies. The rarity of cases has resulted in limited clinical experience, which has hindered understanding, but a few generalizations can be made. First, in the fetus and neonate, atrial fibrillation is almost always associated with an accessory AV connection.[17] In this setting, atrial fibrillation has been postulated to occur as the result of premature atrial stimulation during increased atrial vulnerability associated with increased rate during orthodromic reciprocating tachycardia; the natural history favors spontaneous resolution of tachycardia during the first year of life.[18] A similar mechanism has been proposed for the development of atrial fibrillation during orthodromic tachycardia in adolescents.[19] Second, atrial fibrillation has been reported in association with dilated and hypertrophic cardiomyopathy.[2,20] The precise reason for this association has not been established, but it may be related to other aspects of the heart disease rather than being a consequence of the hemodynamic derangement per se. For example, Spirito et al[20] noted that hypertrophic cardiomyopathy patients with atrial fibrillation usually have the unobstructed type with mild left ventricular hypertrophy. Third, long-standing, severe atrioventricular valve disease is a risk factor for the development of atrial fibrillation. Such problems are uncommon among young people in the industrialized world, but where rheumatic heart disease is prevalent, atrial fibrillation is a common problem in young patients. Finally, in ostensibly normal adolescents, atrial fibrillation rarely develops, but in such cases, hyperthyroidism has been noted.[21] Atrial fibrillation has infrequently been reported in association with intracardiac tumor or muscular dystrophy.

A rather loose definition of atrial flutter in the pediatric patient has led to the terms atrial flutter and intra-atrial reentry being used interchangeably. The mechanism underlying these tachycardias has been best characterized in the survivors of congenital heart disease surgery and appears to be due to reentry within atrial muscle.[3,22–24] The surgical procedures have been shown to have major effects on intra-atrial conduction,[25,26] but the extent to which gross anatomic obstacles such as surgical scar or more microscopic anisotropic structural complexities may be involved in the genesis of reentrant atrial tachycardias in this setting has yet to be determined.[27]

Intra-atrial reentry tachycardia rarely occurs in the nonsurgical patient. During infancy, atrial flutter usually occurs without apparent heart disease,[28] although an association between atrial flutter in infancy and the existence of an AV accessory connection has been reported.[29–30] Beyond infancy, these tachycardias are most commonly seen in the setting of postoperative congenital heart disease, particularly after "atrial" surgery (eg, atrial switch procedures for d-transposition of the great arteries and Fontan operation).[2–5] Among these patients, multiple factors may contribute to the development of atrial dysrhythmias, including atrial scar, ventricular dysfunction, elevated atrial pressures with dilation, or valvular regurgitation. Alternatively, the tendency for dysrhythmia may be another manifestation of the congenital defect. In the postoperative patient, the frequent association with bradycardia may aggravate the development of atrial tachycardia. Although damage to the sinus node was initially hypothesized to result in both bradycardia and tachycardia, alteration in intra-atrial conduction now seems a more plausible explanation.

Some attempts have been made to subdivide ectopic microreentrant foci from tachycardia foci due to abnormal automaticity. Features thought to be suggestive of automatic foci include "warm-up" or tachycardia acceleration at onset, failure to initiate or terminate with extrastimulus testing, and demonstration of the "reset" phenomenon during atrial extrastimuli delivered during tachycardia. Mapping studies have generally identified two regional clusterings of the ectopic foci near the right atrial appendage and near the pulmonary venous connections with the left atrium.[31,32] The anatomic and developmental significance of tissue characteristics at these sites and the natural history of the tachycardia that favors spontaneous termination remain uncertain.[10,11]

The anatomic or functional substrates responsible for chaotic atrial tachycardia remain poorly defined. Whether the rhythm is related to multiple competing automatic foci, multiple reentrant circuits, or triggered mechanisms is uncertain. A similar relationship may be a factor in infancy. While the majority of infants have no major structural heart disease, various cardiac and noncardiac conditions were present among two thirds of patients reviewed by Yeager et al.[14] Nevertheless, the presence of severe and occasionally lethal bradycardias may belie a more fundamental cardiac or autonomic abnormality.

Clinical Features

Atrial tachycardias occur in patients of all ages, and their probability of occurrence is similar from fetal life through adolescence. The clinical features are quite different from those in patients with AV reentrant tachycardia. In the latter, abrupt onset of symptoms is associated with paroxysmal onset of tachycardia at a high heart rate, while patients with atrial tachycardias have an insidious onset of symptoms consisting of malaise, decreased exercise tolerance, palpitations, loss of appetite, and, rarely, peripheral embolic events.

The course of symptom development is consistent with a long duration of tachycardia that gradually results in cardiac dysfunction.

Less frequently, atrial tachycardias result in life-threatening symptoms. In the postoperative patient, atrial tachycardia has been associated with syncope and sudden death,[2,5] but it has been infrequently documented as a cause of cardiac arrest.[33] Another well-described scenario is the young patient with Wolff-Parkinson-White syndrome who develops a life-threatening ventricular response during atrial fibrillation.

Management

The general therapeutic strategies for atrial tachycardias include terminating established tachycardia, preventing recurrences, and minimizing symptoms during recurrences. Management may be complicated by coexisting bradycardia as seen in "sick sinus" or "tachycardia-bradycardia" syndromes, especially in survivors of congenital heart disease surgery.[34] The physician's directive to "first do no harm" is an appropriate consideration in management of atrial tachycardias; when appropriate, the possibility of no or minimal treatment should be a treatment option.

The overall goal in the pediatric patient is maintenance of sinus rhythm. Support for this goal is derived primarily from experience with the late survivors of congenital heart disease. First, cardiac function and exercise tolerance are improved after conversion of atrial tachycardia, even in asymptomatic patients.[35] Second, the risk of sudden death in patients who develop atrial tachycardia is increased compared with those who do not.[5] Finally, among patients who develop atrial tachycardia, the risk of sudden death is increased fourfold in patients who continue to have tachycadia compared with adequately treated patients.[2]

In the acute setting with severe hemodynamic compromise, immediate DC cardioversion remains the treatment of choice. In medically stable patients, termination of atrial fibrillation may be accomplished with digoxin, digoxin and quinidine, or intravenous procainamide. Otherwise, elective DC cardioversion is generally effective for terminating atrial fibrillation. Atrial flutter and intra-atrial reentry may be converted with DC cardioversion, but they may also be terminated with temporary transvenous or transesophageal pacing[36,37] or with an implanted pacemaker.[38] Often, termination occurs as atrial flutter is converted to atrial fibrillation, which is then superseded by sinus rhythm. Pace termination of acute recurrences may be used to acutely terminate infrequent recurrences of well-tolerated atrial tachycardia in lieu of chronic medical therapy.

Because of limited reports in the literature and clinical experience in this age group, questions regarding anticoagulation before pharmacological or electrical cardioversion remain, but if intracardiac thrombi are identified during echocardiography, anticoagulation should be performed before elective conversion.

Medications that seem to be most effective for preventing atrial tachycardia recurrences include class IA drugs, such as quinidine and procainamide, and class III drugs, such as amiodarone and sotalol. Unfortunately, small patient numbers have prevented long-term trials to determine optimal antiarrhythmic drug therapy, and there have been conflicting reports of efficacy. For example, amiodarone has been reported to be both successful[2] and unsuccessful[39] in the treatment of atrial tachycardia in postoperative patients. Class IA medications have anticholinergic effects that potentiate antegrade conduction during atrial flutter or fibrillation and should be coadministered with a medication that offsets this effect, such as digoxin. The efficacy of class IC drugs such as propafenone and flecainide is less well established, and there is some concern that patients with atrial tachycardia may be at increased risk for serious proarrhythmia.[40] The role of permanent atrial pacemakers in preventing tachycardias by preventing bradycardias has not been completely established. It has been generally agreed that patients with symptomatic bradycardia should be treated with a pacemaker. It was previously recommended that patients with tachycardia-bradycardia syndrome requiring antiarrhythmic therapy other than digoxin also be paced, but this has recently been designated a class II pacing indication.[41] In patients with surgically treatable heart disease, the occurrence of atrial tachycardia should be taken as an indication to proceed with surgical treatment.

Patients in whom tachycardia recurrences can be consistently terminated by pacing may benefit from implantable antitachycardia pacemakers as an alternative or adjunct to chronic medical therapy. These may include automatic devices programmed to detect tachycardia and deliver a paced response or standard atrial or AV sequential pacemakers temporarily programmed to AOO or AAT modes for rapid pacing.[38,42] However, antiarrhythmic therapy may still be necessary to prevent rapid conduction to the ventricles during the recurrence.

Medications to slow AV node conduction, including digoxin, β-blockers, and calcium channel blockers, have little effect on preventing recurrences of atrial tachycardia and may aggravate bradycardia. Digoxin and verapamil should be avoided in patients with atrial fibrillation associated with Wolff-Parkinson-White syndrome because of the risk of enhancing antegrade conduction over the accessory connection.

Ablation of the AV node with implantation of a ventricular pacemaker has rarely been advocated. Experience with surgical procedures or radiofrequency ablation of atrial tachycardias has been limited. While the latter technique has been promising for "type I" atrial flutter in adults, it may be less effective in the setting of atrial tachycardia in postoperative congenital heart disease.

Termination by pacing, DC cardioversion, and acute pharmacological suppression are of little benefit for ectopic atrial tachycardia, but sensitivity to adrenergic stimulation may be used to advantage during acute management. Digoxin seems to be relatively ineffective, whereas effective regimens can usually be found among class IA, IC, β-blocking, and class III agents, alone or in combinations. Complete cessation of tachycardia, decrease (normalization) of mean heart rate, slowing of the fastest tachycardia rates, and normalization of associated ventricular dysfunction may all represent appropriate end points of therapy. Careful monitoring during initiation of therapy in these patients is warranted, particularly if ventricular dysfunction coexists with tachycardia. Spontaneous "cures" are common. In medically refractory cases, surgical resection of the automatic focus has been successful.[31] Likewise, radiofrequency ablation has recently been used with excellent short-term success.[32]

General medical treatment strategies for chaotic atrial tachycardia are similar to those outlined for atrial ectopic tachycardias.[12-14,43,44] Drugs that slow the ventricular response during tachycardia, such as verapamil or propranolol, may be sufficient alone, or the tachycardia may usually be completely suppressed with class IA, IC, and III agents or calcium channel blockers. Acute termination attempts with DC cardioversion, pacing, or intravenous agents such as adenosine or verapamil are neither beneficial nor warranted.

Prognosis

Prognosis is dependent in large measure on the extent of underlying disease. This is certainly true for postoperative cardiac lesions with associated AV valve regurgitation and/or reduced ventricular function as well as dilated cardiomyopathy, hypertrophic cardiomyopathy, chronic rheumatic mitral valve disease, hyperthyroidism, and muscular dystrophy.[16]

Atrial flutter in infants without other heart disease is generally a self-limited process, and most patients do not require therapy beyond initial conversion.[28] On the contrary, because of association with sudden death, a consensus has evolved that atrial tachycardia should be aggressively treated in the late survivor of congenital heart disease surgery. The specifics of the treatment have not been universally agreed upon.

Several factors influence the long-term outcome of ectopic atrial tachycardia, including the resolution of ventricular dysfunction, the tendency for spontaneous regression during long-term follow-up, and the possibility of late sequelae due to arrhythmia or its treatment. Thus, the potential (yet undetermined) risks of surgical or transcatheter ablation must be weighed against the potential risks of the antiarrhythmic regimens sometimes necessary to achieve tachycardia control, particularly if ventricular dysfunction is severe. The potential for spontaneous regression may favor medical therapy, whereas the long-term outcome after catheter ablation, if favorable, may prove this approach to be the eventual treatment of choice.

Like automatic atrial tachycardia, chaotic atrial tachycardia frequently regresses within days to months.[12,13] However, sudden death occurred in 17% of the young patients reviewed by Yeager et al,[14] including two witnessed deaths attributed to severe bradycardia. As with other deaths during antiarrhythmic therapy, it is difficult to distinguish deaths occurring as a complication of therapy from those resulting from the tachycardia itself.

References

1. Ko JK, Deal BJ, Strasburger JF, Benson DW Jr. Supraventricular tachycardia mechanisms and their age distribution in pediatric patients. *Am J Cardiol.* 1992;69:1028–1032.
2. Garson A Jr, Bink-Boelkens MTE, Hesslein PS, et al. Atrial flutter in the young: a collaborative study of 380 cases. *J Am Coll Cardiol.* 1985;6:871–878.
3. Gillette PC, Kugler JD, Garson A, et al. Mechanisms of cardiac arrhythmias after the Mustard operation for transposition of the great arteries. *Am J Cardiol.* 1980;45:1225–1230.
4. Bink-Boelkens MTE, Velvis H, van der Heide JJH. Dysrhythmias after atrial surgery. *Am Heart J.* 1983;106:125–130.
5. Flinn CJ, Wolff GS, Dick M II, et al. Cardiac rhythm after the Mustard operation for complete transposition of the great arteries. *N Engl J Med.* 1984;310:1635–1638.
6. Hayes CJ, Gersony WM. Arrhythmias after the Mustard operation for transposition of the great arteries: a long-term study. *J Am Coll Cardiol.*1986;7:133–137.
7. Boineau JP. Atrial flutter: a synthesis of concepts. *Circulation.* 1985;72:249–257.
8. Müller GI, Deal BJ, Strasburger JF, Benson DW Jr. Electrocardiographic features of atrial tachycardias after operation for congenital heart disease. *Am J Cardiol.* 1993;71:122–124.
9. Gillette PC, Garson A Jr. Electrophysiologic and pharmacologic characteristics of automatic ectopic atrial tachycardia. *Circulation.* 1977;56:571–575.
10. Mehta AV, Sanchez GR, Sacks EJ, et al. Ectopic automatic atrial tachycardia in children: clinical characteristics, management and follow-up. *J Am Coll Cardiol.* 1988;11:379–385.
11. von Bernuth G, Engelhardt W, Kramer HH, et al. Atrial automatic tachycardia in infancy and childhood. *Eur Heart J.* 1992;13:1410–1415.
12. Bisset GS III, Seigal SF, Gaum WE, Kaplan S. Chaotic atrial tachycardia in childhood. *Am Heart J.* 1981;101:268–272.
13. Liberthson RR, Colan SD. Multifocal or chaotic atrial rhythm: report of nine infants, delineation of clinical course and management and review of the literature. *Pediatr Cardiol.* 1982;2:179–184.
14. Yeager SB, Hougen TJ, Levy AM. Sudden death in infants with chaotic atrial rhythm. *Am J Dis Child.* 1984;138:689–692.
15. Benditt DG, Benson DW, Dunnigan A, et al. Atrial flutter, atrial fibrillation, and other primary atrial tachycardias. *Med Clin North Am.* 1987;68:895–918.
16. Radford DJ, Izukawa T. Atrial fibrillation in children. *Pediatrics.* 1977;59:250–256.
17. Belhassen B, Pauzner D, Bleiden L, et al. Intrauterine and postnatal atrial fibrillation in the Wolff-Parkinson-White syndrome. *Circulation.* 1982;66:1124–1128.

18. Benson DW Jr, Dunnigan A, Benditt DG. Follow-up evaluation of infant paroxysmal atrial tachycardia: transesophageal study. *Circulation.* 1987;75:542–549.
19. Roark SF, McCarthy EA, Lee KL, Pritchett ELC. Observations on the occurrence of atrial fibrillation in paroxysmal supraventricular tachycardia. *Am J Cardiol.* 1986;57:571–575.
20. Spirito P, Lakatos E, Maron BJ. Degree of left ventricular hypertrophy in patients with hypertrophic cardiomyopathy and chronic atrial fibrillation. *Am J Cardiol.* 1992;69:1217–1222.
21. Perry LW, Hung W. Atrial fibrillation and hyperthyroidism in a 14-year old boy. *J Pediatr.* 1971;79:668–671.
22. Vetter VL, Tanner CS, Horowitz LN. Electrophysiologic consequences of the Mustard repair of d-transposition of the great arteries. *J Am Coll Cardiol.* 1987;10:1265–1273.
23. Vetter VL, Tanner CS, Horowitz LN. Inducible atrial flutter after the Mustard repair of complete transposition of the great arteries. *Am J Cardiol.* 1988;61:428–435.
24. Kurer CC, Tanner CS, Vetter VL. Electrophysiologic findings after Fontan repair of functional single ventricle. *J Am Coll Cardiol.* 1991;17:174–181.
25. Shuman TA, Palazzo RS, Schuessier RB, et al. Characterization of atrial flutter following the Mustard procedure for transposition of the great vessels. *J Am Coll Cardiol.* 1991;17:209A. Abstract.
26. Wittig JH, de Leval MR, Stark J. Intraoperative mapping of atrial activation before, during, and after the Mustard operation. *J Thorac Cardiovasc Surg.* 1977;73:1–13.
27. Spach MS. Anisotropic structural complexities in the genesis of reentrant arrhythmias. *Circulation.* 1991;84:1447–1450.
28. Dunnigan A, Benson DW Jr. Atrial flutter in infancy: diagnosis, clinical features, and treatment. *Pediatrics.* 1985;75:725–729.
29. Johnson WH, Dunnigan A, Fehr P, Benson DW Jr. Association of atrial flutter with orthodromic reciprocating fetal tachycardia. *Am J Cardiol.* 1987;59:374–375.
30. Till J, Wren C. Atrial flutter in the fetus and young infant: an association with accessory connections. *Br Heart J.* 1992;67:80–83.
31. Gillette PC, Wampler DG, Garson A Jr, et al. Treatment of atrial automatic tachycardia by ablation procedures. *J Am Coll Cardiol.* 1985;6:405–409.
32. Walsh EP, Saul JP, Hulse JE, et al. Transcather ablation of ectopic atrial tachycardia in young patients using radiofrequency current. *Circulation.* 1992;86:1138–1146.
33. Silka M, Kron J, McAnulty J. Supraventricular tachyarrhythmias, congenital heart disease, and sudden cardiac death. *Pediatr Cardiol.* 1992;13:116–118.
34. Greenwood RD, Rosenthal A, Sloss LJ, et al. Sick sinus syndrome after surgery for congenital heart disease. *Circulation.* 1975;52:208–213.
35. Wessel HU, Benson DW Jr, Braunlin EA, et al. Exercise response before and after termination of atrial tachycardia after congenital heart disease surgery. *Circulation.* 1989;80:106–111.

36. Butto F, Dunnigan A, Overhold ED, et al. Transesophageal study of recurrent atrial tachycardia after atrial baffle procedures for complete transposition of the great arteries. *Am J Cardiol.* 1986;57:1356–1362.
37. Campbell RM, Dick M II, Jenkins JM, et al. Atrial overdrive pacing for conversion of atrial flutter in children. *Pediatrics.* 1985;75:726–730.
38. Frohlig G, Sen S, Rettig G, et al. Termination of atrial flutter during DDD pacing by rapid overdrive stimulation using the implanted pacemaker lead system. *Am J Cardiol.* 1986;57:483–485.
39. Pongiglione G, Strasburger JF, Deal BJ, Benson DW Jr. Use of amiodarone for short-term and adjuvant therapy. *Am J Cardiol.* 1991;68:603–608.
40. Fish FA, Gillette PC, Benson DW Jr. Proarrhythmia, cardiac arrest and sudden death in young patients receiving encainide and flecainide. *J Am Coll Cardiol.* 1991;18:356–365.
41. Dreifus LS, Fisch C, Griffin JC, et al. Guidelines of implantation of cardiac pacemakers and antiarrhythmia devices. *Circulation.* 1991;84:455–467.
42. Gillette PC, Zeigler VL, Case CL, et al. Atrial antitachycardia pacing in children and young adults. *Am Heart J.* 1991;122:844–849.
43. Zeevi B, Berant M, Sclarovsky S, Blieden LC. Tretment of multifocal atrial tachycardia with amiodarone in a child with congenital heart disease. *Am J Cardiol.* 1986;57:344–345.
44. Sapire DW, Mongkolsmai C, O'Riordan AC. Control of chronic ectopic supraventricular tachycardia with verapamil. *J Pediatr.* 1979;94:312–314.

Chapter 5

Editorial Comments

Arthur Garson, Jr, MD, MPH

As with all arrhythmias, the important questions about atrial tachyarrhythmias in children concern identification, mechanism, pathogenesis, and treatment. As has been well articulated by Dr Benson,[1] even the nomenclature of certain atrial tachyarrhythmias in children is uncertain. It is unlikely that this uncertainty will be resolved until the various patterns on the surface electrocardiogram and even the patterns in the clinical electrophysiology laboratory are associated with an underlying mechanism. Once the mechanism is better understood, it will then be important to understand how these arrhythmias occur, with the long-term goal of prevention; in the short term, the best modes of treatment will need to be determined. These three areas will form the basis for the following discussion.

"Mechanisms" of Atrial Tachyarrhythmias

The area of greatest concern and least knowledge is in postoperative atrial tachyarrhythmias. In patients after the Mustard operation, the rapid and constant atrial rate led to the label "atrial flutter".[2] However, typical flutter waves are absent, and there is usually not an isoelectric baseline. In patients after the Fontan operation, at least three atrial tachyarrhythmias can be recognized on the surface electrocardiogram: one with a relatively constant atrial rate that responds to cardioversion, one with a variable atrial rate that responds to cardioversion, and one with a variable atrial rate that does not respond to cardioversion.[3]

Are these tachyarrhythmias after atrial surgery all the same mechanism or different mechanisms? Does it matter? The atrium

From DiMarco JP, Prystowsky EN (eds): *Atrial Arrhythmias: State of the Art.* Armonk, NY, Futura Publishing Company, Inc., © 1995.

after congenital heart surgery is an extremely complex structure. There are areas of fibrosis both related and unrelated to suture lines; different parts of the atrium may be under different hemodynamic conditions (the Fontan atrium with a lateral tunnel may have part of the right atrium under high pressure and part under low pressure); and atrial tissue may be exposed to hemodynamic stresses for which the atrium was not intended. There is no particular reason to think that these complex anatomic and physiological derangements should always produce the same mechanism. It seems likely that, especially in the Fontan patient, there are different tachyarrhythmias, some perhaps even resulting from injury in the same general area of the atrium and some at other sites as well. In the postoperative Mustard and Senning patient, the anatomy is much more similar from patient to patient, and it seems more likely that this reentrant tachyarrhythmia previously labeled as atrial flutter has a similar mechanism from patient to patient.

The distinction among mechanisms matters for several reasons. First, if an arrhythmia is due to a macroreentrant circuit around large areas of scar, the catheter treatment for this arrhythmia will be different than if the arrhythmia involves a microreentrant circuit in a relatively small area with atrial activation spreading passively from this area.[4] These distinctions are not made simply in the complex postoperative atrium, and further research in this area would be extremely illuminating and practical in terms of treatment. The distinction of these reentrant arrhythmias from a presumably focal automatic arrhythmia would also be important, since it is possible that the optimal type of catheter treatment for the focal arrhythmia may be different from that for the reentrant arrhythmia. The second reason relates to drug treatment. While catheter treatment eventually may be the optimal method of treating all these tachycardias, at present, drug treatment remains an option. If the "mechanism" for these arrhythmias were better known, the likelihood of successful drug treatment could be improved. The third reason for understanding the mechanism involves eventual prevention. This is considered in the next section.

Pathophysiology and Potential Prevention

It is known that many adults with ostium secundum atrial septal defect eventually develop atrial flutter and atrial fibrillation without any heart surgery at all.[5] However, it is unquestioned that patients after the Mustard, Senning, Fontan, and even atrial septal defect operations develop atrial tachyarrhythmias much sooner than the natural history would predict.[2] Therefore, it is likely that the surgery and its resultant scarring contribute significantly to the development of these atrial arrhythmias. If it could be understood exactly how atrial scarring contributes to these arrhythmias, perhaps they could be prevented. In our experimental laboratories, we have performed atriotomies and ventriculotomies in a number of different animal models and have found that the morphology and the composition of the scar are at least partially dependent on the hemodynamics present at the time of scarring.[6] The ratio of dense collagen to adipose tissue in scars is much higher in scars that heal under high pressure than those that heal under low pressure. In growing animals, the length of the scar increases in proportion to the growth of the atrium: animals in whom scars were placed early in life had a 200% increase in the length of the scar after 5 months of growth, while scars made in adults decrease in length. Exactly how these changes related to the genesis of arrhythmias is unknown. The questions in this area are similar to those following myocardial infarction with remodeling of the infarct scar. However, the complexity is increased in that growth is also occurring. If the specific anatomic and physiological conditions necessary to produce an arrhythmogenic scar were known, perhaps they could be avoided or at least modified. While the Mustard and Senning operations are essentially no longer being performed, cardiac transplantation in the very young produces some suture lines not dissimilar to the those from the Mustard and Senning operations. Therefore, the study and understanding of these arrhythmias may have important future implications.

Treatment

In 1984, a large study of "atrial flutter" in 380 children and young adults was undertaken by the pediatric electrophysiology group.[2] One of the findings of that study was that the risk of sudden death in patients with atrial flutter was four times higher in those in whom the atrial flutter continued (despite a "controlled" ventricular rate) than in those in whom episodes no longer occurred.[2] There were similar findings for nonsudden death. It was therefore recommended that all attempts be made to eliminate episodes of atrial flutter in children, especially those with congenital heart disease. Since that time, Herculean efforts have been made to achieve this end, including use of class IA agents (with their potential for torsade de points), class IC agents (with their potential for proarrhythmia), class III agents (with their potential for bradycardia and systemic toxicity), antibradycardia pacemakers, antitachycardia pacemakers, AV node ablation, and direct catheter ablation. It remains to be demonstrated whether in the 10 years since 1984, with all of these "advances," the mortality of patients who have atrial flutter is any different. Such a study is currently under way. While it is likely that catheter ablation is an extremely attractive option for the treatment of these patients, the technical problems in achieving catheter access to some areas of these atria may make ablation difficult or in some cases impossible. For example, in some individuals with a Fontan operation, blood draining from both venae cavae drains directly into the pulmonary arteries. Access to most of the atrial mass is restricted. While it may be possible to place a single catheter through a sheath that has made a hole in prosthetic material, it is not likely that the multiple catheters potentially necessary for adequate mapping could be placed in this manner. While repeat open-heart surgery could be done for such patients, the potential risks of that procedure could be considerable.

It remains, therefore, that for some of these patients, drug and/or pacing treatment for postoperative atrial tachyarrhythmias will be the only option. It is likely that the only way to demonstrate the optimal treatment for these patients (including no aggressive treatment at all) will be to perform a prospective randomized controlled trial. We know that certain subsets of patients with these arrhythmias have a high mortality, and there are a number of options for treatment. We must now demonstrate in appropriately controlled studies that suppression of the arrhythmia leads to improved quality of life and improved survival. If it does not, cardiac transplantation may be the only option for those at highest risk.

Unlike in older adults, atrial tachyarrhythmias in children and young adults are associated with significant morbidity and mortality. As the answers to these questions become increasingly available, the long-term outlook for infants born with heart disease should improve markedly.

References

1. Benson DW. Atrial tachycardias in pediatric patients. This volume.
2. Garson A, Bink-Boelkens MTE, Hesslein PS, et al. Atrial flutter in the young: a collaborative study of 380 cases. *J Am Coll Cardiol*. 1985;6: 871–878.
3. Porter CJ, Garson A, Puga F. Right ventriculotomy: does it cause right bundle branch block? *Pediatr Res*. 1988;23:233A.
4. Perry JC, Nihill MR, Ludomirsky A, Ott DA, Garson A. The pulmonary artery lasso: epicardial pacing lead causing right ventricular outflow tract obstruction. *PACE Pacing Clin Electrophysiol*. 1991;14:1019–1023.
5. Brandenburg RO, Homes DR, McGoon DC. Clinical follow-up study of supraventricular tachyarrhythmias after operative repair of a secundum type atrial septal defect in adults. *Am J Cardiol*. 1983;51:273–276.
6. Denfield SW, Kearney DL, Michael L, Gittenberger-de Groot A, Garson A. Developmental differences in canine cardiac surgical scars. *Am Heart J*. 1993;126:382–389.

Chapter 6

Nonuniform Anisotropic Cellular Coupling as a Basis for Reentrant Arrhythmias

Madison S. Spach, MD

Introduction

Clinical electrophysiologists generally agree that the vast predominance of atrial and ventricular tachycardias are due to some type of reentry.[1] During the past decade, major attention has been focused on ventricular rather than atrial tachyarrhythmias, presumably because of the immediate life-threatening danger of ventricular fibrilliation. However, many clinical services encounter atrial tachyarrhythmias as a very great problem, and atrial fibrillation in particular, with its attendant complications, may be even more common than ventricular tachycardia (J.C. Greenfield, Jr, personal communication). Because it is known that there are differences in the sarcolemmal membrane ionic currents of atrial and ventricular myocytes as well as differences in the fibers of the specialized ventricular conduction system, drug therapy has generally been designed to be different for tachyarrhythmias of ventricular and atrial origin. The currently known proarrhythmic effects of sodium channel blocking drugs that slow conduction also make it clear that the same drug therapy can produce different responses in different patients.[2] In contrast, catheter devices may offer other alternatives. The application of radiofrequency ablation techniques has resulted in considerable progress in the therapy of tachyarrhythmias by removing a selective part of a reentrant circuit,[3]

This work was supported by U.S. Public Health Service Grant HL 50537.

From DiMarco JP, Prystowsky EN (eds): *Atrial Arrhythmias: State of the Art*. Armonk, NY, Futura Publishing Company, Inc., © 1995.

especially in patients with atrial tachyarrhythmias due to atrioventricular (AV) bypass tracts and AV nodal tachycardias as well as in some patients with ventricular tachycardias. All of these clinical developments during the past decade emphasize the need to develop a framework of the underlying mechanisms of reentry that can be applied to all reentry circuits yet are detailed enough to account for the underlying complex interactions that result in the marked differences in the behavior of different types of reentrant tachycardias.

Essential Requirement for Reentry: Nonuniformity of the Conduction Medium

The single general requirement to initiate reentry in any tissue is the presence of a nonuniformity that results in functionally different conduction pathways. A spatial nonuniformity is necessary because it creates spatial asymmetry in the ability of the membrane to supply enough current to depolarize itself and to supply the necessary current to charge the capacitance of the neighboring tissue that has yet to depolarize. Reentry can be initiated only by stimuli that initiate wave fronts that propagate into tissue before its return of partial or full excitability (during the absolute or relative refractory periods). If the underlying nonuniformities are of sufficient magnitude, they further alter the diminished excitatory currents of the excitation waves in a spatially nonuniform manner to create functionally different pathways. In effect, a nonuniformity must be present to produce spatial asymmetry of the safety factor of conduction so that conduction block occurs in one pathway that has a longer effective refractory period while stable (usually slow) propagation is maintained in a second pathway that has a shorter refractory period.

Before we analyze the events that initiate reentry in different circuits, it is useful to apply the above general principles to two situations in which reentry cannot occur:

First, normal beats cannot produce reentry because the action potentials at all sites are initiated after full recovery of the excitatory (sodium) current,[4] ie, during phase 4 recovery at a normal resting potential. During normal beats, the wave fronts spread away from a single site of origin and propagate through fully excitable tissues until conduction is abolished by termination at the boundaries of the structure or by collisions. That is, normal repetitive beats are associated with the conduction of impulses at the maximal available safety factor in each area of the heart.

Second, a continuous medium that has no resistive discontinuities or other inhomogeneities, such as spatial differences in the membrane ionic currents, is a highly idealized model that is often applied to the analysis of propagating impulses in cardiac muscle. In such an idealized medium, reentry cannot occur when premature action potentials are initiated at a single site. In this case, premature action potentials propagate into regions before there is full recovery of the sodium current, eg, an early premature stimulus in the relatively refractory period during the repolarization phase of the previous action potential. Propagation of the premature impulse in relatively refractory tissue results in the excitation wave having decreased excitatory currents, decreased $\dot{V}_{max}$, decreased safety factor, and decreased conduction velocity. Even though the sarcolemmal membrane currents are decreased in this idealized medium, the excitatory currents are the same at all sites, and the resistance of the medium is also uniform and continuous (the structure is similar to that of a continuous cable in all directions). Thus, once stable propagation is established, even though the excitatory current is diminished, there is nothing in the medium to change the conduction of the excitation wave until it is extinguished by the boundaries of the structure or by collisions.

It is well known that healthy people have occasional atrial or ventricular premature beats that do not lead to tachycardia. From the above general information, one or all of the following many prevent a premature beat from initiating reentry: (1) The intrinsic nonuniformities in the atria and ventricles may be sufficiently small in magnitude that the inhomogeneities have minimal effects on the premature excitation waves that conduct with reduced excitatory current. (2) The time interval between the normal beat (S_1) and the premature stimulus (S_2) may be long enough to allow sufficient recovery of the excitatory sodium current to override the effects of any underlying nonuniformities. (3) The location of the site of the premature stimulus may produce a sequence of excitation spread that prevents the underlying nonuniformities from altering conduction of the premature impulse.[5] For example, premature stimuli originating near the top of the right atrium in the medial portion of the crista terminalis near the sinus node do not produce conduction block in the crista terminalis [Fig 1B(1)]. This is because the dura-

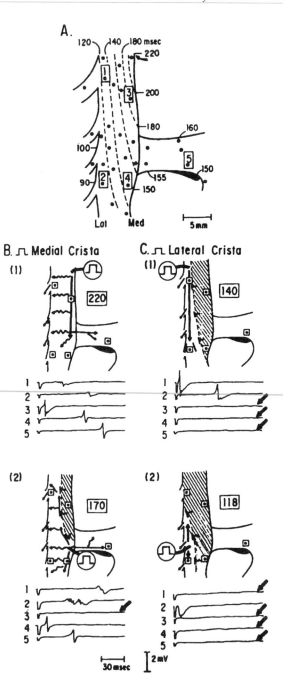

tion of the action potential and the effective refractory period decrease as one moves from the medial to the lateral border of the crista and from the top (sinus node area) to the bottom (AV node area) of the right atrium, as illustrated in Fig 1A. However, when an early premature stimulus originates in the lateral or inferior portions of the crista terminalis, conduction block occurs.[6] This is because early premature impulses conducting medially or in the superior direction now encounter increasing refractory tissue due to the longer action potentials in the medial and upper crista (Fig 1B and 1C).

These considerations demonstrate that only stimuli that produce action potentials that enter regions before the return of normal excitability set the stage for the underlying nonuniformities to significantly alter the depolarizing current in a spatially asymmetrical manner. The development of reentry, therefore, should be very sensitive to the initial conditions of the location and timing of the

◄───

FIGURE 1. *Propagation of premature impulse from different sites in relation to the anisotropic distribution of refractory periods in the crista terminalis of the canine right atrium. A, Two-dimensional repolarization map of the effective refractory periods measured at the sites indicated by solid circles. Isochrone (dashed) lines were drawn by interpolating the values of the refractory periods at each measurement site. Numbers in boxes indicate the locations of the unipolar extracellular recording electrodes for the waveforms shown with each sequence in B and C. In A, the arrow indicates where atrial excitation was initiated spontaneously from invasion of the sinus node impulse. In B and C, the number in the large rectangle with each sequence indicates the premature interval (msec) of the accompanying excitation sequence and set of waveforms. The darkened areas superimposed on the excitation patterns indicate the distribution of refractory periods that were the same as or greater than the associated premature interval. The pattern of conduction is indicated by lines with arrows: straight lines signify longitudinal propagation, and irregular curved lines signify transverse propagation. The "T" symbols at the border of the light and dark areas indicate the approximate area where propagation failed (conduction block); the small boxes with solid circles in each drawing represent the sites of the recording electrodes shown in A. The solid arrows on some of the premature waveforms indicate sites at which no local excitation occurred. Reproduced with permission from Reference 6.*

premature impulse. That is, to develop reentry secondary to a premature impulse, there are important interactions that must occur, depending on the magnitude of the spatial nonuniformities and the degree to which the excitatory depolarizing current is decreased below that produced by fully excitable membranes.

Finally, from the above it is apparent that to fully understand the origin of reentry, one has to consider the mechanisms that cause premature excitation of the membrane as well as the manner in which spatial nonuniformities influence the propagation of premature impulses. This chapter will not consider the mechanisms that generate premature excitation of the sarcolemmal membrane. However, it should be emphasized that current evidence indicates that a major cause of premature beats in abnormal conditions is afterpotentials or afterdepolarizations, which occur following interventions that enhance calcium overload of cardiac myocytes (eg, ischemia[6] and digitalis glycosides[7]). Here, we limit our considerations to how premature impulses initiate reentry by identifying nonuniformities that produce functionally different pathways that have different effective refractory periods, the singular requirement to initiate circus movement reentry (also known as reentrant excitation, circulating wave fronts, circulating excitations, spiral waves, and rotors).[8]

Spatial Nonuniformities that Lead to Reentry

To place the underlying known causes of reentry in a contemporary perspective, it useful to consider in isolation each of the general mechanisms that have been shown to produce conduction abnormalities leading to reentry. Thus far, only three types of nonuniformities have been shown to produce the functionally different pathways required to initiate reentry.[8] These spatial inhomogeneities will be considered in the chronological order in which each concept was developed and applied to reentry in cardiac muscle.

Continuous Isotropic Media with Intrinsic Repolarization Inhomogeneities

It was long held that an anatomic obstacle was necessary for reentry to occur.[9] Then, in 1964, Moe et al introduced a computer model of atrial fibrillation that demonstrated that an anatomic obstacle was not necessary to generate reentrant circuits.[10] The authors' model was based on a two-dimensional continuous sheet that contained intrinsic repolarization inhomogeneities. They noted that "inhomogeneity [inhomogeneity of repolarization] was clearly necessary for the induction of self-sustained activity in the model and must be responsible for continued turbulence." The authors also mentioned anisotropic conduction velocity differences by commenting that "this feature would probably be of little significance in the model."

Experimental verification of a functional central obstacle during reentrant excitation was achieved in 1977 by Allessie et al[11] with in vitro experiments in atrial muscle. Reentry was induced by an early premature stimulus (S_2) delivered after a series of stimuli at normal intervals (S_1) at the same location. The authors noted that the initiation of circulating wave fronts was very sensitive to the location of the site of the premature stimulus. During the reentrant tachycardia, the fibers at the center of the circulating wave fronts were not activated. The inactivation was caused by these fibers being held above threshold potential because of the electronic effects of the circulating excitations. Allessie et al[11] observed that "In this way the center is functionally inexcitable, and the activation wave will travel around this functional obstacle." Because of the electronic effects of the circulating wave front on the central area (vortex), the authors referred to this model as the "leading-circle concept," now considered to be an essential feature of many reentrant circuits.

The major features of the leading-circle concept presented by Allessie et al[11] are the following:

1. The events that initiate the reentrant circuit are due to the "electrophysiological properties" of the tissue. The electrophysiological properties that create the spatial inhomogeneities that alter conduction are due to spatial nonuniformities in the kinetics of the membrane ionic repolarization currents. The structure is considered to be continuous and isotropic.

2. The action potentials circulate around a functional central obstacle, which is created by the electronic effects of the circulating excitation waves (the "leading circle").

3. There is no fully excitable gap in the reentrant circuit of the leading-circle model because the excitatory impulse propagates in the relative refractory period of the preceding action potential (crest and tail[11]). Consequently, the smallest circuit is one in which the

excitatory current of the propagating impulse is just enough to excite the "downstream" tissue, which is in its relative refractory period. If the action potential duration increases, the size of the circuit increases, and vice versa. A change in size of the reentrant circuit can occur because the length of the reentrant circuit is determined by the effective refractory period and the average conduction velocity. That is, this model assumes that the circuit wavelength = (velocity) × (refractory period).[9]

4. The experimental results of Allessie et al[11] indicated that a minimum area of 30 to 50 mm² was necessary for reentrant circuits based on the leading-circle concept.

Continuous Isotropic Media Free of Inhomogeneities in Which Transient Nonuniformities of Repolarization Are Induced

In 1980, van Capelle and Durrer[12] demonstrated in a computer model that reentry could be initiated in a continuous isotropic medium in the absence of any intrinsic inhomogeneity. The maneuver used to create the nonuniformities of repolarization necessary to induce reentry in such a medium was that the normal S_1 and premature S_2 stimuli were delivered at different locations. The S_1 stimulus was delivered along an extensive straight line to produce regular beats, and the S_2 stimulus was delivered at a distant site along a short straight line to initiate premature excitation.

Transient nonuniformities of refractoriness are created in a homogeneous medium by the above maneuver by the following sequence of events.[12] Regular beats (S_1) initiated along an extensive straight line produce planar excitation wave fronts. In a uniform medium, the propagation of excitation as a plane wave is followed by a plane wave of repolarization, which is associated with the zones of complete and partial refractoriness oriented along straight lines. When the premature stimulus (S_2) is delivered along a short line located within the lengthy partially refractory zone, the resultant premature excitation waves propagate differently in different directions[8]: (1) Antegrade conduction occurs into the zone of complete refractoriness, which results in conduction block. (2) Propagation in the opposite direction (away from the lengthy refractory zone) results in stable retrograde conduction because the action potentials in the area proximal to the refractory zone are generated by membrane in which normal excitability has returned. (3) Simultaneously, in a small area at the end of the short S_2 stimulus line, the wave front bends. The bending wave front eventually leads to reentry, after which the reentrant excitation wave can continue to move around a functional obstacle (vortex).

The computer simulations of van Capelle and Durrer[12] demonstrated that electrotonic interactions provide the mechanism by which circulating excitations (spiral waves) generate inactivated vortices. The results also showed that the essential requirement to initiate reentry in an intrinsically uniform continuous isotropic medium is that the excitation wave has to encounter nonuniform regions of repolarization. It does not matter whether the repolarization nonuniformity is intrinsic to the medium or whether the repolarization inhomogeneity is induced transiently by delivering the S_1 and S_2 stimuli at different locations. Finally, the authors' model demonstrated that in a continuous isotropic medium, a large area is required to initiate reentry due to repolarization nonuniformities; ie, an area approximating 20 resting space constants is required.[12] On the basis of a typical space constant of 1.5 mm measured in small ventricular trabeculae,[13] an area of 900 mm^2 would be required to develop a reentrant circuit. An interesting experimental fact is that numerous reentrant circuits have been verified that occupy much less than the estimated 900 mm^2 required for reentry in an isotropic medium with a resting space constant of 1.5 mm.[8]

Experimental verification of the induction of reentry under uniform conditions in which repolarization nonuniformities are created transiently was achieved by Frazier et al[14] in 1989 in the in vivo normal dog ventricle. Their experimental setup for delivering the normal S_1 and premature S_2 stimuli was similar to that of the van Capelle and Durrer model; ie, the S_1 and S_2 stimuli were delivered along lines that were positioned at different locations. After the S_2 stimulus, an inactive area developed at the end of the short line along which the premature stimulus was delivered, and reentrant excitation occurred because of rotation of the wave front around the inactive area, which the authors called the "critical point."[14]

It should be pointed out that once a reentrant circuit is established by the mechanism of inducing transient spatial nonuniformities of repolarization, the original delivery of the S_1 and S_2 stimuli at different locations does not affect the maintenance or creation of new inactive vortices. That the intrinsic nonuniformities of the tissue have their usual influence during subsequent spiral waves (multiple reentry episodes) was demonstrated recently by Davidenko et al,[15] who used optical mapping to study isolated sheep ventricular muscle. These authors initiated reentry under the same initial uniform repolarization conditions using different S_1 and S_2 stimulation locations as done in the van Capelle and Durrer[12] simulations. Once repeated spiral waves occurred, the vortices of depolarized tissue (3 × 5 mm) moved about and continued to change in location (as predicted by the van Capelle and Durrer[12] model results). Also, the spatial inhomogeneity of repolarization increased with multiple reentrant episodes. Davidenko et al[15] suggested that uniform and nonuniform anisotropy may contribute to the initiation, location, and size of the central inactivated area (vortices). The authors thereby provided important questions about the role of anisotropic propagation in the behavior of spiral waves.

Discontinuous Anisotropic Media With Nonuniformities of Electrical Load

In the above considerations of nonuniformities of repolarization, cardiac muscle was assumed to behave as a continuous isotropic structure. This assumption was based on the interpretation of measurements of the passive cable properties at a macroscopic size scale in small cardiac bundles.[13] When small currents are injected into one end of a small trabeculum, the potential across the membrane (V_m) decreases over a distance of 1 to 2 mm. This falloff in V_m with distance is fit well by a single exponential function, which is characteristic of the change in V_m when small currents are injected into an electrically uniform continuous one-dimensional cable. In this type of medium, the production of conduction disturbances that lead to reentry is limited to spatial variations in the kinetics of the membrane repolarization currents. Spatial nonuniformities of repolarization alter the depolarization phase of premature action potentials differently in different areas (pathways) by producing differences in takeoff potentials. The differences in takeoff potential result in spatially nonuniform decreases in $\dot{V}_{max}$ that, in turn, result in conduction failure in one pathway while stable conduction continues in another pathway.

A perplexing problem has been that it is not possible to explain the occurrence of reentry within small areas of cardiac muscle on the basis of the mechanism of nonuniformities of repolarization. As demonstrated by van Capelle and Durrer,[12] a large area is required to initiate reentry on the basis of repolarization inhomogeneities in continuous isotropic media (approximately 20 space constants). Also, Allessie et al[11] showed experimentally that a surface area of at least 30 to 50 mm² is necessary for reentrant excitation to occur, according to the leading-circle concept.

A new and different type of spatial nonuniformity that occurs at a microscropic level was discovered in 1981. In atrial and ventricular muscle, anisotropic conduction was found to be discontinuous in nature because of recurrent resistive discontinuities created by the cellular connections.[16] The associated electrophysiological nonuniformity is a spatial variation in electrical load produced by the nonuniform distribution of the electrical connections between cells. Nonuniformities of electrical load were apparent from the fact that different values of $\dot{V}_{max}$ occurred with different directions of conduction in the presence of constant membrane properties. $\dot{V}_{max}$ was lower during fast conduction along the long axis of the fibers (longitudinal conduction) and higher during slow conduction across the fibers (transverse conduction).[16] The variations in conduction velocity can be explained by differences in effective axial resistance of a continuous medium. In a continuous medium, however, differences in axial resistance do not alter the time course of depolarization. Also, a decrease in $\dot{V}_{max}$ with an increase in conduction velocity is just the opposite of what occurs in a continuous isotropic medium. The cause for this inverted relationship was considered to be that conduction in cardiac muscle is discontinuous in nature due to the connections between cells producing discontinuities of intracellular resistance that, in turn, affect the membrane depolarization currents, $\dot{V}_{max}$, and the safety factor of conduction.[16]

Recent extensive experimental measurements have shown marked effects on $\dot{V}_{max}$ of microscopic electrical boundaries (discontinuities) because of the complex geometry of individual cardiac myocytes and the associated nonuniform arrangement of their interconnections.[17] Discontinuities of internal resistance produce boundary effects that result in spatial variations of the electrical load on each small area of the sarcolemmal membrane. The variations in electrical load at a microscopic level alter the maximal rate of rise of the action potential. That is, $\dot{V}_{max}$ decreases at sites at which the downstream load becomes greater and , conversely, $\dot{V}_{max}$ increases at sites at which the downstream load is diminished. That cardiac muscle is composed of microscopic discontinuities that produce nonuniformities of electrical load is further evidenced by the variation in $\dot{V}_{max}$ from site to site within small areas in which the membrane properties are the same.[17] These differences in $\dot{V}_{max}$ at different microelectrode impalement sites are explained by differences in the spatial relationships between the cellular couplings and the membrane at the microelectrode impalement site in different cells.[17]

From analysis of extracellular potential waveforms and their derivatives during transverse propagation, it soon became apparent that there are two types of anisotropic electrical properties: uniform and nonuniform anisotropy.[18] As shown in Fig 2A, smooth extracellular waveforms occur during transverse conduction in tissues with uniform anistropic properties in which there is extensive electrical coupling between the cells in all directions. However, with the development of nonuniform anisotropy, complex multiphasic waveforms occur during transverse propagation (Fig 2B), which provide the electrophysiological basis for identifying nonuniform anisotropic electrical properties. Nonuniform anisotropic electrical properties are caused by a sparseness of side-to-side electrical connections between individual cells and/or small groups of cells in the presence of tight electrical coupling between cells along the long axis of the fibers. Thus far, measurement of extracellular potential waveforms has provided the only method to distinguish between uniform and nonuniform anisotropic cardiac bundles. For example, it has not been possible to distinguish between the two by injecting small currents and measuring the falloff of V_m with distance.[13]

A change from uniform to nonuniform anisotropic properties occurs normally because of electrical uncoupling of side-to-side fiber connections in atrial bundles at different ages. Such changes occur within a few months immediately after birth with growth and developmental (Fig 2)[18] and over a much longer period with aging in people >50 years old.[19] Abnormal states such as chronic hypertrophy[20] also are associated with the development of nonuniform anisotropic properties. The multiphasic extracellular waveforms during transverse conduction correlate histologically with the development of small longitudinally oriented collagenous septa that encircle individual myocytes and small groups of myocytes (Fig 2B).[18–20] This microfibrosis provides a histological basis for identi-

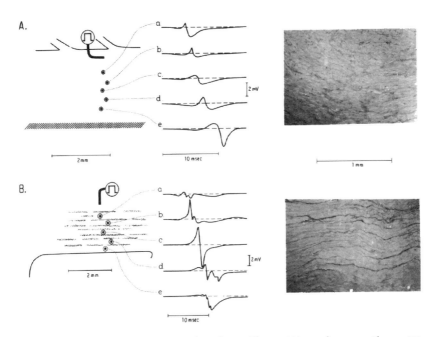

FIGURE 2. *Transverse propagation in uniform (A) and nonuniform (B) anisotropic canine atrial muscle bundles. The two preparations were from the same atrium of a puppy 1 week after birth. A shows crista terminalis; B shows limbus of the fossa ovalis. The unipolar extracellular waveforms recorded during transverse propagation are shown in the middle of the figure. Smooth single deflections occurred with uniform anisotropy (A), and irregular multiphasic waveforms occurred with nonuniform anisotropy (B). The associated microscopic structure of uniform versus nonuniform anisotropy is shown on the right. With uniform anisotropy, collagenous tissue is distributed among the myocytes in a scattered and irregular manner (A). With nonuniform anisotropy, collagenous tissue is organized into fine connective-tissue septa (microfibrosis), which appear as wavy horizontal lines that separate individual myocytes and groups of myocytes along the long axis of the fibers (B). By adulthood in dogs, many areas of the atrium, including the crista terminalis, demonstrate nonuniform anisotropic properties with microfibrosis and multiphasic extracellular waveforms similar to those in B. Reproduced with permission from Reference 19.*

fying preparations with the electrical properties of "fine" nonuniform anisotropy. A "gross" type of nonuniform anisotropy develops in the ventricle after myocardial infarction. Wit et al[21] demonstrated very prominent irregularities in the extracellular waveforms during transverse conduction in tissues of healed infarcts. In the postinfarcted ventricle, there is also very prominent connective tissue accumulation between groups of fibers. We use the term "gross" nonuniform anisotropy for such tissues in which considerably greater fibrotic areas occur than with the microfibrosis of bundles with "fine" nonuniform anisotropic properties.

In nonuniform anisotropic tissues, fast longitudinal conduction with a lower $\dot{V}_{max}$ should be more vulnerable to decreases in the excitatory depolarizing current than is slow transverse propagation with a higher $\dot{V}_{max}$.[16] This inverted relationship suggested that at most sites, the current load on the membrane is greater during longitudinal than transverse conduction. We therefore considered that premature action potentials should continue to propagate in the transverse direction after conduction block would occur in the longitudinal direction, with resultant reentry. This prediction of anisotropic reentry was confirmed in 1981 when premature stimuli were induced within a single canine atrial bundle.[16] An important feature of this new type of reentry is that neither intrinsic nor induced repolarization nonuniformities are involved (previously, they had been considered necessary for premature impulses to initiate reentry).

Refractory Periods in Fast and Slow Pathways Are Determined by the Distribution of Cellular Coupling in Nonuniform Anisotropic Cardiac Muscle

Perhaps the most fundamental change produced by the demonstration of anisotropic reentry is that the effective refractory period is determined independently by a new and different mechanism: the nonuniform anisotropic distribution of the electrical coupling between cardiac myocytes. In the past, spatial differences in the effective refractory period have been considered to be caused solely by spatial nonuniformities in the excitability of the membrane that, in turn, are determined by the time course of decay of the repolarizing currents and reactivation of the depolarizing (sodium) current. Now it can be seen that there is a "passive" structural mechanism that also determines the effective refractory period because of microscopic nonuniformities of electrical load created by the distribution of the cellular couplings.

Conduction velocity curves, the reciprocal of conduction time curves, are graphs of the values of conduction time per unit distance; they show the effective conduction velocity within an area located between two monitoring electrodes (Fig 3). Moe et al[22,23] demonstrated that when a discontinuity occurs in a conduction time curve of the AV node, the discontinuity (sudden jump) in conduction time indicates the presence of at least two underlying functionally different pathways. A discontinuity in a conduction time or velocity curve is caused by the effective refractory period of one pathway being longer than that of another pathway. Accordingly, the conduction of premature impulses can continue in the pathway with the shorter refractory period after the premature stimulus interval is decreased to less than that of the pathway with the longer refractory period. As noted previously, this phenomenon is the singular functional requirement to initiate reentry.

On the basis of discontinuities in conduction time curves, Moe et al[22,23] proposed that in the AV node, there are dual pathways with different properties. Slow conduction occurs in one AV nodal pathway with a short effective refractory period, and fast conduction occurs in another pathway with a longer refractory period.

The conduction velocity curves of Fig 3 demonstrate that dual pathways with these properties are not limited to the AV node. In fact, they are a general property of cardiac bundles that develop nonuniform anisotropic properties. The conduction velocity curves shown are representative of those obtained in previously reported experiments in human and canine atrial and ventricular preparations.[18,20] Twenty-three velocity curves were obtained in uniform anisotropic bundles, and 54 velocity curves were obtained in nonuniform anisotropic preparations. The measurements were performed as illustrated by the drawing in the upper part of Fig 3A. One pair of recording unipolar electrodes was located along the longitudinal axis of the fibers and another pair along the transverse axis. A single electrode was used to deliver the normal and premature stimuli, and each premature impulse was delivered after 10 regular stimuli, which occurred at cycle lengths between 600 and 800 msec. The conduction velocity at each premature interval was determined by dividing the distance between the two electrodes of each pair by the time of conduction of the extracellular potential between the two electrodes.

It is apparent from Fig 3 that the effects of decreasing the premature interval on anisotropic conduction are quite different in uniform (A) versus nonuniform (B) anistropic preparations. When the premature interval is shortened in uniform anistropic bundles, the conduction velocities decrease in the fast longitudinal and slow transverse pathways until propagation ceases simultaneously in both pathways. Thus, in uniform anisotropic bundles, the effective refractory period is the same in all conduction pathways.

In the nonuniform anisotropic bundles, however, reducing the premature interval results in discontinuities in the conduction velocity curves (Fig 3B). Specifically, different effective refractory periods occur in different pathways in relation to the direction of propagation with respect to the orientation of the fibers. As the premature interval is gradually decreased, fast longitudinal conduction suddenly stops (vertical dashed line in Fig 3B). With further reduction of the premature interval, slow conduction continues in the transverse pathway in the absence of fast longitudinal conduction. In the 54 velocity curves with discontinuities we have obtained thus far in nonuniform anisotropic preparations, the differences in the effective refractory periods of the fast longitudinal and slow transverse pathways have varied from 25 to 45 msec. These values are similar to the differences in the effective refractory periods reported for "fast" and "slow" AV nodal pathways (up to approximately 55 msec).[24]

The above differences in effective refractory periods in different pathways of cardiac bundles with nonuniform anisotropic properties cannot be explained by differences in repolarization time. The site of the stimulating electrode could be shifted in any direction in each nonuniform anisotropic preparation, and the same result occurred with respect to the orientation of the fibers: the slow transverse conduction pathway had a shorter effective refractory period than the fast longitudinal pathway. In each case, there was multidimensional propagation in a two- or three-dimensional network of cells. Therefore, the sudden shift in conduction from fast longitudinal to slow transverse conduction cannot be accounted for by electronic spread of currents across an isolated area of block. In one-dimensional structures, "jumps" in conduction time across an ischemic gap were demonstrated by Antzelevitch and Moe[25] and across a sucrose gap by Jalife.[26]

The following can be concluded from the above: (1) Disconti-

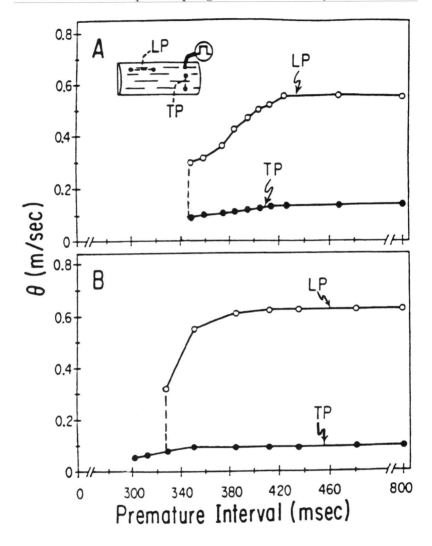

FIGURE 3. *Typical anisotropic velocity curves in uniform (A) and nonuniform (B) human atrial bundles. Conduction velocities during propagation in the longitudinal and transverse directions (LP and TP, respectively) were measured simultaneously with the electrode arrangement shown at the top of A. Premature action potentials were introduced after every 10th stimulus at a basic cycle length of 800 msec. The preparation in A was from a 12-year-old patient, and the preparation in B was from a 62-year-old patient. Reproduced with permission from Reference 21 in modified form.*

nuities in conduction time or velocity curves are a general property of nonuniform anisotropic cardiac muscle. (2) "Dual pathways" are not limited to AV nodal conduction; rather, they are a general property of any cardiac bundle that develops nonuniform anisotropic cellular coupling. (3) In the fast and slow pathways of nonuniform anisotropic muscle, the underlying differences in the effective refractory periods are due to microscopic nonuniformities of electrical load which, in turn, are created by the nonuniform anisotropic distribution of electrical coupling between cells.

Microreentry Due to Nonuniform Anisotropic Cellular Coupling

An additional major feature of conduction associated with the presence of nonuniform anisotropic cellular coupling in otherwise normal cardiac bundles is that the effective conduction velocity along the transverse axis of the fibers decreases to the range of "very slow" conduction in the AV node (<0.1 m/s). In a series of nonuniform anisotropic human atrial bundles, we found the average effective conduction velocity in the transverse direction to be 0.04 m/s.[20] A major implication of these very low effective conduction velocities is that they should provide a means for reentry to occur within very small areas. The following demonstrates that such is the case.

Fig 4 shows an example of anisotropic reentry occurring within a single human pectinate bundle with markedly nonuniform anistropic electrical properties. In the drawing of the reentrant circuit at the lower right, it can be seen that the circuit had the shape of a rectangle that was elongated along the long axis of the fibers. The maximum width of the circuit was 0.6 mm, and the maximum length was 2.6 mm. These dimensions resulted in the reentrant circuit occupying a surface area of 1.6 mm², with a perimeter of 6.4 mm. In this human atrial bundle, the intrinsic sarcolemmal membrane ionic properties were normal, as indicated by the occurrence of normal action potentials with fast upstrokes when the preparation was paced at cycle lengths between 300 and 1000 msec.[20]

Analysis of this small reentrant circuit demonstrates that the length (perimeter) of the circuit can be smaller than the wavelength of refractoriness, which is estimated by using the widely applied formula originated by Wiener and Rosenblueth[9]: "wave length" = (velocity) × (refractory period). In Fig 4, the minimum effective

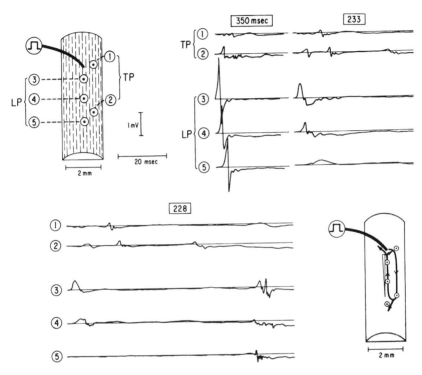

FIGURE 4. *Microreentry in response to premature action potentials in a human nonuniform anisotropic pectinate muscle bundle. Results were obtained at a cycle length of 350 msec; a premature stimulus was introduced every 10th beat at the interval shown in the box above each group of waveforms. Drawing at upper let shows locations at which each waveform was recorded. Drawing at lower right shows the perimeter of the reentrant circuit, which is indicated by solid lines with arrows. In the drawing, the open elongated triangle indicates initial decremental longitudinal conduction to block. Shaded region denotes surrounding areas in which extracellular waveforms were measured at 16 sites; at each of these peripheral sites, local excitation occurred after that of sites confined to the perimeter of the reentrant circuit for the corresponding area. This confirmed that the circuit that initiated reentry was limited to the region marked by solid lines with arrows. Reproduced with permission from Reference 21.*

refractory period in the area of microreentry was 223 msec. In this small circuit, we were not able to obtain reliable estimates of the velocity throughout the perimeter of 6.4 mm. We therefore used the above formula to estimate the average velocity, which was 0.028 m/s. This average velocity is considerably less than the very low velocities encountered in the normal AV node. In Fig 4, the marked irregularities of the extracellular waveforms indicate that there were multiple localized delays of conduction during the anisotropic microreentry. Consequently, delays of conduction at a microscopic level due to a nonuniform anisotropic distribution of the cellular couplings can reduce the perimeter of a reentrant circuit to less than the wavelength of refractoriness. It is interesting that in 1966 Krinski[27] demonstrated in a theoretical model that localized conduction delays, which were produced in the model by impulses entering a region of increased refractoriness, reduce the perimeter of a reentrant circuit. With multiple delays, the perimeter of the circuit "may be considerably less than the wavelength of refractoriness . . . ."[27]

In all of the nonuniform anisotropic preparations in which we have encountered anisotropic reentry, the reentry has developed after a discontinuity has occurred in the conduction time (velocity) curves due to initial failure of fast longitudinal conduction. Recently, we collaborated with Josephson to determine whether the AV node of the rabbit has nonuniform anisotropic conduction properties during antegrade propagation of normal action potentials.[8] The results demonstrated that the transitional region of the AV node has markedly nonuniform anisotropic conduction properties. On the basis of the above considerations of the effects of nonuniform anisotropy on conduction within small areas, we proposed that (1) AV nodal "fast" and "slow" pathways are a result of nonuniform anisotropic cellular coupling in the transitional region of the node and (2) AV nodal "dual pathways" and reentry need to be reevaluated in terms of the nonuniform anisotropic properties of this region of the AV node.[8]

Determinants of the Effective Refractory Period

At this point, it is worthwhile to view measurements of the effective refractory period under different experimental conditions in a new light. In a small isolated patch of membrane, the effective refractory period is identified as the shortest premature interval at which an action potential upstroke can be generated. In this case, a membrane action potential is generated without conduction of the excitatory impulse; ie, the patch remains isopotential throughout the time course of the action potential. For a stimulus to produce depolarization of the membrane from any takeoff potential, the inward depolarizing current not only must depolarize the capacitance of the membrane but also must exceed any repolarizing currents that are present. Consequently, in isolated small patches of membrane, the only way to change the effective refractory period is to alter the kinetics of the membrane repolarization and depolarization ionic currents.

In multicellular preparations, however, the effective refractory period is identified as the shortest interval at which a conducted impulse occurs. For stable (nondecremental) conduction to occur, each small patch of membrane within a cell not only must supply enough current to depolarize itself but also must supply sufficient current downstream to charge the capacitance of the neighboring tissue that has yet to depolarize. In anisotropic cardiac muscle, a nonuniform distribution of resistive discontinuities is created by the cellular interconnections. In turn, the periodic resistive discontinuities encountered during conduction create microscopic differences in the downstream load, ie, differences in current required for each patch to discharge the downstream capacitance. The greater the load, the lower the value of $\dot{V}_{max}$ and the greater the amount of current that must be generated for stable conduction to continue.[17] Also, the downstream load on a given patch of membrane changes when the direction of conduction is altered.[16] This occurs because, when there is a change in the pattern of current flow, there is a change in the relative position of each patch of membrane with respect to the surrounding "upstream" and "downstream" resistive boundaries (cell borders and gap junctions).[17]

The term "safety factor" has been used to compare the maximum current a patch of membrane can supply with the current required to bring it to threshold.[8] If the ratio is >1, stable conduction will occur. If the ratio is <1 decremental conduction and failure (block) will occur. During conduction, the local electrical circuit requires the excitatory current of each membrane patch to supply downstream current through the interconnections of multiple cells. Hence, it might be expected that variations in the distribution of cellular coupling could affect the downstream load, change cell-to-cell current flow, and independently alter the safety factor of conduction, which, in turn, would affect the effective refractory period.

To summarize: A single "active" mechanism resulting from the kinetics of the membrane ionic currents determines the effective refractory period in isopotential patches of membrane that generate membrane action potentials. But in multicellular preparations, the effective refractory period is determined by two mechanisms: (1) an "active" mechanism resulting from the kinetics of the membrane depolarization and repolarization currents and (2) a "passive" structural mechanism resulting from nonuniformities of electrical load produced by the nonuniform anisotropic distribution of the cellular couplings.

Conclusions

This chapter establishes cellular coupling as a basis for arrhythmias by placing a new type of inhomogeneity, nonuniform anisotropic cellular coupling, in an overall perspective with the widely known repolarization nonuniformities that lead to reentrant arrhythmias. This new nonuniformity produces microscopic inhomogeneities of electrical load due to resistive discontinuities created by the cellular couplings. The distribution of the cellular interconnection is characterized electrically by sparse side-to-side coupling between cells and between small groups of cells. Bundles with nonuniform anisotropic properties are marked histologically by the presence of fine collagenous septa along the course of the fibers (microfibrosis).

Until recently, the nonuniformities necessary to initiate reentry were considered to be limited to two types of media: (1) continuous isotropic media with intrinsic repolarization nonuniformities and (2) continuous isotropic media without intrinsic inhomogeneities in which repolarization nonuniformities are introduced transiently. Review of theoretical and experimental models of reentry as they were developed chronologically produces the following picture: as the conduction velocity decreases, reentrant circuits become small in size, and the nonuniformities necessary to initiate reentry are provided by nonuniform anisotropic cellular coupling.[8] Repolarization nonuniformities (eg, the leading-circle model) create relatively large reentrant circuits (>30 to 50 mm^2). Nonuniform anisotropic cellular coupling, which is associated with microfibrosis,[8] makes it possible for reentry to occur within small areas (<10 to 15 mm^2).

A general property of nonuniform anisotropic bundles is the presence of functionally different pathways in the absence of intrinsic repolarization nonuniformities. Fast longitudinal conduction occurs in one pathway with a longer effective refractory period, and slow (<0.1 m/s) transverse conduction occurs in another pathway with a shorter refractory period. Preceding the onset of reentry within nonuniform anisotropic bundles, there are "discontinuities" in the velocity (conduction time) curves due to differences in the effective refractory periods in the longitudinal and transverse directions with respect to the orientation of the fibers.

Discontinuous anisotropic conduction is quite different from conduction in a continuous anisotropic medium, and it requires new ways of thinking about propagation in cardiac muscle. There is asynchrony of firing of adjacent fibers, which is indicated at a microscopic level by multiple notches in the derivatives of the extracellular waveforms.[17] When the membrane excitability is decreased, conduction delays at the junctions between cells are markedly increased. Most importantly, the enhanced delays at the junctions are associated with a relative increase in the nonuniformities of electrical load, which lead to unidirectional block and reentry within small areas in nonuniform anisotropic bundles. Consequently, nonuniform anisotropic cellular coupling provides a previously unrecognized basis for reentrant arrhythmias.

References

1. Josephson ME, Buxton AE, Marchlinski FE, et al. Sustained ventricular tachycardia in coronary artery disease: evidence for reentrant mechanism. In: Zipes DP, Jalife J, eds. *Cardiac Electrophysiology and Arrhythmias.* New York, NY: Grune and Stratton; 1985:409–418.
2. Podrid PJ. Aggravation of arrhythmia: a complication of antiarrhythmic drugs. *J Cardiovasc Electrophysiol.* 1993;4:311–319.
3. Kalbfleisch SJ, Langberg JJ. Catheter ablation with radiofrequency energy: biophysical aspects and clinical applications. *J Cardiovasc Electrophysiol.* 1992,3:173–186.
4. Luo C-H, Rudy Y. A model of the ventricular cardiac action potential: depolarization, repolarization, and their interaction. *Circ Res.* 1991;68: 1501–1526.
5. Spach MS, Dolber PC, Heidlage JF. Interaction of inhomogeneities of

repolarization with anisotropic propagation in dog atria: a mechanism for both preventing and initiating reentry. *Circ Res.* 1989;65:1612–1631.

6. Clusin WT, Bristow MR, Karagueuzian HS, et al. Do calcium-dependent ionic currents mediate ischemic ventricular fibrillation? *Am J Cardiol.* 1982;49:606–612.

7. Leder WJ, Tsien RW. Transient inward current underlying arrhythmogenic effects of cardiotonic steroids in Purkinje fibers. *J Physiol.* 1976; 273:73–100.

8. Spach MS, Josephson ME. Initiating reentry: the role of nonuniform anisotropy in small reentry circuits. *J Cardiovasc Electrophysiol.* In Press.

9. Wiener N, Rosenblueth A. The mathematical formulation of the problem of conduction of impulses in a network of connected excitable elements, specifically in cardiac muscle. *Arch Inst Cardiol Mexico.* 1946; 16:205–265.

10. Moe GK, Rheinboldt WC, Abildskov JA. A computer model of atrial fibrillation. *Am Heart J.* 1964:67:200–220.

11. Allessie MA, Bonke FIM, Schopman FJG. Circus movement in rabbit atrial muscle as a mechanism of tachycardia, III: the "leading circle" concept: a new model of circus movement in cardiac tissue without the involvement of an anatomical obstacle. *Circ Res.* 1977;41:9–18.

12. van Capelle FJL, Durrer D. Computer simulation of arrhythmias in a network of coupled excitable elements. *Circ Res.* 1980;47:454–466.

13. Weidmann S. Electrical constants of trabecular muscle from mammalian heart. *J Physiol (Lond).* 1970;210:1041–1054.

14. Frazier DW, Wolf PD, Wharton JM, et al. Stimulus-induced critical point: mechanism for electrical initiation of reentry in normal canine mycardium. *J Clin Invest.* 1989;83:1039–1052.

15. Davidenko JM, Kent PF, Chialvo DR, et al. Sustained vortex-like waves in normal isolated ventricular muscle. *Proc Natl Acad Sci USA.* 1990; 87:8785–8789.

16. Spach MS, Miller WT III, Geselowitz DB, et al. The discontinuous nature of propagation in normal canine cardiac muscle: evidence for recurrent discontinuities of intracellular resistance that affect the membrane currents. *Circ Res.* 1981;48:39–45.

17. Spach MS, Heidlage, JF, Darken ER, et al. Cellular $\dot{V}_{max}$ reflects both membrane properties and the load presented by adjoining cells. *Am J Physiol.* 1992;263:H1855-H1863.

18. Spach MS, Miller WT III, Dolber PC, et al. The functional role of structural complexities in the propagation of depolarization in the atrium of the dog: cardiac conduction disturbances due to discontinuities of effective axial resistivity. *Circ Res.* 1982;50:175–191.

19. Spach MS, Dolber PC. Relating extracellular potentials and their derivatives to anisotropic propagation at a microscopic level in human cardiac muscle: evidence for electrical uncoupling of side-to-side fiber connections with increasing age. *Circ Res.* 1986;58:356–371.

20. Spach MS, Dolber PC, Heidlage JF. Influence of the passive anisotropic properties on directional differences in propagation following modification of the sodium conductance in human atrial muscle: a model of

reentry based on anisotropic discontinuous propagation. *Circ Res.* 1988;62:811–832.

21. Wit AL, Dillon S, Ursell PC. Influences of anistropic tissue structure on reentrant ventricular tachycardia. In: Brugada P, Wellens HJJJ, eds. *Cardiac Arrhythmias: Where To Go From Here?* Mount Kisco, NY: Futura Publishing Co; 1987:27–50.

22. Moe GK, Preston JM, Burlington H. Physiologic evidence for a dual AV transmission system. *Circ Res.* 1956;4:357–375.

23. Mendez C, Moe GK. Demonstration of a dual AV conduction system in the isolated heart. *Circ Res.* 1966;19:378–393.

24. Wu D. Dual atrioventricular nodal pathways: a reappraisal. *PACE Pacing Clin Electrophysiol.* 1982;5:72–89.

25. Antzelevitch C, Moe GK. Electrotonically mediated delayed conduction and reentry in relation to "slow response" in mammalian ventricular conducting tissue. *Circ Res.* 1981;49:1129–1139.

26. Jalife J. The sucrose gap preparation as a model of AV and nodal transmission: are dual pathways necessary for reciprocation and AV nodal "echoes"? *PACE Pacing Clin Electrophysiol.* 1983;6:1106–1122.

27. Krinski VI. Spread of excitation in an inhomogeneous medium (state similar to cardiac fibrillation). *Biofizika.* 1966;11:676–683.

Chapter 6

Editorial Comments

Yoram Rudy, PhD

Introduction

The preceding chapter discussed the role of cellular coupling in cardiac arrhythmias of the reentry type. The structural complexity of the myocardium as an assembly of discrete cells separated by a periodic intercalated disk structure was established in 1954. Until recently, however, propagation of the action potential in cardiac muscle has been characterized as though it occurred in a syncytium. The characteristics of action potential propagation were associated with membrane properties alone, ignoring structural effects arising from the anatomic complexity of the myocardium. Historically, conduction disturbances leading to arrhythmias were thought to result from altered membrane characteristics (eg, reduced excitability) and, in particular, from nonuniformities of membrane properties (eg, spatial dispersion of repolarization). This view reflected the "syncytium hypothesis," which neglected the architectural complexities of the tissue.

Recent experimental studies have demonstrated the important role of the anatomic structure in causing conduction abnormalities such as slow conduction, conduction block, and reentry. There is accumulating evidence that these conduction disturbances that lead to reentrant arrhythmias can result from structural changes and that membrane effects (altered or depressed transmembrane potentials, nonuniform distribution of membrane refractoriness) may not always be necessary for abnormal conduction to occur.

In these comments, we summarize theoretical principles that characterize structural effects on propagation of excitation and reentry in cardiac tissue. These observations are based on computer

From DiMarco JP, Prystowsky EN (eds): *Atrial Arrhythmias: State of the Art.* Armonk, NY, Futura Publishing Company, Inc., © 1995.

models that were used to examine the effects of the discrete cellular structure of the myocardium on propagation of the action potential. The focus is on cellular level discontinuities rather than on more global structural discontinuities (eg, fiber bundles separated by connective tissue septa). We emphasize the effects of changes in the degree of cell-to-cell coupling at gap junctions. A high degree of cellular uncoupling has been demonstrated in cardiac tissue under experimental ischemic conditions[1-3] and in association with various types of injury.[4] An increased degree of separation between fibers has been observed in the setting of infarction.[5] In the model simulations, we attempted to cover the normal physiological range of gap junction resistance, the transition to increased degree of cellular decoupling, and the pathological range of high degree of decoupling between cells whose upper bound is complete separation. We studied the role of these changes in the development of conduction abnormalities such as slow conduction, conduction block, and reentry. We also examined the reflection of the discrete cellular structure and the discontinuous nature of propagation in computed extracellular potential waveforms. Details can be found in previous publications.[6-11]

Discontinuous Propagation

The following observations were based on a theoretical model of propagation in a multicellular one-dimensional fiber that consists of 100 individual cells of realistic dimension (100 μm long and 16μm in diameter) connected to each other by gap junctions.[6-8]

1. Propagation is a discontinuous process at the cellular level, exhibiting local propagation delays at gap junctions that are very significant compared with the conduction time through the cell. This is true even for longitudinal propagation in a tightly coupled tissue. For normal, well-coupled tissue, the propagation delay at the gap junction is roughly equal to the propagation time through the entire cell.

2. The discontinuous behavior becomes progressively more pronounced with increasing degrees of decoupling between cells. For a 10-fold increase in decoupling relative to the typical value under normal, well-coupled conditions, the gap junction delays are

very long (300 μsec) compared with the propagation time through the cell, which is practically negligible. Under these conditions, conduction velocity is determined by the gap junction delays.

3. The discontinuous nature of propagation is not revealed in global measurements (eg, macroscopic conduction velocity, temporal extracellular potential waveforms) unless cells become highly uncoupled. For high degrees of uncoupling, the discontinuous behavior is reflected in the global conduction velocity, which decreases faster with increased gap junction resistance than the inverse square root relations of a continuous syncytium, and in the occurrence of decremental conduction and conduction block even when the membrane (action potential) is normal and fully excitable. For high degrees of uncoupling, the discontinuous structure is also reflected as irregularities (foot potentials, notches) in the action potential and in the extracellular potential waveforms.

4. Extracellular potential measurements with microscopic spatial resolution reveal nonuniformities in the local (microscopic) conduction velocity even when the tissue is well coupled.

5. Important characteristics of the propagating action potential are influenced by the discrete structure of the myocardium. Importantly, $(dV/dt)_{max}$, the maximum rate of rise of the action potential, displays a nonmonotonic behavior as a function of conduction velocity when velocity is reduced by decreasing the degree of coupling between cells (increasing gap junction resistance). The behavior implies that $(dV/dt)_{max}$ cannot be used as an index of conduction velocity when structural changes (decoupling) are involved. Also, slow conduction can occur with normal or even high $(dV/dt)_{max}$ when decoupling is involved.

Reentry

The following observations were based on computer simulations of propagation in a ring-shaped fiber model. This model represents a fixed reentry pathway. It consists of up to 1500 cells of realistic dimensions, connected to each other by gap junctions.[9-11]

1. Conduction disturbances that lead to reentry, such as slow conduction, decremental conduction, and conduction block, can be caused by decreased intercellular coupling alone and do not neces-

sarily involve membrane changes in all cases. In particular, decreased coupling in our model can bring about a 20-fold reduction in conduction velocity before conduction block occurs. In comparison, reduced membrane excitability can reduce velocity to only one third of its normal value before block occurs. Therefore, cellular uncoupling probably plays a very important role in causing slow conduction, a necessary condition for reentry.

2. A "window of vulnerability" exists in the refractory period of a propagating action potential. It is defined as a window during which unidirectional block can be induced by a premature stimulus. Outside this window, it is impossible to induce unidirectional block; an action potential induced by a premature stimulus either propagates or blocks in both directions, and reentry cannot be established. Thus, the vulnerable window is the basis for unidirectional block and reentry, and the size of the window represents the inducibility of unidirectional block and reentry by premature stimuli. The wider the window, the more vulnerable is the tissue to unidirectional block and reentry.

3. A uniform increase in the degree of cellular decoupling results in a greater vulnerability to the induction of unidirectional block and reentry. For normal cellular coupling, the vulnerability is only about 0.5 msec. Very precise timing (better than 0.5 msec) of a premature stimulus is required for induction of reentry. In contrast, for high degrees of cellular decoupling, the vulnerability is increased to 30 msec. For such a wide window, reentry can be easily induced. This simulation demonstrates that induction of reentrant arrhythmias by a stimulation protocol is not an all-or-none phenomenon but rather constitutes a probabilistic event. For normal tissue with a normal degree of cellular coupling, the probability of hitting the narrow vulnerable window (<0.5 msec) is extremely small, and inducing reentry is practically impossible. For abnormal tissue with increased cellular decoupling, the probability of inducing reentry is increased, and for a high degree of uncoupling, the size of the vulnerable window (>30 msec) makes it highly probable that a premature stimulus will hit the window, thereby inducing reentry.

4. A uniformly high degree of cellular decoupling creates conditions that favor sustained reentry. In our simulations, for a gap junction resistance of 20 $\Omega \cdot cm^2$ (a typical value for normal tissue with normal cellular coupling), reentry is not sustained in a 2-cm-long reentry pathway. For a high degree of cellular uncoupling (gap

junction resistance of 50 $\Omega \cdot$ cm^2), reentry in the same pathway is sustained.

5. A uniform decrease throughout the entire reentry pathway in membrane excitability (sodium channel conductance) results in slow conduction with slightly decreased vulnerability to the induction of reentry (in contrast to increased vulnerability with reduced velocity caused by uniform increase in gap junction uncoupling as described in paragraph 3 above). The reduced vulnerability reflects increased symmetry in the state of the membrane at the vicinity of the vulnerable window.

6. The observations in the previous five paragraphs were based on simulations conducted in a homogeneous (uniform) reentry pathway with uniform membrane properties (ie, refractory period and excitability), uniform geometry (ie, fiber cross section), and uniform distribution of gap junction resistances. In general, inhomogeneities in any of these parameters bring about a large increase in vulnerability. The increase in vulnerability is proportional to the degree of inhomogeneity. In the presence of membrane inhomogeneities, reentry can be induced by applying both the primary and premature stimuli at the same site (in the homogeneous pathway, the stimulation sites must be different). In the presence of structural inhomogeneities (ie, segments with different cross sections, segments with different degrees of cellular coupling), reentry can be induced by a single stimulus, without the need for a premature stimulus following the primary stimulus.

Concluding Remarks

The theoretical observations summarized above demonstrate the importance of the microscopic cellular structure in determining propagation of the excitation process in cardiac tissue. They also suggest that modulation of cellular coupling caused by pathology, such as decreased coupling due to ischemia and infarction, can result in conduction disturbances and reentrant arrhythmias. This implies that approaches to arrhythmia therapy and arrhythmia management (eg, antiarrhythmic drugs) should take into consideration structural factors and the effects of the intervention on the properties of gap junctions.

References

1. Kleber AG, Riegger CB, Janse MJ. Electrical uncoupling and increase of extracellular resistance after induction of ischemia in isolated, arterially perfused rabbit papillary muscle. *Circ Res.* 1987;51:271–279.
2. Yan G, Cascio W, Kleber A. Evidence for inhomogeneous cellular uncoupling in ventricular muscle during ischemia. *Circulation.* 1988;78 (suppl II):II–639. Abstract.
3. Wu J, McHowat J, Saffitz JE, Yamada KA, Corr PB. Inhibition of gap junctional conductance by long-chain acylcarnitines and their preferential accumulation in junctional sarcolemma during hypoxia. *Circ Res.* 1993;72:879–889.
4. DeMello WC. Intercellular communication in cardiac muscle. *Circ Res.* 1982;51:1–9.
5. Janse MJ, Wit AL. Electrophysiological mechanisms of ventricular arrhythmias resulting from myocardial ischemia and infarction. *Physiol Rev.* 1989;69:1049–1152.
6. Rudy Y, Quan W. A model study of the effects of the discrete cellular structure on electrical propagation in cardiac tissue. *Circ Res.* 1987;61:815–823.
7. Rudy Y, Quan W. The effects of the discrete cellular structure on propagation of excitation in cardiac tissue: a model study. In: Sperelakis N, Cole W, eds. *Cell Interactions and Gap Junctions.* Boca-Raton, Fl: CRC Press; 1989;2:123–141.
8. Rudy Y, Quan W. Propagation delays across cardiac gap junctions and their reflection in extracellular potentials: a simulation study. *J Cardiovasc Electrophysiol.* 1991:2:299–315.
9. Quan W, Rudy Y. Unidirectional block and reentry of cardiac excitation: a model study. *Circ Res.* 1990;66:367–382.
10. Rudy Y, Quan W. Reentry of cardiac excitation: a simulation study. In: Sideman S, Beyar R, Klebar A, eds. *Cardiac Electrophysiology, Circulation, and Transport.* Boston, Mass: Kluwer Academic Publishers; 1991:63–72.
11. Quan W, Rudy Y. Termination of reentrant propagation by a single stimulus: a model study. *PACE Pacing Clin Electrophysiol.* 1991;14:1700–1706.

Chapter 7

Electrophysiological Mechanisms of Atrial Fibrillation

M. Allessie, MD, PhD; K. Konings, MD; and M. Wijffels, MD

In this chapter, we focus on two recent studies performed in our institution that provide some new insights into the electrophysiological mechanisms of atrial fibrillation (AF).[1,2]

Mapping of Atrial Fibrillation in Humans

In the first study, by Konings et al,[1] the electrical activation of the free wall of the right atrium was mapped during electrically induced AF in 25 patients with Wolff-Parkinson-White syndrome. The patients (16 men, 9 women) underwent surgical interruption of their accessory pathway for symptomatic or drug-refractory tachycardias. No cardiac abnormalities other than the Wolff-Parkinson-White syndrome were found in any of the patients. High-density mapping of the free wall of the right atrium was performed with a spoon-shaped mapping electrode (diameter, 3.6 cm; interelectrode distance, 2.25 mm) positioned manually on the atrial wall. Two hundred forty-four unipolar electrograms were recorded simultaneously with a large silver plate in the thoracic cavity as indifferent electrode. The excitation pattern of the right atrium was mapped during sinus rhythm, rapid pacing, and electrically induced AF before the patients were put on cardiopulmonary bypass and before cryoablation of the accessory pathway(s).

In 8 patients, the free wall of the left atrium was also mapped during AF. During sinus rhythm and rapid atrial pacing (330 beats

From DiMarco JP, Prystowsky EN (eds): *Atrial Arrhythmias: State of the Art.* Armonk, NY, Futura Publishing Company, Inc., © 1995.

per minute), in all patients, the free wall of the right atrium was activated by a single broad, uniformly propagating wave of depolarization. The conduction velocity of this depolarization wave was 73 ± 5 cm/s during sinus rhythm and 68 ± 3 cm/s during rapid pacing. No areas of slow conduction or conduction block were found. In each patient, during AF, a time window of 4 to 12 seconds was selected for analysis. The first and last 12 seconds of an episode of AF were excluded. In each patient, only one episode of AF was analyzed. The average duration of the episodes of AF selected for analysis was 173 ± 154 seconds.

In the 25 patients, during AF, a wide spectrum of atrial activation patterns was found. In an attempt to classify AF, three different categories of activation patterns were defined, based on the degree of complexity of activation. All maps of AF(n=1500) were classified into one of the following categories:

Type I :   In type I, the surface of the right atrium was activated by a single wave front propagating uniformly or with minor local conduction delay not disturbing the main course of the activation wave.

Type II: During type II, the area under the mapping electrode was activated either by a single wave front showing marked local conduction delays or by two different activation waves separated by a line of functional conduction block.

Type III: During type III, the right atrium was activated by multiple wavelets (three or more) separated by multiple lines of conduction block or areas of slow conduction (<10 cm/s).

In Fig 1, the three different patterns of activation during AF are shown. If >50% of the "beats" were of type I, II, or III, the episode of AF was classified as AF of type I, II, or III, respectively. By these criteria, 10 of the 25 patients were classified as type I fibrillation (40%), 8 patients as type II (32%), and 7 patients as type III (28%). There was no statistically significant difference between the three groups with respect to age, sex, location of the accessory pathway(s), incidence of documented AF, or the duration of electrically induced episodes of AF. Also, the conduction velocity of uniformly propagating activation waves during sinus rhythm, rapid atrial pacing, or fibrillation did not differ in patients with type I, II, or III fib-

Three types of atrial fibrillation

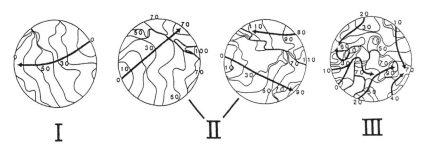

FIGURE 1. *Examples of the different patterns of activation of the free wall of the right atrium during atrial fibrillation. The diameter of the mapped area was 3.6 cm. The spatial resolution of the electrodes was 2.25 mm. Isochrones have been drawn at 10-msec intervals. During type I fibrillation, the mapped area is activated by a rapidly propagating activation wave with only small areas of local conduction delay. In contrast, during type III, the same area was activated by multiple activation waves (three or more) propagating in different directions. During type II, either a single activation wave with larger areas of conduction block was present or the area under the mapping electrode (10 cm²) was activated by two separate activation waves. Reproduced with permission from Reference 1.*

rillation. However, there was no clear correlation between the type of fibrillation and the AF rate. In the group of patients showing type I fibrillation, the average mean AF interval was 174 ± 28 msec, whereas in types II and III AF, the median fibrillation intervals were 150 ± 14 and 136 ± 16 msec, respectively (P<.05). The average conduction velocity during AF was considerably lower than during sinus rhythm or rapid regular pacing. During type I fibrillation, the average median conduction velocity was still relatively high (61 ± 6 m/s). However, during types II and III AF, the average conduction velocity was clearly depressed (54 ± 4 and 38 ± 10 m/s, respectively). Also, the time that no propagation waves were present in the mapped area became markedly shorter with increasing complexity of activation. In type I, most beats were separated by a clear diastolic period, and $42 \pm 11\%$ of the time, no depolarization waves were present in the free wall of the right atrium. During type II, electrical activity was absent $21 \pm 4\%$ of the time, whereas during type

III fibrillation, the mapped area was electrically inactive only $8 \pm 4\%$ of the time. Thus, during type III fibrillation, the free wall of the right atrium was activated by continuous electrical activity most of the time. Also, the incidence of local reentry was different in the three types of AF. Whereas during type I fibrillation, complete reentrant circuits in the free wall of the right atrium were rare, during type II fibrillation, functionally determined reentry was more common. In contrast, during type III fibrillation, complete local reentrant circuits were the rule rather than an exception, and during $66 \pm 29\%$ of the "beats," a shifting leading circle should be identified.

In 8 of the 25 patients, we also succeeded in mapping the free wall of the left atrium during the same episode of AF (Fig 2). In 5 of these 8 patients, the right and left atria showed the same type of AF. In 2 patients, activation of the left atrium was more fragmented than the right, whereas in 1 patient, the right atrium showed type III fibrillation, compared with type II in the left atrium. No local differences in fibrillation interval or variation in fibrillation intervals were found between the right and left atria.

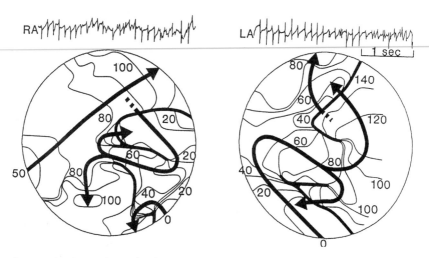

FIGURE 2. *Maps from the free wall of the right (RA) and the left (LA) atrium recorded successively during the same episode of atrial fibrillation. As can be seen, both atria are activated by multiple reentering activation waves (type III fibrillation).*

Electrical Remodeling by Atrial Fibrillation

To investigate whether AF, in addition to being the result of electrophysiological or structural abnormalities of the atria, also may cause electrical or structural changes of the atria, we developed the following chronic goat model of AF.[2]

Female goats (42.4 ± 4.9 kg) were anesthetized with nestonyl (10 mg $\cdot$ kg $-$ 1) and ventilated by halothane (1% to 2%) and a 2:1 mixture of O_2 and N_2O_2. The thorax was opened by a left intercostal thoracotomy, and after a pericardial cradle was made, three silicon strips (Silastic, Dow Corning) containing a total of 27 unipolar platinum electrodes (1.5-mm diameter, 6- 10-mm interelectrode distance) were sutured to the epicardium of the atria. One electrode strip containing 11 electrodes was positioned on Bachmann's bundle, running all the way from the left to the right atrial appendage. The other two, each containing eight electrodes, were sutured to the free wall of the right and left atria. The thorax was closed, and the electrode leads were tunneled subcutaneously to the neck and and exteriorized by a 30-pin connector (10-mm outer diameter; Lemosa). Three subcutaneous silver plates (25-mm diameter) were left to serve as reference electrodes and for recording of precordial electrocardiograms. One week after surgery, the goats were connected to an external automatic fibrillator. This device continuously analyzed a bipolar electrogram recorded from the left atrium and automatically detected the moments of spontaneous termination of fibrillation. As soon as fibrillation terminated and the goat returned to sinus rhythm, the automatic fibrillator reinduced AF by delivering a 1-second burst of electrical stimuli (biphasic, 50 Hz, 4 times threshold). In this way, AF could be maintained 24 hours a day, 7 days a week.

Several interesting observations were made in these chronically instrumented goats.

1. While at the beginning, episodes of electrically induced AF were of very short duration (<10 seconds), artificial maintenance of AF by a fibrillation pacemaker within a few days led to a marked prolongation of the duration of paroxysms of AF. Typically, after 2 to 3 days, AF continued for several hours instead of a few seconds, whereas after 1 to 2 weeks, in the majority of goats, the episodes of induced AF persisted for >24 hours.

2. During the first 24 to 48 hours of AF, the average AF interval progressively shortened from 150 to about 100 msec.

3. Intra-atrial conduction velocity did not decrease during the first 48 hours of AF.

4. The atrial refractory period shortened markedly. During the first 24 hours of AF, the effective refractory period (ERP) during regular pacing at 400-msec intervals gradually decreased from 151 ± 12 to 93 ± 20 msec (-38%).

5. Since the shortening of atrial ERP by fibrillation was more marked during slow pacing than during rapid pacing, the adaptation of the refractory period to changes in heart rate was completely changed. Instead of a prolongation of the ERP at slower heart rates, now the atrial refractory period became shorter at slower pacing rates (inverse rate adaptation).

6. In three goats, the atrial refractory period during sinus rhythm was measured after cardioversion of AF that had persisted for >4 weeks. A surprisingly and dangerously short refractory period of <60 msec was measured during sinus rhythm with a spontaneous interval of 600 msec.

These preliminary results of the recently developed goat model of chronic AF may have important implications for prevention and treatment of clinical AF in patients. The observed marked shortening of the atrial refractory period during the first 24 to 48 hours of AF offers a good explanation for the increased stability and prolonged duration of AF. It may also explain why in human patients, AF of longer duration is more difficult to defibrillate either electrically or by intravenous administration of drugs. The extremely short refractory period found during sinus rhythm directly after cardioversion leaves the atria extremely vulnerable to reinitiation of AF. This may be the reason why defibrillation may be unsuccessful or why so many patients have a recurrence of AF shortly after cardioversion.

Another clinically important implication may be that antifibrillatory drugs act differently in patients with prolonged AF. Because of the electrical remodeling of the atrial myocyte caused by AF, the refractory period and thus the repolarization phase of the action potential becomes markedly shortened. This means that the ion channels responsible for repolarization must have been changed or a new channel must have been formed. In this case, drugs that under normal circumstances are effective in prolonging the action potential by blockade of one or more of the ion channels involved in repolarization may lose their effectiveness after several days of fibrillation. If, on the other hand, a new ion channel has indeed been formed or has become operative, new drugs that normally would not affect the repolarization may exert a specific effect during sustained AF. In general, this study made us realize that the electrophysiological properties of the heart may change dramatically within a time frame of only hours or days. Although the mechanisms involved in this electrical remodeling are still incompletely understood, we strongly believe that such electrical remodeling of the heart may have important clinical consequences.

References

1. Konings KTS, Kirchhof JHJ, Smeets JRLM, Wellens HJJ, Penn OC, Allessie MA. High-density mappings of electrically induced atrial fibrillation in humans. *Circulation.* 1994;89:1665–1680.
2. Wijffels MCEF, Kirchhof CJHJ, Boersma LVA, Dorland R, Allessie MA. Atrial fibrillation begets atrial fibrillation. In: Allessie M, Campbell R, Olsson B, eds. *Atrial Fibrillation–Mechanisms and Therapeutic Strategies.* Armonk, NY: Futura Publishing Co; 1994.

Chapter 7

Editorial Comments

Michael R. Rosen, MD

Over the years, Allessie and colleagues have performed a tour de force in their studies of atrial fibrillation (for example, References 1 and 2). Recently, in human subjects with Wolff-Parkinson-White syndrome, they demonstrated three patterns of atrial fibrillation.[3] Type I (40% of patients) manifests single, broad wave fronts uniformly propagating across the right atrium; type II (32%) has one or two wave fronts, indicating nonuniformity; and type III (28%) shows highly fragmented activation of the right atrium. In going from type I to type III, both the frequency and irregularity of atrial fibrillation increase, as do the incidences of continuous electrical activity and reentry, while the conduction velocity decreases. Hence, it is stated that three types of atrial fibrillation can be identified in humans, with each having different numbers of intra-atrial circuits and different dimensions of these circuits.[3]

It is of immediate interest to compare the results of these mapping studies with those of Wells et al,[4] conducted after open-heart surgery. A major difference between the two reports is the inclusion of only patients with Wolff-Parkinson-White syndrome and presumably otherwise healthy atria in the present study. In contrast, Wells et al reported on a variety of cardiac lesions, whose basic cause was largely rheumatic heart disease or coronary artery disease.

Despite this different patient population and the use of different recording techniques (Wells et al[4] used a single bipolar atrial electrogram; Konings et al[3] mapped 244 points on the right atrial free wall), there are more similarities than dissimilarities between the two studies. In Wells' type I atrial fibrillation, there were discrete atrial complexes having variable morphology but with a clearly

From DiMarco JP, Prystowsky EN (eds): *Atrial Arrhythmias: State of the Art.* Armonk, NY, Futura Publishing Company, Inc., © 1995.

definable baseline (Konings' type I has broad, rapidly propagating wave fronts with essentially normal conduction).

Wells' type II was similar to his type I except that the baseline showed continuous perturbations (Konings' type II showed more delayed conduction and intra-atrial conduction block than type I). In Wells' type III, the atrial electrograms were highly fragmented, with no discrete complexes or intra-atrial intervals (Konings' type III showed three or more wavelets reentering themselves or each other in a highly complex pattern). Wells also identified a type IV, which incorporated properties of the other three.

Hence, whether we are dealing with the Wolff-Parkinson-White syndrome and otherwise apparently normal hearts or with other disease processes and overtly diseased hearts, there are similar rather than dissimilar patterns of fibrillation. This may be troubling, since one might think that with increasing atrial dilatation and cellular pathological lesions, there would be an increase in the disorganization of conducting pathways, fragmentation of electrograms, and severity of arrhythmias. However, we are told by Konings et al[3] that their three groups had comparable pathological features. Yet did they? One way to explore this question is by considering the ages of Konings' patients in light of their documentation of spontaneous (as opposed to induced) atrial fibrillation. Admittedly, it is unfair to use sporadic recordings to test the presence or absence of a spontaneous arrhythmia; yet, making the assumption that comparable efforts were made to record atrial arrhythmias from all 25 patients, we can assume that any error induced by the sporadic nature of the recordings was random across all 25. Of 7 patients who had spontaneous atrial fibrillation, one was a 12-year-old child. If this one is discarded from the analysis, then the remaining patients with spontaneous atrial fibrillation averaged 41.5 years of age. Of the 18 patients without spontaneous fibrillation, one was a 16-year-old child. If this one is discarded from analysis, then the average age of those who did not fibrillate spontaneously was 31 years, a decade younger than those who fibrillated spontaneously. Whether the occurrence of spontaneous fibrillation here reflects the longer persistence of their primary disease and intercurrent arrhythmias and/or the evolution of other diseases (including atherosclerosis) is impossible to state, but this possibility should be kept in mind.

This brings us to Dr Allessie's discussion of the goat model of atrial fibrillation,[5] in which the acute, electrically induced arrhythmia terminates rapidly but in which 1 to 2 weeks of artificially maintained atrial fibrillation leads to a state of chronic fibrillation, associated with about a one-third shortening of the atrial refractory period. This leads Dr Allessie to generalize that "atrial fibrillation begets atrial fibrillation."

In fact, some rather old data[6] can be brought to bear on the pathogenesis of atrial fibrillation in the goat and in human subjects. The authors studied 121 patients, of whom 23 had atrial fibrillation. The lesion in 17 was rheumatic heart disease, with others having coronary artery disease, atrial septal defect, pulmonary atresia, tetralogy of Fallot, or mitral valve prolapse. Fibrillation occurred only in the older age range, the mean being 50 ± 18 years ($\pm$ SD).

The authors believed it would be useful to test whether clinical data available for the patients might be predictive of all atrial arrhythmias, including fibrillation. They therefore devised a prognostic index incorporating sex, age, diagnosis, atrial size, atrial pressure, digitalis therapy, and P-wave duration in sinus rhythm. They used a logistic discrimination method with a stepwise variable selection procedure and found that the most important parameters (in decreasing order of importance) were P-wave duration, cyanosis, and digitalis therapy. For atrial fibrillation but not other atrial arrhythmias, atrial pressure alone was an important determinant.

The formula described was

$$LDF = 0.067 \text{ age} + 0.994 \text{ atrial size} + 2.65 \text{ cyanosis} - 6.49$$

where LDF is linear discriminant function.

When tested in 29 patients not previously analyzed, the error rate for the equation was 10% and the predictive value, 75%.

Because of the importance of atrial pressure in atrial fibrillation, the correlation between atrial pressure and maximum diastolic potential (MDP) was tested, the assumption being that cells with lower membrane potentials would have more slowly propagating action potentials. As shown in Fig 1, there was a significant correlation between membrane potential and pressure. Fig 2 relates atrial pressure, atrial size, and MDP. Although atrial pressure is the variable best correlated with MDP, the addition of atrial size improves the correlation. Moreover, as shown in Table 1, there is a good correlation between atrial size in its own right and MDP.

Finally, ultrastructural studies were done in which intercalated disk changes and cellular degeneration were related to electrical

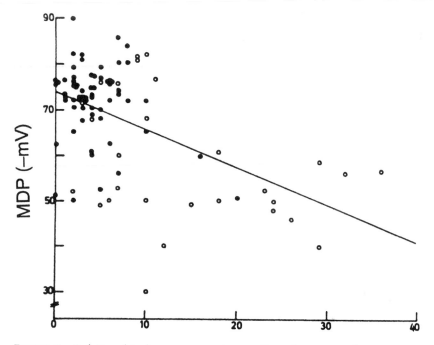

FIGURE 1. *Relationship between maximum diastolic potential (MDP) (in mV: vertical axis) and atrial pressure in mm Hg; horizontal axis). The solid circles refer to normal or moderately dilated atria, whereas the open circles refer to markedly dilated atria. The correlation coefficient, r, is .52 (P<.05). Reproduced with permission from Reference 6.*

function. Cellular degeneration was more prominent in older (mean, 49.6 years) than younger (mean, 21.1 years) patients and was further in evidence in more dilated atria and at higher atrial pressures. The group showing cellular degeneration had significantly longer P waves (118 vs 90 msec), lower MDP (-58 vs -75 mV), and lower $\dot{V}_{max}$ of phase 0 (90 vs 162 V/s) than the others. The relationship of degeneration and disk changes to clinical data and MDP are shown in Table 2.

The occurrence of ultrastructural changes, too, could be predicted from a linear discriminant function (Table 3). From the equation in Table 3, the ultrastructure could be predicted with an error rate of 5.4%.

Where does this information lead us? It appears from the data

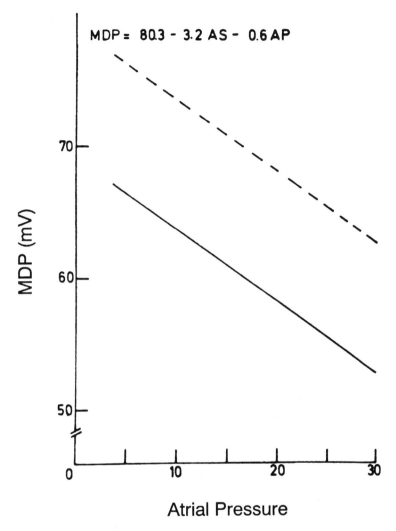

Atrial Pressure

FIGURE 2. *Relationship between maximum diastolic potential (MDP), atrial pressure (AP), and atrial size (AS). The broken line describes the relationship expected in atria of normal size between MDP and atrial pressure. The solid line represents the same relationship in severely dilated preparations. Atrial pressure is the variable best correlated with MDP, but the addition of AS significantly improves the correlation (r=.59). The lines differ significantly (P<.05). Reproduced with permission from Reference 6.*

TABLE 1. Relationship of Atrial Size in MDP

Atrial Size	n	MDP (-mV)
+	39	73.1 ± 8.2
++	29	72.3 ± 7.0
+++	16	69.5 ± 9.2
++++	33	59.8 ± 13.7*

MDP = maximum diastolic potential; n = number of observations; + = atria of normal size; ++ = atria slightly dilated; +++ = atria moderately dilated; ++++ = atria markedly dilated. *$P<.001$ compared with (+ to +++) atria.
Reproduced with permission from Reference 6.

of Konings et al[3] in humans that the occurrence of atrial fibrillation in Wolff-Parkinson-White syndrome is related to the age of the patient. Other aspects of atrial pathological feature that might have been considered are not reported. It is clear from the goat data that artificial maintenance of the fibrillatory site in otherwise normal goats results in the occurrence of chronic fibrillation. Not long ago, Karpawich et al[7] reported that neonatal canine hearts chronically paced from the ventricle showed marked disorder of myofibrillar structure. Judging from the work of Karpawich et al in ventricle, it would be fascinating to see whether there is structural disorganization in the goat atrium as a result of chronic pacing. Finally, the data of Mary-Rabine et al[6] indicate that on the basis of clinical and historical evidence obtained, the likelihood of fibrillation and changes in ultrastructure and cellular electrophysiology is predictable.

TABLE 2. Regression Equations Relating MDP, Degenerative Changes, and Clinical Data

(1) MDP = 80.3 - 3.24 AS - 0.56 AP (r=.59)
(2) MDP = 87.1 - 0.60 AP - 0.14 P dur (r=.61)
(3) DC = 0.017 P dur + 0.059 AP - 1.45 (r = .66)
(4) MDP = 74.1 - 2.2 disk changes - 4.9 DC (r=.72)

MDP = maximum diastolic potential; AS = atrial size; AP = atrial pressure, P dur = P-wave duration; and DC = degenerative changes.
Reproduced with permission from Reference 6.

TABLE 3. Discriminant Analysis of Clinical and Electrical Variables Related to Cellular Ulstrastructure

LDF = 0.24 MDP + 0.029 P dur + 0.085 age + 0.585 AP
$+ \begin{cases} 8.63 \text{ for nonrheumatic heart disease} \\ 3.90 \text{ for rheumatic heart disease} \end{cases}$

	Allocated Group	
	I	II
Real group		
I	46	1
II	3	24

LDF = linear discriminant function; group I = normal ultrastructure; and group II = abnormal ultrastructure. AP = atrial pressure; P dur = P-wave duration; MDP = maximum diastolic potential.
Reproduced with permission from Reference 6.

References

1. Allessie MA, Rensma PL, Lammers WJEP, Kirchhof CJHJ. The role of refractoriness, conduction velocity, and wavelength in initiation of atrial fibrillation in normal conscious dogs. In: Attuel P. Coumel P, Janse ML eds. *The Atrium in Health and Disease.* Mt Kisco, NY: Futura Publishing Co; 1989:27–41.
2. Allessie MA, Kirchhof CJHJ, Scheffer GJ, Chorro F, Brugada J. Regional control of atrial fibrillation by rapid pacing in conscious dogs. *Circulation.* 1991;84:1689–1698.
3. Konings KTS, Kirchhof CJHJ, Smeets JRLM, Wellens HJJ, Penn OC, Allessie MA. High-density mapping of electrically induced atrial fibrillation in humans. *Circulation.* 1994;89:1665–1680.
4. Wells JL, Karp RB, Kouchoukos NT, Maclean WAH, James TN, Waldo AL. Characterization of atrial fibrillation in man: studies following open heart surgery. *PACE Pacing Clin Electrophysiol.* 1979;1:426–438.
5. Allessie M, Konings K, Wijffels M. Electrophysiological mechanisms of atrial fibrillation. In: DiMarco JP, Prystowsky EN, eds. *Atrial Arrythmias: State of the Art.* Armonk, NY: Futura Publishing Co; 1995.
6. Mary-Rabine L, Albert A, Pham TD, Hordof A, Fenoglio JJ, Malm JR, Rosen MR. The relationship of human atrial cellular electrophysiology to clinical function and ultrastructure. *Circ Res.* 1983;52:188–199.
7. Karpawich PP, Justice CD, Cavitt DC, Chang CH: Developmental sequelae of fixed-rate ventricular pacing in the immture canine heart: an electrophysiologic, hemodynamic, and histopathologic evaluation. *Am Heart J.* 1990;119:1077–1083.

Chapter 8

Role of Sodium and Potassium Channels in Atrial Electrogenesis and Their Blockade by Antiarrhythmic Drugs

David W. Whalley, MD; and Augustus O. Grant, MD

Introduction

Normal excitability and conduction in the atrium result from the movement of Na^+, K^+, Ca^{2+}, and Cl^- ions through a variety of voltage- and ligand-operated ion channels.[1] Membrane transport processes, eg, the Na^+–K^+ pump, play a secondary role by maintaining the ionic gradients and producing small currents as a result of net ion movement. Cardiac arrhythmias necessarily result from the function of these channels. Other factors, however, such as derangements of the structural organization of cells or changes in autonomic tone, may play a critical role in arrhythmogenesis. These factors are discussed in other chapters of this book. In this chapter, we focus on the ion channels. An overview of the currents underlying the action potential is presented. This is essential so as to put the individual ion channels into perspective. We omit any discussion of the ionic currents underlying the normal pacemaker function in the sinus node. The mechanisms by which antiarrhythmic drugs block their target ion channels is discussed, with a focus on

This work was supported in part by National Heart, Lung, and Blood Institute grants HL-32708 and HL-17670. Dr Whalley is an Overseas Research Fellow of the National Heart Foundation of Australia.

From DiMarco JP, Prystowsky EN (eds): *Atrial Arrhythmias: State of the Art*. Armonk, NY, Futura Publishing Company, Inc., © 1995.

the implication of these actions for the antiarrhythmic and toxic effects of these agents.

Ion Channels and Currents Underlying the Atrial and Ventricular Action Potentials

Analysis of the membrane currents underlying the action potential is most complete for the ventricle. These ionic currents will be described first and contrasted with those present in the atria.

Ventricular Action Potential

Fig 1 illustrates the ion channels and electrogenic (voltage-generating) membrane transport processes underlying the resting membrane potential (RMP) and action potentials in ventricular and atrial cells.

Ventricular cells maintain a stable RMP of approximately -80 to -85 mV. This RMP is determined primarily by the selective permeability of the sarcolemmal membrane to K^+ and the transmembrane K^+ gradient, which, in turn, is maintained by the Na^+–K^+ pump. The predominant K^+ conductance at the RMP is the inwardly rectifying K^+ current (I_{K1}), so called because it passes inward current readily at voltages negative to the equilibrium potential for K^+ (E_K) but passes little outward current at depolarized potentials during the plateau phase of the action potential. The RMP is typically slightly positive to E_K by virtue of a small inward depolarizing current carried primarily by Na^+ ions.

The action potential in ventricular cells is typically characterized by four phases. Depolarization to threshold potential activates a regenerative inward Na^+ current (I_{Na}) that drives the membrane potential (V_m) to approximately +30 to +40 mV: (phase 0 = action potential upstroke). The maximum rate of rise of the action potential upstroke (V_{max}) is an important determinant of the velocity of impulse conduction. The increase in Na^+ conductance is brief (<1 to 2 msec) and is terminated by voltage-dependent inactivation of Na^+ channels (I_{Na}) at depolarized potentials.[2]

The peak of the action potential upstroke is followed by a phase

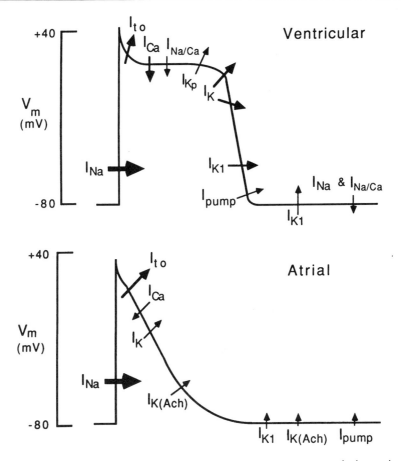

FIGURE 1. *Schematic representation of membrane currents underlying the action potential in ventricular and atrial myocytes. I_{Na}=fast Na^+ current: Ito=transient outward current; I_{Ca}=L-type Ca^{2+} current; $I_{Na/Ca}$=Na^+-Ca^2 exchange current; I_{Kp}=plateau K^+ current; I_K=delayed rectifier; I_{K1}= inwardly rectifying K^+ current; I_{pump}=Na^+-K^+ pump current; $I_{K(Ach)}$ =acetylcholine-activated K^+ current.*

of rapid repolarization (phase 1). This rapid repolarization is due to inactivation of I_{Na} together with activation of the transient outward current (I_{to}). In several mammalian species, I_{to} consists of two components.[3,4] I_{to1} is a voltage-activated K^+ current. It undergoes time- and voltage-dependent inactivation and may be a determinant of rate-dependent changes in action potential duration (APD).[5] I_{to2} is a Ca^{2+}-activated Cl^- current (inward flow of Cl^-).[6] Differences in the prominence of phase 1 repolarization between endocardial and epicardial ventricular cells have been ascribed to variation in the density of I_{to} channels in the two regions.[7] During the plateau phase (phase 2), membrane resistance is high, and net transmembrane current is small by virtue of a delicate balance between inward (depolarizing) and outward (hyperpolarizing) currents. The depolarizing currents contributing to this phase include the L-type Ca^{2+} current [$I_{Ca(L)}$], Na^+–Ca^{2+} exchange current, and possibly a slowly inactivating ("late") Na^+ current.[8] The delayed-rectifier K^+ current (I_K) is the predominant outward current during this phase, although a recently described K^+ conductance that activates rapidly at plateau potentials (I_{Kp}) may also contribute.[9] In several species, including the guinea pig, I_K has two components.[10–12] I_{Kr} is the smaller, more rapidly activating component of I_K (time constant $\approx$100 to 500 msec) and shows inward rectification. It is the only delayed rectifier current found in the rabbit and cat. I_{Ks} is larger in amplitude, activates with a slower time course (several seconds), and shows minimal or absent rectification. The distribution of delayed rectifier K^+ channels in the human ventricle remains to be clearly defined.

With time, the inactivation of $I_{Ca(L)}$ and progressive activation of I_K results in an increasing outward current that terminates the plateau phase and initiates the phase of rapid repolarization: phase 3.

As V_m repolarizes further, I_{K1} becomes activated and is the predominant current responsible for the final phase of repolarization back to the RMP.[13] The Na^+–K^+ pump, which extrudes three intracellular Na^+ ions in exchange for two extracellular K^+ ions, generates a small outward current that contributes to action potential repolarization and maintenance of the RMP. Under physiological conditions, the time course of recovery of Na^+ channels from inactivation and hence the return of membrane excitability parallels action potential repolarization. During the action potential plateau and early phase of repolarization, almost all Na^+ channels are in the inactivated state and unable to open in response to an excitatory stimulus. This defines the absolute refractory period. As V_m repolarizes further, an increasing fraction of Na^+ channels recover from inactivation. If an impulse encounters the cell during this period of relative refractoriness, it may either fail to elicit a response or generate an action potential with reduced V_{max} and amplitude. Full recovery of excitability occurs shortly after V_m returns to its resting potential.

This relationship between repolarization and membrane excitability forms the basis for understanding the antiarrhythmic properties of drugs that block the Na+ channel (class I agents) and prolong APD (class III agents). Both classes of agents may prolong refractoriness but do so via different mechanisms (see Fig 2).[14] Class I agents change the relationship between membrane voltage and Na+ channel availability, ie, the voltage dependence of recovery of Na+ channels from inactivation. The result is that at any given membrane potential during the repolarization process, fewer Na+ channels have recovered from inactivation in the presence of drug than in the drug-free state. It follows that the critical degree of Na+ channel recovery that will allow a propagated response occurs at a more hyperpolarized potential and hence later in the repolarization process, thereby prolonging refractoriness.

Drugs that purely prolong the ADP without directly affecting Na+ channel function increase the duration of refractoriness by delaying the time taken for V_m to reach the value associated with recovery from inactivation.

Atrial Action Potential

Several features distinguish the atrial action potential from its ventricular counterpart (see Fig 1). In general, the atrial action potential has a decreased amplitude, overshoot potential, V_{max}, plateau phase, and APD compared with ventricular cells.[15-17]

The predominant resting K+ conductance in working atrial cells is I_{K1}, although it is much smaller than in ventricular cells,[15,16] resulting in a high membrane resistance at the normal RMP (typically $\approx$ 1GΩ compared with 30 to 50 MΩ in ventricular cells).

The acetylcholine (Ach)-activated K+ current $[I_{K(Ach)}]$ also contributes to the resting K+ conductance. It is an inwardly rectifying current activated by the binding of acetylcholine to the muscarinic (M2) receptor.[18] $I_{K(Ach)}$ activation will hyperpolarize the RMP and markedly shorten the atrial ADP. This current is also activated by the binding of adenosine to purinergic (P$_2$) receptors.

The kinetics of the I_{Na} that underlies phase 0 of the atrial action potential are similar to those in ventricular myocytes.[19] V_{max}, however, may be slightly reduced in atrial cells if the action potential arises from a more depolarized RMP and/or the density of Na+ chan-

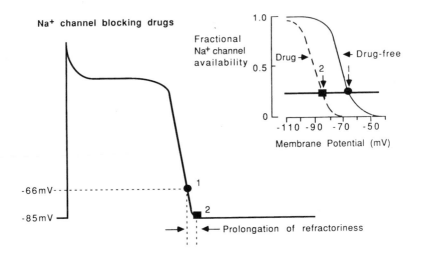

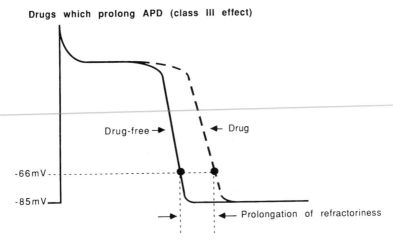

FIGURE 2. *Mechanisms of increased refractoriness by Na⁺ channel block-ade (upper panels) and action potential prolongation (lower panel). Upper panel: Inset shows the fraction of Na⁺ channels that are available for excitation (noninactivated) as a function of membrane potential. The heavy horizontal line indicates the critical level of Na⁺ channel avail-ability needed to permit propagated excitation (here arbitrarily set at 0.25). The potential at which this critical level of availability is reached is shifted in a negative direction from (1) −66 mV in the drug-free state to (2) −85 mV in the presence of a Na⁺ channel blocking drug. As shown in the schematic action potential, this shift in voltage dependence will*

nels in the sarcolemma is lower than that in ventricular cells. The phase of rapid repolarization following the upstroke is more pronounced in the atria than in the ventricles, reflecting the dominant role of I_{to} in repolarization of atrial myocytes.[15,20] The plateau phase is shorter and less clearly defined in atrial cells and merges with a slower terminal phase of repolarization. A relatively small I_{Ca} in combination with a large I_{to} probably accounts for this configuration. There is considerable interspecies variability in the size of the delayed rectifier currents in atria. In guinea pigs, the atrial I_K is large, and both rapidly and slowly activating components exist.[10] In human and rabbit atria, however, I_K is very small, and its kinetics have not been clearly defined.[15,20,21] Finally, the $I_{K(Ach)}$ current, which contributes to basal K^+ conductance in the atrium, also participates in repolarization of the atrial action potential and modulates APD in response to changing autonomic tone.

Mechanisms of Antiarrhythmic Drug Action

It is customary to discuss antiarrhythmic drugs grouped into classes, the most widely applied scheme being that proposed by Vaughan Williams[22]: (1) blockade of ion channels (Na^+, K^+, and Ca^{2+} channel blockers) and (2) blockade of membrane surface receptors (β-adrenergic blockers). However, the various classes represent ways in which drugs may act. They should not be construed as specific categories to which particular drugs belong. The recent cloning and sequencing of most membrane ion channels have emphasized the remarkable similarity of the structure of Na^+, Ca^{2+}, and K^+ channels.[23] It is hardly surprising that most antiarrhythmic drugs block *all* ion channels. Agents differ in the specificity of blockade of a given class of channels. In this review, we retain the structure of the analysis of drug-blocking mechanisms based on the presumed classes (I, II, III, IV) of action. However, it should be emphasized

---

prolong the refractory period. Lower panel: Drugs that exert a pure class III effect do not change the potential associated with recovery from inactivation (eg, −66 mV) but prolong refractoriness by increasing the time taken to achieve this potential. ADP - action potential duration. Modified from Reference 14 with permission.

that the apparent secondary actions (blockade of other ion channels or receptors) may be critically important in their therapeutic or toxic potential. For example, the K^+ blocking properties of the class I (Na^+ channel) blocking agents quinidine and disopyramide have important implications in their effect on sinus rate, atrioventricular (AV) node conduction, and the induction of torsade de pointes by action potential prolongation.Quinidine, disopyramide, and its *N*-monodealkylated metabolite exert their anticholinergic effect by blockade of the K^+ channel activated by acetycholine.[24,25] They prolong the action potential by blocking other K^+ channels that control repolarization (discussed below).

Sodium Channel Blocking Agents

Local anesthetic–class antiarrhythmic agents are assumed to act by blocking the inward Na^+ current. They induce block of conduction in diseased tissue in which conduction is partially slowed. Inasmuch as conduction of normal impulses may also be slowed, there is a window during which drug action is antiarrhythmic and one in which drug action is proarrhythmic. The separation of these two regions of drug action is critical to specificity of an antiarrhythmic action. However, all these agents retain a proarrhythmic potential.

Central to an understanding of the mechanism of drug action is the observation that drug effects depend on the frequency of stimulation. At normal heart rates, little or no channel blockade is evident. Repetitive excitation is required for the occurrence of blockade.[26] This property of frequency- or use-dependent block provides a mechanism for antiarrhythmic specificity. Impulses arising at the heart rates of normal sinus rhythm are hardly affected. However, the rapid succession of impulses during tachycardia is strongly suppressed. The observation that repetitive depolarization favors block suggests that channel states occupied during depolarization have an enhanced affinity for Na^+ channel blocking drugs. The focus of the studies in the basic laboratory has been an analysis of the channel states that are blocked by specific drugs, the differing kinetics of block, and the implications of these differences for the therapeutic and toxic action of these local anesthetic-class agents.

Fig 3 outlines a general scheme of drug interaction with a recep-

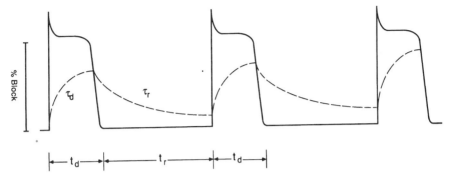

FIGURE 3. *Use-dependent block during repetitive stimulation. The continuous line shows consecutive action potentials of duration t_d elicited by pulses with an interstimulus interval ($t_d + t_r$). The broken line shows the fraction of blocked channels as a function of time. During the action potential, net binding of drug occurs to its receptor with time constant τ_d. In the interval between action potentials (t_r), net unbinding occurs with time constant τ_r. If $t_r < 4\tau_r$, block accumulates.*

tor site on the Na$^+$ channel.[27] Drug binding is phasic. During the action potential, net binding occurs with a time constant τ_d. In the interval between action potentials, partial recovery from block occurs with a recovery time constant τ_r. If the interval between action potentials (t_r) is less than 4 times τ_r, block accumulates during repetitive depolarization. Eventually, a nonequilibrium steady state is reached in which block acquired during the action potential is equal to that dissipated between action potentials. The various models of drug interaction with the Na$^+$ channel specify the states that are blocked during each phase of the cardiac cycle. The clinical profile of blockade is reflected in the kinetics (τ_d and τ_r) of blockade.

The modulated receptor model makes the simplest assumption concerning the states blocked by local anesthetic-class drugs.[28,29] It assumes that all channel states, resting, open, and inactivated, are susceptible to blockade. The open and inactivated states have much higher affinity for drug than the resting state. Data demonstrating the specific states that are blocked by a given agent have been difficult to derive experimentally. Table 1 summarizes some of the available data.[30] The data are most convincing for the open-state blockers. The open state can be uniquely defined by single channel

TABLE 1. Principal States Blocked by Specific Drugs

Drug	Open State	Inactivated State
Disopyramide	+++	++
Procainamide		++
Quinidine	++	
Amiodarone		++
Lidocaine		+++
Mexiletine		+++
Phenytoin		+++
Tocainide		++
Encainide	++	
Ethmozine		++
Flecainide	++	
Propafenone	+++	

Modified from Reference 30.

recordings. Evidence for blockade such as reduction in single-channel open time or single-channel conductance is readily apparent from experimental records.[31-35] Molecular modeling of Na^+ channel blockers suggests that the occlusion of open channels by blocking drugs is related to molecular dimensions, drugs have x-y dimensions greater than a certain value being effective open channel blockers.[36] The other channel states, resting and inactivated, are nonconducting. Therefore, their blockade can only be inferred indirectly from the behavior of the remaining conducting channels.

The kinetics of block development and recovery have been examined systematically by Campbell[37-39] and Weirich et al.[40] The experimental paradigm is illustrated in Fig 4. Upstroke velocity V_{max} measurements are obtained from guinea pig papillary muscles during control and exposure to concentrations of class I drugs that produce equivalent depression of the maximum upstroke velocity. In the absence of drugs, there is no depression of V_{max} during trains of depolarization at an interstimulus interval of 300 msec. The pattern of decline of V_{max} varies markedly between drugs. In the case of lidocaine, steady-state block is achieved after one or two depolarizations. During exposure to encainide, steady-state block required >60 beats. With disopyramide, the rate of block development is intermediate. The rate of recovery from block can be determined by first inducing block with trains of action potentials and testing the rate of recovery by introducing pulses after varying rest intervals. Onset rates are highly correlated with rates of recovery from block. Since the rates of recovery from block are relatively dose-independent, they provide a more convenient measure of the kinetics of the blocking action of drugs.

The diastolic (rest) intervals between action potentials may not be the only time that drug dissociation may occur during the cardiac cycle. If the pattern of excitation is changed abruptly, eg, at the termination of a tachycardia, the rate at which the new equilibrium level of block is approached depends on the final excitation pattern.[41–43] This is illustrated for the class IC drug flecainide in Fig 5. Block of Na$^+$ conductance was induced by 20-Hz trains of pulses. In the absence of stimulation (rest recovery), recovery from block occurs with a time constant of 12.9 seconds. However, if stimulation (of 5 Hz) is maintained after the blocking pulse train, recovery from block is much more rapid. This phenomenon is called use-dependent unblocking. It has been suggested that this process may be much more relevant as a recovery mechanism during the normal use of the drug.

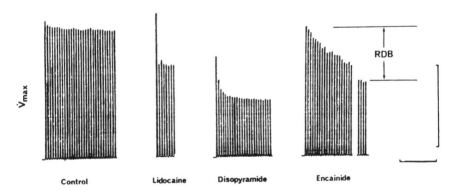

FIGURE 4. *Kinetics of the onset of use-dependent block during control and exposure to lidocaine (2×10^{-4} mol/L, disopyramide (10^{-4} mol/L), and encainide (3×10^{-6} mol/L). Stimulus pulses were applied at a cycle length of 300 msec. There was minor rate-dependent reduction of maximum upstroke velocity ($\dot{V}_{max}$) during control. Block developed rapidly with lidocaine and slowly with encainide. For encainide, the first 20 and the last 4 beats of the train are shown. With disopyramide, the rate of onset of block was intermediate. The calibrations are 200 V/s and 5 seconds. RDB=rate-dependent block. Reproduced with permission from Reference 39.*

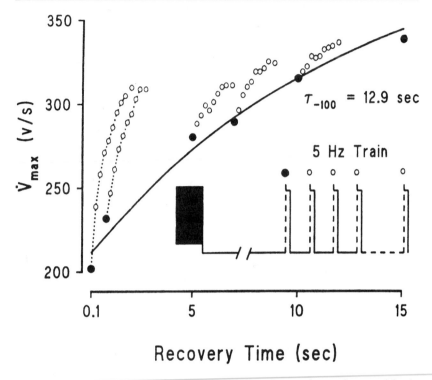

Recovery Time (sec)

FIGURE 5. *Comparison of rest recovery and use-dependent unblock. Block was induced by a 20-Hz pulse train during exposure to flecainide. Recovery from block was assessed with single pulses after a varying recovery interval (solid circles) or with a 5-Hz pulse train (open circles). Rest recovery occurred with a time constant of 12.9 seconds. In contrast, at any point in the recovery interval, the process could be speeded up by application of a train of pulses. Reproduced with permission from Reference 43.*

The local anesthetic-class drugs fall into three broad groups based on their kinetics of recovery from block: (1) Group IB agents have rapid recovery from block, with $\tau_r < 1$ second. Conduction velocity and QRS duration are unchanged at normal heart rates. However, closely coupled extrasystoles are strongly suppressed. (2) Group IC agents have very slow kinetics of recovery from block, with $\tau_r \geq 12$ seconds. Conduction velocity is slowed and QRS duration is prolonged at normal heart rates. (3) Group IA agents have intermediate kinetics, with $1 < \tau_r \leq 12$ seconds. Although conduction slowing and QRS prolongation are minimal at normal heart rates, these may become substantial during tachycardia.

The subclassification into subgroups IA, IB, and IC as originally proposed by Harrison[44] also used other considerations, such as drug effects on the ADP. Alternative bases for the subclassification of class I agents have been proposed, eg, that of Weirich and Antoni.[40] However, they have not yet received widespread application. As pointed out by Campbell,[45] the essence of the subclassification scheme is that there are drugs with relatively fast dissociation kinetics that produce equilibrium block rapidly at increasing heart rates and drugs that produce block slowly at rapid heart rates.

Determinants of the kinetics of drug dissociation from the Na^+ channel include the physicochemical properties of the drug and the channel milieu. Fast drug dissociation is correlated with small molecular dimension.[46,47] Low pK_a and high lipid solubility play a lesser role.[48-50] It is not clear that these structure-activity data have been used in the design of newer agents. Low extracellular pH slows the dissociation of local anesthetic-class drugs from the Na^+ channel.[51] However, drug association rate is also slowed. It is only when low pH is combined with membrane depolarization that greater block is observed.[52] The combination of low pH and membrane depolarization may occur during myocardial ischemia.

Clinical Implications of the Different States Blocked by Drugs and the Kinetics of Block

APD is shorter in the atrium than in the ventricle (see Fig 1). Na^+ channels are primarily in the inactivated state during the action potential. Therefore, inactivated-state blockers like lidocaine have less time for binding to atrial myocardium compared with ventricular myocardium (Fig 6). This may be one reason that lidocaine is relatively ineffective in the treatment of atrial arrhythmias. For agents with slow binding and unbinding characteristics, eg, flecainide, similar levels of steady-state block would be anticipated in the atria and ventricles. These agents are highly effective against atrial arrhythmias.

Differences in the states blocked by antiarrhythmic agents provide a rationale for using these drugs in combination. Because of its

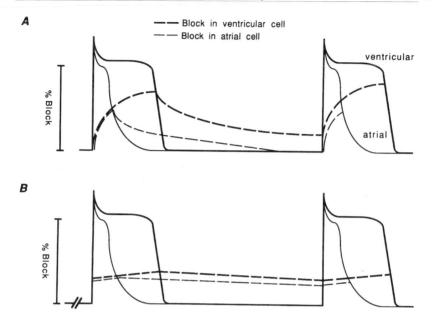

FIGURE 6. *Use-dependent blockade in atrial and ventricular myocardium during exposure to drugs with fast (panel A) or slow (panel B) kinetics of interaction with the Na⁺ channel. The continuous lines show overlapping atrial and ventricular action potentials. The atrial action potential is of shorter duration. For an inactivated-state blocker, less block (broken lines) develops during the shorter action potential. At a fixed interstimulus interval, there is more time for unblock during diastole in the atrium. The level of block falls to zero before the next action potential. In contrast, more block develops in the ventricle, and there is less time for dissociation between action potentials. Residual block is present at the onset of the second action potential, and block accumulates. For a drug with slow kinetics (or for an open-state blocker), there is little difference in the level of block achieved in the atrium and ventricle.*

K⁺ channel blocking action, one drug, eg, quinidine, may prolong the APD. By this mechanism, it may increase the amount of time available for blockade by an agent (eg, mexiletine) that interacts with inactivated Na⁺ channels. The combination of the two drugs may be synergistic, with a smaller dose of each drug being more effective in combination therapy.[53] Amiodarone is unique in that prolongation of APD as a result of its class III action enhances its inactivated-state blockade of the Na^+ channel.[54] Although the principle of synergistic drug combinations has been well documented as a therapeutic approach to ventricular arrhythmias, treatment with combinations of local anesthetic-class drugs has not been widely applied in the management of atrial arrhythmias.

Because of their slow kinetic interaction with the Na^+ channel, therapeutic concentrations of class IC agents produce substantial slowing of conduction. This may result in an important atrial proarrhythmic response with these agents. By slowing the atrial rate of atrial flutter or atrial tachycardia, they may enhance the AV conduction ratio and cause a substantial increase in the ventricular response. The enhanced conduction ratio occurs even though the drugs actually increase the A-H interval.[55] Functional bundle block may result from the increase in ventricular rate. This mechanism may have been operative in the group of patients (10 percent) that experienced an atrial proarrhythmic response while receiving the class IC drugs flecainide or encainide.[56] For this reason, combination therapy with an AV nodal blocking agent, eg, a β-adrenergic or Ca^{2+} channel blocker, is recommended.

Sympathetic Modulation of Sodium Channel Function

The sympathetic nervous system plays an important role in the genesis of cardiac arrhythmias. β-Adrenergic receptor activation has also been reported to reverse the effects of local anesthetic-class drugs.[57-59] A proarrhythmic response to these drugs may be precipitated by exercise.[60]. Proarrhythmic drug effects may be reversed by β-adrenergic blockade.[61] The mechanisms of those potentially important effects are uncertain. The effects of β-adrenergic receptor activation on many ionic currents, eg, the L-type calcium channel current, have been well characterized. However, its effects on the sodium channel are controversial.

β-Adrenergic receptor activation decreases V_{max} at reduced membrane potentials in the K^+-depolarized guinea pig heart.[36,62,63] The strategy of elevating $[K^+]$ to reduce the membrane potential may accentuate the nonlinear relationship between V_{max} and available sodium conductance. Direct voltage clamp experiments have yielded divergent results. Schubert et al[64,65] and Ono et al[66] showed that isoproterenol decreases the sodium current at low membrane potentials. The reduction results from a shift in the voltage dependence of inactivation to more negative potentials.[67,68] In contrast, Matsuda et al[69] report an enhancement of the sodium current by β-receptor activation without any shift in the voltage dependence of channel gating. This question remains unresolved. The confounding influence of time-dependent changes in sodium channel gating makes the resolution of this issue difficult. Further, the response to β-adrenergic receptor activation may be dependent on the state of other second messenger systems, eg, protein kinase C activity.[70]

Potassium Channel Blocking Agents

K^+ channel blocking agents represent a diverse group of compounds that share the common property of prolonging APD and hence myocardial refractoriness. In recent years, there has been a major shift in focus at both the experimental and clinical levels away from drugs whose primary mode of action is to slow conduction (class I effect) to those that prolong refractoriness by prolonging APD (class III effect). This is due in part to a growing awareness of the inefficacy and proarrhythmic potential of class I agents, especially when they are used in the context of previous myocardial infarction.[71,72] It also results from accumulating evidence that class III agents may be more effective than class I agents in treating a range of atrial and ventricular arrhythmias[73-76] and have favorable effects on hemodynamic parameters[77] and defibrillation thresholds.[78]

The majority of drugs that prolong APD do so by blocking repolarizing K^+ currents. It should be noted, however, that APD may also be prolonged by increasing inward current carried by Na^+, or Ca^{2+} at plateau potentials. Indeed, a drug currently under investigation, ibutilide, exerts its class III effect by activating a slow plateau Na^+ current.[79] The present discussion focuses on the mechanisms by which drugs interact with the voltage-sensitive K^+ channels and the relationship between channel block, action potential prolongation, and the antiarrhythmic and proarrhythmic potential of these agents.

Table 2 lists the drugs with K^+ channel blocking properties that are approved for general clinical use in the United States and some of those currently undergoing investigation. It is important to note that although the class IA and IC agents are defined by their Na^+

TABLE 2. Specificity of K+ Channel Blocking Drugs

Drug	I_K	I_{K1}	I_{to}
Class IA			
Quinidine	+	+	+
Disopyramide	+	+	+
Class IC			
Flecainide	+	−	−
Encainide	+	−	−
Class III			
Sotalol	+	+	+
Amiodarone	+	+	−
Bretylium	+	−	+
E-4031*	+	−	−
Dofetilide*	+	−	−
Risotilide*	+	−	−
Almokalant*	+	−	−
Sematilide*	+	−	−
Ambasilide*	+	−	−
Terikalant*	−	+	+
Tedisamil*	+	−	+
RP58866*	−	+	−

I_K=delayed rectifier; I_{K1}=inward rectifier; I_{to}=transient outward current; + denotes block of channel by drug. *Investigational agent. Modified from Reference 12.

channel blocking properties, they also block K+ channels with vary-ing selectivity. The class III agents sotalol, bretylium, and amio-darone are relatively nonselective, having effects on at least two of the three major voltage-sensitive K+ channels. In contrast, the newer investigation agents are more selective for the individual K+ chan-nel subtypes. Most recent effort has been directed toward the devel-opment of selective blockers of the delayed rectifier channel, I_K. Such agents include E-4031, dofetilide, and sematilide. Rationales for developing agents that specifically target I_K include, first, the important role played by this current in terminating the action potential and initiating the phase of rapid repolarization in ventric-ular myocardium; second, its slow deactivation kinetics, which should result in accumulation of channels in the open state at short cycle lengths, thereby facilitating use-dependent drug block; and third, its inwardly rectifying properties, which may accentuate drug block in partially depolarized (eg, ischemic) tissue.[12,80] There is mounting evidence that the selective I_K blockers are effective against a range of atrial and ventricular tachycarrhythmias.[73] However, it remains to be established whether the theoretical benefits of K^+ channel specificity will translate into greater efficacy and reduced potential for proarrhythmia compared with the relatively nonselective agents now in clinical use.

I_{to} has also been proposed as a suitable target for the development of selective channel blockers.[81] Such agents would be expected to be most effective against supraventricular arrhythmias, since I_{to} is the dominant repolarizing current in the atria. Their effect on arrhythmias arising from ventricular muscle or the Purkinje system would probably be less impressive because the complex secondary effects of I_{to} blockade on I_K may result in either no change of APD or even shortening of APD and refractoriness in these tissues.[7,82]

Mechanisms of K^+ Channel Block

As previously discussed, the class I drugs block Na^+ channels and decrease V_{max} in a use-dependent manner such that block increases at faster heart rates. Analogously it has been suggested that the "ideal" class III agent should exert minimal effects on APD at physiological heart rates while prolonging repolarization and refractoriness preferentially at rates encountered during atrial and ventricular tachyarrhythmias.[83] In contrast to this "ideal" behavior, most K^+ channel blocking agents, including the more selective investigational agents, prolong the APD maximally at slow heart rates and have a progressively diminishing effect at faster rates[83–86] (see Fig 7). This phenomenon, called "reverse use dependence" by Hondeghem and Snyders,[83] probably limits the antiarrhythmic efficacy of these agents during sustained tachycardia and predisposes to the development of triggered arrhythmias such as torsade de pointes by excessively lengthening APD and QT_c at long cycle lengths. Reverse use dependence was initially believed to reflect a preferential block of I_K channels in their closed (rested) state and diminishing block during depolarization when channels have entered the open state. According to this scheme, at slow heart rates, the relatively long diastolic interval would favor block of the closed channel and APD prolongation. At faster rates, abbreviation of diastole would limit the development of block and hence APD prolongation. This hypothesis was supported by experimental observations of the I_K blocking behavior of quinidine.[87] Further support was provided by the demonstration

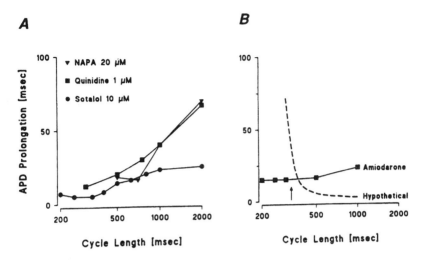

FIGURE 7. *Rate-dependent effects on action potential duration (APD) of several class III agents. Data have been redrawn by Hondeghem and Snyders[83] from Reference 85 for N-acetylprocainamide (NAPA). Reference 84 for quinidine, Reference 86 for sotalol, and Reference 91 for amiodarone. A: As heart rate increases (cycle length shortens), the magnitude of APD prolongation diminishes—"reverse use dependence." B: The dashed line represents the response of APD to a hypothetical "ideal" class III agent. Prolongation of APD is minimal at normal cycle lengths (600 to 1000 msec) but increases rapidly at cycle lengths shorter than 500 msec (120 beats per minute). The arrow indicates a rate of 180 beats per minute. Note that the response of amiodarone is relatively rate-independent. Reproduced with permission from reference 83.*

that reverse use dependence of APD prolongation could be accounted for by use of a modulated receptor model of K^+ channel block and assuming preferential binding of drug to the closed state. Modeling of open channel block predicted minimal lengthening of APD at normal heart rates but marked prolongation at short cycle lengths—the more desirable electrophysiological response.[83]

Although preferential block of the closed state provided an attractive explanation for the rate-dependent effects of K^+ channel blockers on APD, more recent studies suggest that most drugs, including amiodarone, quinidine, dofetilide, E-4031, and flecainide, are actually open channel blockers of I_K and show "normal" use dependence.[11,88–90] This has led some investigators to suggest that the term "reverse use dependence" may be inappropriate when describing the rate-dependent effects of drugs on the APD, since use dependence strictly applies to phenomena at the channel level.[82]

If drug binding to the I_K channel is use-dependent, then why do the majority of these agents have a "reverse use-dependent" effect on APD? The answer to this question remains unclear; however, Colatsky et al[12] suggested that it may relate in part to a disproportionality between I_K block and APD prolongation such that at higher rates the influence of other channels [eg, $I_{Ca(L)}$ inactivation] may assume a more dominant role in repolarization and overshadow the contribution of I_K.

There are two notable exceptions to the phenomenon of "reverse use dependence" of APD prolongation. Amiodarone, when given chronically, prolongs APD to a similar degree over a wide range of cycle lengths.[91] Indeed, this rate independence of APD prolongation may partially explain the greater antiarrhythmic efficacy and lower potential for proarrhythmia observed with amiodarine compared with other antiarrhythmic agents.[75,92] Perhaps surprisingly, the only convincing demonstration of tachycardia-dependent APD prolongation has been with the class IC agent flecainide. Wang et al[93] reported that the prolongation of APD and effective refractory period induced by flecainide in atrial tissue increases progressively with heart rate, ie, shows "normal use dependence." This was in sharp contrast to the effects of quinidine on APD, which diminished markedly at faster rates. The rate-dependent effects of flecainide on atrial APD and refractoriness therefore most closely approximate the properties of an "ideal" antiarrhythmic drug for reentrant arrhythmias.[83] If, as suggested by Wang et al, the ionic mechanisms underlying these desirable properties of flecainide could be identified and dissociated from its potent Na^+ channel blockade, it might be possible to develop a safer and more effective agent against atrial fibrillation.[93]

Mechanisms of Arrhythmia Termination by Agents With Class III Properties

Several potential mechanisms may underlie the antiarrhythmic effect of class III agents on reentrant tachyarrhythmias.[80,92] The initiation and maintenance of circus-movement reentry require slow conduction of an impulse around a zone of unidirectional block. The path of slow conduction must be sufficiently long to allow recovery of excitability in tissue proximal to the zone of block and hence reentrant penetration. The wavelength of the reentrant circuit is given by the product of the conduction velocity (CV) and refractory period (RP): wavelength=CV×RP. The wavelength represents the minimum circuit length that can support reentry and has been suggested to be an important predictor of susceptibility to reentrant atrial arrhythmias.[94] The success of antiarrhythmic drug therapy has also been closely correlated with the effect of a particular drug on wavelength. Rensma et al[94] found that in the canine heart, short wavelengths favored the induction of atrial flutter and fibrillation, whereas prolongation of wavelength by drug therapy (quinidine or d-sotalol) prevented arrhythmia induction. In contrast, the class IC drug propafenone, by virtue of its combined depression of conduction velocity and modest prolongation of refractoriness, had minimal effect on wavelength and did not significantly alter the inducibility of atrial fibrillation. The importance of prolonging atrial refractoriness in the termination and prevention of atrial flutter and fibrillation has been confirmed by several other groups.[76,95]

Prolongation of refractoriness without a change in conduction velocity, ie, a pure class III effect, should increase the reentrant wavelength and render initiation of a stable circuit more difficult. In addition, an increase in refractoriness should (1) prolong the cycle length of an established tachycardia, (2) prevent its degeneration into atrial or ventricular fibrillation, and (3) favor extinction of the circuit by decreasing the amount of potentially excitable tissue between the advancing head of the reentrant impulse and its refractory tail—the excitable gap.[80,92,96] A schema of reentrant tachycardia termination based on abolition of the excitable gap is illustrated in Fig 8. Inoue et al[96] tested this paradigm in a canine model of atrial flutter caused by reentry. They found that the class III agent E-4031 terminated atrial flutter by abolishing the excitable gap, whereas class I agents disopyramide, flecainide, and propafenone terminated tachycardia by depressing conduction to a critical point beyond which reentry could no longer be sustained. Although this apparent discrimination between class I and class III mechanisms of terminating tachycardia is appealing, it may be too simplistic, since sotalol has also been reported to terminate atrial flutter without abolishing the excitable gap,[97] whereas flecainide may exert its therapeutic effect in atrial fibrillation by prolonging refractoriness.[95]

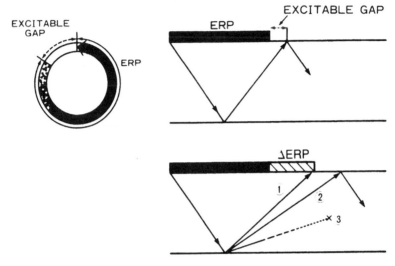

FIGURE 8. *Possible mechanisms of termination of reentry in atrial flutter. Upper panels: The flutter cycle length consists of the atrial effective refractory period (ERP) and an excitable gap. Lower panel: After administration of a class III agent, the ERP is prolonged to a greater extent than conduction is slowed (1). The wave front collides with its refractory tail, abolishing the excitable gap and terminating atrial flutter. If conduction is slowed to a greater extent than the ERP is prolonged, reentry persists (2). If conduction is suppressed to a critical point (eg, by a class IC agent), impulse propagation ceases and tachycardia terminates (3). Reproduced with permission from Reference 96.*

Proarrhythmia With K⁺ Channel Blocking Agents

The characteristic manifestation of proarrhythmia in patients treated with agents that prolong the APD (class IA and III) is the development of polymorphic tachycardia in the form of torsade de pointes. This arrhythmia is associated with prolongation of the QT interval and is typically related to bradycardia or an abrupt increase in cycle length (eg, a postextrasystolic pause).[98] Electrolyte abnormalities such as hypokalemia and hypomagnesemia are also important contributing factors. The cellular mechanisms underlying the development of drug-induced torsade de pointes remain somewhat controversial,[99] although the weight of present evidence suggests that triggered activity due to early afterdepolarizations (EADs) possibly originating in the Purkinje fiber system may be responsible.[98,100] According to this hypothesis, induction of triggered activity is initiated by APD prolongation. Reactivation of channels carrying inward current [eg, $I_{Ca(L)}$ and/or the slowly inactivating Na^+ current] then causes depolarization of V_m during the action potential plateau or phase 3 repolarization.[101] The initial therapy of torsade de pointes (after the precipitating drug is suspended) is to increase heart rate and thereby shorten the APD and QT interval. This may be achieved either by overdrive pacing ($\approx$90 to 100 beats per minute) or with isoproterenol. Electrolyte abnormalities should be corrected, and supplemental Mg^{2+} may be helpful even in the absence of hypomagnesemia.

Singh et al[92] have highlighted some important differences in the incidence and presentation of torsade de pointes between the K^+ channel blocking drugs. Of particular note is the apparently low incidence of this arrhythmia with amiodarone therapy (<1%) in comparison with both sotalol ($\approx$3% to 5%) and quinidine (3% to 8%). This may relate in part to the Ca^{2+} and Na^+ channel blocking actions of amiodarone in light of the probable role of these channels in the generation of EADs. It is also noteworthy that in contrast to quinidine, which usually produces torsade de pointes at plasma concentrations within or below the therapeutic range, sotalol-induced torsade appears to be dose related, occurring most frequently at high (or toxic) concentrations.[102] A recent study suggests that differences in the dose dependence of APD prolongation and EAD induction between the two agents may be responsible.[103]

Conclusions

Drug treatment of atrial arrhythmias poses a dilemma for the clinician. Although the arrhythmias may be associated with significant symptoms and morbidity, they are rarely life-threatening. By the nature of their mechanism of action, the class I antiarrhythmic drugs have an inherent proarrhythmic and lethal potential. Available data identify certain patient groups who may be at higher risk, eg, patients with a prior history of myocardial infarction.[72] For a substantial proportion of patients with atrial arrhythmias, there is no underlying heart disease, or the risk associated with drug treatment in the presence of disease is unknown.

Does the study of the mechanisms of atrial arrhythmias and the action of drugs that terminate or prevent them offer the prospect of agents with substantially less risk than those currently available? The human Na^+ channel and several K^+ channels have been cloned and their sequences inferred from the respective cDNA. Informed guesses of the likely three-dimensional structure of these channel proteins are possible. Within the next decade, the crystal structure of the smallest channel protein should be available. Then, it should be possible to effect more specific drug design. The prospects are better for the class III agents. Of all the ion channels, the K^+ channels have the smallest subunits.[104] They would be most amenable to molecular analysis. It is our guess that the development of K^+ blocking agents that prolong the APD with the normal pattern of use dependence, possibly combined with some Ca^{2+} channel blocking action, is more likely to provide effective agents with low proarrhythmic potential than the development of other agents with local anesthetic class/Na^+ channel blocking action. Given the rapid pace of advances in membrane biophysics and molecular biology in the past decade, there is good reason to be optimistic about significant progress in drug design in the next decade and beyond.

References

1. Katz AM. Cardiac ion channels. *N Eng J Med.* 1993;328:1244–1251.
2. Gettes LS, Reuter H. Slow recovery from inactivation of inward currents in mammalian myocardial fibres. *J Physiol (Lond).* 1974;240: 703–724.
3. Coraboeuf E, Carmeliet E. Existence of two transient outward currents in sheep cardiac Purkinje fibers. *Pflugers Arch.* 1982;392:352–359.
4. Tseng G-N, Hoffman BF. Two components of transient outward current in canine ventricular myocytes. *Circ Res.* 1989;64:633–647.
5. Fermini B, Wang Z, Duan D, et al. Differences in rate dependence of transient outward current in rabbit and human atrium. *Am J Physiol.* 1992;263:H1747-H1754.
6. Zygmunt AC, Gibbons WR. Calcium-activated chloride current in rabbit ventricular myocytes. *Circ Res.* 1991;68:424–437.
7. Litovsky SH, Antzelevitch C. Transient outward current prominent in

canine ventricular epicardium but not endocardium. *Circ Res.* 1988;62: 116–126.

8. Patlak JB, Ortiz M. Slow currents through single sodium channels of adult rat heart. *J Gen Physiol.* 1985;86:89–104.

9. Yue DT, Marban E. A novel cardiac potassium channel that is active and conductive at depolarized potentials. *Pflugers Arch.* 1988;413:127–133.

10. Sanguinetti MC, Jurkiewicz NK. Two components of cardiac delayed rectifier K+ current. *J Gen Physiol.* 1990;96:195–215.

11. Balser JR, Bennett PB, Hondeghem LM et al. Suppression of time-dependent outward current in guinea-pig ventricular myocytes: actions of quinidine and amiodarone. *Circ Res.* 1991;69:519–529.

12. Colatsky TJ, Follmer CH, Starmer CF. Channel specificity in antiarrhythmic drug action: mechanism of potassium channel block and its role in suppressing and aggravating cardiac arrhythmias. *Circulation.* 1990;82:2235–2242.

13. Shimoni Y, Clark RB, Giles WR. Role of an inwardly rectifying potassium current in rabbit ventricular action potential. *J Physiol (Lond).* 1992;448:709–727.

14. Roden DM. Treatment of cardiovascular disorders: arrhythmias. In: Melmon KL, Morrelli HF, Hoffman BB, Nierenberg DW, eds. *Clinical Pharmacology: Basic Principles in Therapeutics.* New York, NY: McGraw-Hill, Inc; 1992:151–185.

15. Giles WR, Imaizumi Y. Comparison of potassium currents in rabbit atrial and ventricular cells. *J Physiol (Lond).* 1988;405:123–145.

16. Heidbuchel H, Vereecke J, Carmeliet E. Three different potassium channels in human atrium. *Circ Res.* 1990;66:1277–1286.

17. Hume JR, Uehara A. Ionic basis of the different action potential configurations of single guinea-pig atrial and ventricular myocytes. *J Physiol (Lond).* 1985;368:525–544.

18. Kurachi Y, Nakajima T, Sugimoto T. Acetylcholine activation of K+ channels in cell-free membrane of atrial cells. *Am J Physiol.* 1986;251: H681-H684.

19. Gilliam FR III, Starmer CF, Grant AO. Blockade of rabbit atrial sodium channels by lidocaine: characterization of continuous and frequency-dependent blocking. *Circ Res.* 1989:65:723–739.

20. Escande D, Coulombe A, Faivre J-F, et al. Two types of transient outward currents in adult human atrial cells. *Am J Physiol.* 1987;252:H843-H850.

21. Shibata EF, Drury T, Refsum H, et al. Contributions of a transient outward current to repolarization in human atrium. *Am J Physiol.* 1989; 257:H1773-H1781.

22. Vaughn Williams EM. Classification of antiarrhythmic drugs. In: Sandoe E, Flensted-Jensen E, Olsen EH, eds. *Symposium on Cardiac Arrhythmias.* Denmark: Astra; 1970:449–501.

23. Cattarall WA. Structure and function of voltage-sensitive ion channels. *Science.* 1988;242:50–61.

24. Baines MW, Davies JE, Kellett DN, et al. Some pharmacological effects of disopyramide and a metabolite. *J Int Med Res.* 1976;4:5–12.

25. Nakajima T, Kurachi Y, Ito H, et al. Anticholinergic effects of quinidine, disopyramide, and procainamide in isolated atrial myocytes: mediation by different molecular mechanisms. *Circ Res.* 1989;64:297–303.
26. Johnson EA, McKinnon MG. The differential effect of quinidine and pyrilamine on the myocardial action potential at various rates of stimulation. *J Pharmacol Exp Ther.* 1957;120:460–468.
27. Starmer CF, Grant AO. Phasic ion channel blockade: a kinetic and parameter estimation procedure. *Mol Pharmacol.* 1985;28:348–356.
28. Hille B. Local anesthetics: hydrophilic and hydrophobic pathways for the drug-receptor reaction. *J Gen Physiol.* 1977;69:497–515.
29. Hondeghem LM, Katzung BG. Time- and voltage-dependent interactions of antiarrhythmic drugs with cardiac sodium channels. *Biochim Biophys Acta.* 1977;472:373–398.
30. Snyders DJ, Bennett PB, Hondeghem LM. Mechanism of drug-channel interaction. In: Fozzard HA, et al, eds. *The Heart and Cardiovascular System.* New York, NY: Raven Press Ltd; 1992:2165–2193.
31. Kohlhardt M, Fichtner H, Froebe U, et al. On the mechanism of drug-induced blockade of Na$^+$ current: interaction of antiarrhythmic compounds with DPI-modified single cardiac Na$^+$ channels. *Circ Res.* 1989;64:867–881.
32. Yazuto Y, Kaibata M, Ohara M, et al. An improved method for isolating cardiac myocytes useful for patch-clamp studies. *Jpn J Physiol.* 1990;40:157–163.
33. Benz I, Kohlhardt M. Responsiveness of cardiac Na$^+$ channels to antiarrhythmic drugs: the role of inactivation. *J Membr Biol.* 1991;12:267–278.
34. Benz I, Kohlardt M. Differential response of DPI-modified cardiac Na$^+$ channels to antiarrhythmic drugs: no flicker blockade by lidocaine. *J Membr Biol.* 1992;126:257–263.
35. Grant AO, Wendt DJ, Zilberter Y, et al. Kinetics of interaction of disopyramide with the cardiac sodium channel: fast dissociation from open channels at normal rest potentials. *J Memb Biol.* In press.
36. Courtney KR. Why do some drugs preferentially block open sodium channels? *J Mol Cell Cardiol.* 1988;20:461–464.
37. Campbell TJ: Resting and rate-dependent depression of maximum rate of depolarization (V_{max}) in guinea pig ventricular action potentials by mexiletine, disopyramide and encainide. *J Cardiovasc Pharmacol.* 1983; 5:291–296.
38. Campbell TJ, Vaughn Williams EM. Voltage- and time-dependent depression of maximum rate depolarization of guinea-pig ventricular action potential by two new antiarrhythmic drugs, flecainide and lorcainide. *Cardiovasc Res.* 1983;17:251–258.
39. Campbell TJ. Kinetics of onset of rate-dependent effects of class 1 antiarrhythmic drugs are important in determining their effects on refractoriness in guinea pig ventricle, and provide a theoretical basis for their subclassification. *Cardiovasc Res.* 1983;17:344–352.
40. Weirich J, Antoni H. Differential analysis of the frequency-dependent effects of class 1 antiarrhythmic drugs according to periodic ligand

binding. implications for antiarrhythmic and proarrhythmic efficacy. *J Cardiovasc Pharmacol.* 1990;15:998–1009.

41. Gintant GA, Hoffman BF. Use-dependent block of cardiac sodium channels by quaternary derivatives of lidocaine. *Pflugers Arch.* 1984; 400:121–129.

42. Carmeliet E. Activation block and trapping of penticainide, a disopyramide analogue, in the Na^+ channel of rabbit cardiac Purkinje fibers. *Circ Res.* 1988;63:50–60.

43. Anno T, Hondeghem LM. Interaction of flecainide with guinea pig cardiac sodium channels: importance of activation unblocking to the voltage dependence of recovery. *Circ Res.* 1990;66:789–803.

44. Harrison DC. Symposium on perspectives on treatment of ventricular arrhythmias: introduction. *Am J Cardiol.* 1983;52:1C–2C.

45. Campbell TJ. Subclassification of class 1 antiarrhythmic drugs: enhanced relevance after CAST. *Cardiovasc Drug Ther.* 1992;6:519–528.

46. Courtney KR. Interval-dependent effects of small antiarrhythmic drugs on excitability of guinea-pig myocardium. *J Mol Cell Cardiol.* 1980; 12:1273–1286.

47. Courtney KR. Sodium channel blockers: the size/solubility hypothesis revisited. *Mol Pharmacol.* 1990;37:855–859.

48. Courtney KR. Fast frequency-dependent block of action potential upstroke in rabbit atrium by small local anesthetics. *Life Sci.* 1979;24: 1581–1588.

49. Moorman JR, Yee R, Bjornsson T, et al. pKa does not predict pH potentiation of sodium channel blockade by lidocaine and W6211 in guinea-pig ventricular myocardium. *J Pharmacol Exp Ther.* 1986;238:159–166.

50. Broughton A, Grant AO, Starmer CF, et al. Lipid solubility modulates pH potentiation of local anesthetic block of V_{max} reactivation in guinea-pig myocardium. *Circ Res.* 1984;55:513–523.

51. Grant AO, Strauss LJ, Wallace AG, et al. The influence of pH on the electrophysiological effects of lidocaine in guinea pig ventricular myocardium. *Circ Res.* 1982;47:542–550.

52. Wendt DJ, Starmer CF, Grant AO. pH dependence of kinetics and steady-state block of cardiac sodium channels by lidocaine. *Am J Physiol.* 1993;264:H1588-H1598.

53. Duff HJ, Roden D, Primm RK, et al. Mexiletine in the treatment of resistant ventricular arrhythmias: enhancement of efficacy and reduction of dose related side effects of combination with quinidine. *Circulation.* 1983;67:1124–1128.

54. Mason JW, Hondeghem LM, Katzung BG. Block of inactivated sodium channels and of depolarization-induced automaticity in guinea pig papillary muscle by amiodarone. *Circ Res.* 1984;55:277–285.

55. Olsson SB, Edvardsson N. Clinical electrophysiologic study of antiarrhythmic properties of flecainide: acute intraventricular delayed conduction and prolonged repolarization in regular paced and premature beats using intracardiac monophasic action potentials with programmed stimulation. *Am Heart J.* 1981;102:864–871.

56. Feld GK, Peng-Sheng C, Nicod P, et al. Possible atrial proarrhythmic

effects of class 1C antiarrhythmic drugs. *Am J Cardiol.* 1990;66:378–383.
57. Morady F, Kou WH, Kadish AH, et al. Antagonism of quinidine's electrophysiologic effect by epinephrine in patients with ventricular tachycardia. *J Am Coll Cardiol.* 1988;12:388–394.
58. Jazayeri MR, Van Wyhe G, Akhtan M. Isoproterenol reversal at antiarrhythmic effects in patients with inducible sustained tachyarrhythmias. *J Am Coll Cardiol.* 1989;14:705–711.
59. Markel ML, Miles WM, Luck JC, et al. Differential effects of isoproterenol on sustained ventricular tachycardia before and during procainamide and quinidine antiarrhythmic drug therapy. *Circulation.* 1993;87:783–792.
60. Ranger S, Talagic M, Lemery R, et al. Amplification of flecainide-induced ventricular conduction slowing by exercise. *Circulation.* 1989; 79:1000–1006.
61. Myerburg R, Kessler KM, Cox MM, et al. Reversal of proarrhythmic effects of flecainide acetate and encainide hydrochloride by propranolol. *Circulation.* 1989;80:1571–1579.
62. Hisatome I, Kiyosue T, Imanishi S, et al. Isoproterenol inhibits residual fast channel via stimulation of β-adrenoceptors in guinea-pig ventricular muscle. *J Mol Cell Cardiol.* 1985;17:657–665.
63. Gillis AM, Kohlhardt M. Voltage-dependent V_{max} blockade in Na^+-dependent action potentials after β_1 and H_2-receptor stimulation in mammalian ventricular myocardium. *Can J Physiol.* 1988;66:1291–1296.
64. Schubert B, VanDongen AMJ, Kirsh GE, et al. Inhibition of cardiac Na^+ currents by isoproterenol. *Am J Physiol.* 1990;258:H977-H982.
65. Schubert B, VanDongen AMJ, Kirsh GE, et al. β-Adrenergic inhibition of cardiac sodium channels by dual G-protein pathways. *Science.* 1989;245:516–519.
66. Ono K, Kiyosue T, Arita M. Isoproterenol. DBcAMP and forskolin inhibit cardiac sodium current. *Am J Physiol.* 1989;256:C1131–C1137.
67. Ono K, Fozzard HA, Hanck D. On the mechanism of cAMP-dependent modulation of cardiac sodium channel current kinetics. *Circ Res.* 1993;72:807–815.
68. Kirstein M, Eickhorn R, Langfeld H, et al. Influence of β-adrenergic stimulation of the fast sodium current in the intact rat papillary muscle. *Basic Res Cardiol.* 1991;86:441–448.
69. Matsuda JJ, Lee H, Shibata EF. Enhancement of rabbit cardiac sodium channels by β-adrenergic stimulation. *Circ Res.* 1992;70:199–207.
70. Ming L, West JW, Numann R, et al. Convergent regulation of sodium channels by protein kinase C and cAMP-dependent protein kinase. *Science.* 1993;261:1439–1442.
71. Teo K, Yusuf S, Furberg C. Effect of antiarrhythmic drug therapy on mortality following myocardial infarction. *Circulation.* 1990;82(suppl III):III–197. Abstract.
72. CAST Investigators. Preliminary report: effect of encainide and flecainide on mortality in a randomized trial of arrhythmia suppression after myocardial infarction. *N Engl J Med.* 1989;321:406–412.

73. Lynch JJ Jr, Sanguinetti MC, Kimura S, et al. Therapeutic potential of modulating potassium currents in the diseased myocardium. *FASEB J.* 1992;6:2952–2960.
74. Mason JW. A comparison of seven antiarrhythmic drugs in patients with ventricular tachyarrhythmias. *N Engl J Med.* 1993;329:452–458.
75. Burkart F, Pfisterer M, Kiowski W, et al. Effect of antiarrhythmic therapy on mortality in survivors of myocardial infarction with asymptomatic complex ventricular arrhythmias: basal antiarrhythmic study of infarct survival (BASIS). *J Am Coll Cardiol.* 1990;16:1711–1718.
76. Feld GK, Venkatesh N, Singh BN. Pharmacologic conversion and suppression of experimental canine atrial flutter: differing effects of d-sotalol, quinidine and lidocaine and significance of changes in refractoriness and conduction. *Circulation.* 1986;74:197–204.
77. Josephson MA, Singh BS. Hemodynamic effects of class III antiarrhythmic agents. In: Singh BN, ed. *Control of Cardiac Arrhythmias by Lengthening Repolarization.* Mt Kisco, NY: Futura Publishing Co; 1988: 153–174.
78. Echt DS, Black JN, Barbey JT, et al. Evaluation of antiarrhythmic drugs on defibrillation energy requirements in dogs: sodium channel block and action potential prolongation. *Circulation.* 1989;79:1106–1117.
79. Lee KS. Ibutilide, a new compound with potent class III antiarrhythmic activity, activates a slow inward Na current in guinea-pig ventricular cells. *J Pharmacol Exp Ther.* 1992;262:99–108.
80. Janse MJ. To prolong refractoriness or to delay conduction (or both)? *Eur Heart J.* 1992;13(suppl F):14–18.
81. Hondeghem LM. Development of class III antiarrhythmic agents. *J Cardiovasc Pharmacol.* 1992;20(suppl 2):S17–S22.
82. Carmeliet E. K+ channels and control of ventricular repolarization in the heart. *Fundam Clin Pharmacol.* 1993;7:19–28.
83. Hondeghem LM, Snyders DJ. Class III antiarrhythmic agents have a lot of potential but a long way to go. *Circulation.* 1990;81:686–690.
84. Roden DM, Hoffman B. Action potential prolongation and induction of abnormal automaticity by low quinidine concentrations in canine Purkinje fibers. *Circ Res.* 1985;56:857–867.
85. Dangman KH, Miura DS. Effects of therapeutic concentrations of procainamide on transmembrane action potentials of normal and infarct zone Purkinje fibers and ventricular muscle cells. *J Cardiovasc Pharmacol.* 1989;13:846–852.
86. Strauss HC, Bigger JT, Hoffman BF. Electrophysiological and beta-receptor blocking effects of MJ1999 on dog and rabbit cardiac tissue. *Circ Res.* 1970;26:661–678.
87. Roden DM, Bennett PB, Snyders DJ, et al. Quinidine delays I_K activation on guinea pig ventricular myocytes. *Circ Res.* 1988;62:1055–1058.
88. Carmeliet E. Voltage- and time-dependent block of the delayed K+ current in cardiac myocytes by dofetilide. *J Pharmacol Exp Ther.* 1992; 262:809–817.
89. Snyders DJ, Knoth KM, Roberds SL, et al. Time-, voltage-, and state-dependent block by quinidine of a cloned human cardiac potassium channel. *Mol Pharmacol.* 1992;41:322–330.

90. Follmer CH, Cullinan CA, Colatsky TJ. Differential block of cardiac delayed rectifier current by class IC antiarrhythmic drugs: evidence for open channel block and unblock. *Cardiovasc Res.* 1992;26:1121–1130.
91. Anderson KP, Walker R, Dustman T, et al. Rate-related electrophysiologic effects of long-term administration of amiodarone on canine ventricular myocardium in vivo. *Circulation.* 1989;79:948–958.
92. Singh BN, Sarma JSM, Zhang Z-H, et al. Controlling cardiac arrhythmias by lenthening repolarization: rationale from experimental findings and clinical considerations. *Ann N Y Acad Sci.* 1992;644:187–207.
93. Wang Z, Pelletier LC, Talajic M, et al. Effects of flecainide and quinidine on human atrial action potentials. *Circulation.* 1990;82:274–283.
94. Rensma PL, Allessie MA, Lammers WJEP, et al. Length of excitation wave and susceptibility to reentrant atrial arrhythmias in normal conscious dogs. *Circ Res.* 1988;62:395–410.
95. Wang Z, Page P, Nattel S. Mechanism of flecainide's antiarrhythmic action in experimental atrial fibrillation. *Circ Res.* 1992;71:271–287.
96. Inoue H, Yamashita T, Nozaki A, et al. Effects of antiarrhythmic drugs on canine atrial flutter due to reentry: role of prolongation of refractory period and depression of conduction to excitable gap. *J Am Coll Cardiol.* 1991;18:1098–1044.
97. Spinelli S, Hoffman BF. Mechanisms of termination of reentrant atrial arrhythmias by class I and class III antiarrhythmic agents. *Circ Res.* 1989;65:1565–1579.
98. Roden D, Thompson KA, Hoffman BF, et al. Clinical features and basic mechanism of quinidine-induced arrhythmias. *J Am Coll Cardiol.* 1986;8:73A–78A.
99. Surawicz B. Electrophysiologic substrate of torsade de pointes: dispersion of repolarization or early afterdepolarizations? *J Am Coll Cardiol.* 1989;14:172–184.
100. Nattel S, Quantz MA. Pharmacological response of quinidine induced early afterdepolarizations in canine cardiac Purkinje fibres: insights into underlying ionic mechanisms. *Cardiovasc Res.* 1988;22:808–817.
101. January CT, Riddle JM, Salata JJ. A model for early afterdepolarizations: induction with the Ca^{2+} channel agonist Bay K 8644. *Circ Res.* 1988;62:563–571.
102. Want T, Bergstrand RH, Thompson KA, et al. Concentration-dependent pharmacologic properties of sotalol. *Am J Cardiol.* 1986;57:1160–1165.
103. Wyse KR, Ye V, Campbell TJ. Action potential prolongation exhibits simple dose-dependence for sotalol, but reverse dose-dependence for quinidine and disopyramide: implications for proarrhythmia due to triggered activity. *J Cardiovasc Pharmacol.* 1993;21:316–322.
104. Philipson LH, Miller RJ. A small K^+ channel looms large. *Trends Pharmacol Sci.* 1992;13:8–11.

Chapter 8

Editorial Comments

Dan M. Roden, MD

Whalley and Grant[1] outline the important principles in the genesis of the cardiac action potential and the way in which block of atrial sodium or potassium channels may result in antiarrhythmic or proarrhythmic effects. This commentary is intended to expand on their presentation. The emphasis is on specific points that may be important for a molecular and cellular framework within which to consider atrial arrhythmogenesis and its management; in addition, directions for future research in this area are outlined.

Heterogeneity of Action Potential Configurations

Whalley and Grant point out that the atrial action potential is different from the ventricular action potential and outline the concept that differences in the number or function of the ion channels that sustain these action potentials are responsible. It appears self-evident that region-specific expression of specific ion channel genes accounts for these differences, although very little is known about the regulation of such expression in health and disease. The notion that atrial and ventricular action potentials differ and that action potentials vary among species is but a first step in the recognition of heterogeneity of the cardiac action potential. Within the ventricle, it is now well recognized that epicardial, midmyocardial, and endocardial action potentials display differing configuration.[2-4] The prominent phase 1 notch or "spike and dome" in the epicardial action potential is absent in the endocardial ones, probably reflecting a larger transient outward current in epicardial cells. This may

From DiMarco JP, Prystowsky EN (eds): *Atrial Arrhythmias: State of the Art.* Armonk, NY, Futura Publishing Company, Inc., © 1995.

be modified in disease. For example, Lue and Boyden[5] showed that epicardial cells isolated from the border zone of a 5-day-old myocardial infarction in dogs lack a notch and show markedly reduced transient outward current. Since, as pointed out by Whalley and Grant, the transient outward current "sets" the plateau potential and hence may control intracellular calcium and action potential duration, these changes may be of importance in infarct-related arrhythmogenesis. One possible explanation is that changes in expression of gene(s) that encode the transient outward behavior may well be perturbed following coronary occlusion; alternatively, ischemia itself may damage ion channel proteins. Similarly, recent data suggest decreased expression of genes encoding transient outward currents in humans with heart failure[6]; it is conceivable that these changes may contribute to arrhythmias in this setting.

Species variability in action potential presumably also reflects variability in the expression of ion channel genes. The discussion of I_{Kr} is an example: In some preparations, such as cat ventricular myocytes[7] or cultured mouse atrial cells (AT-1 cells),[8] I_{Kr} is the major repolarizing current. In other species, I_{to} (rabbit)[9,10] or I_{Ks} (guinea pig)[11,12] contributes. I_{Kr} has not yet been directly observed in human ventricular tissue, but the fact that the "highly specific" I_{Kr} blockers, listed in Table 2 of Whalley and Grant, prolong QT[13] indicates that the gene encoding I_{Kr} behavior is expressed in at least some human ventricular, Purkinje, and/or M cells. In human atria, both I_{to} and I_{Kr} have been identified.[14] Importantly, there is substantial heterogeneity among atrial cells in the extent to which these two behaviors are observed, moving the concept of heterogeneity of cardiac electrophysiology to a new, cell-to-cell, level even under apparently "physiological" conditions.

Which Genes Encode Which Current?

A major challenge in molecular electrophysiology is the attempt to correlate expression of ion channel genes with currents in native myocytes. This problem is being attacked by use of both electrophysiological and molecular biological approaches. From the electrophysiological point of view, a difficulty in correlating individual channel expression with native currents is the problem of "contamination" of individual current phenotypes by multiple channel behaviors. Thus, for example, at least two types of inactivating channels, with different permeation characteristics and regulatory features, contribute to the phenotype called "I_{to}."[15,16] Obviously, attempts to understand which ion channel genes "encode" I_{to} must first isolate the specific transient outward current of interest. Similarly, studies of "the" cardiac delayed rectifier must recognize that this current has at least two components with different permeation characteristics, rectification characteristics, regulatory features, and drug block: I_{Kr} and I_{Ks}.[11,12] Studies in which the multicomponent nature of "I_K" are not recognized run the risk of providing incomplete or misleading data. Our own initial study,[17] which reported closed-state block of I_K by quinidine, is one example; follow-up studies suggest open-channel block, at least of I_{Ks}.[18] Similarly, multiple subtypes of cardiac calcium current,[19] and more recently multiple sodium channel genes,[20-22] have been identified. In fact, it is not yet clear that all or even a majority of the proteins involved in cardiac electrogenesis have been cloned. The initial potassium channel cDNA was cloned from the *Drosophila* fruit fly *Shaker* mutant,[23] and most cardiac potassium channel cDNAs reported to date have been isolated by homology screening using *Shaker*-derived probes.[24] If there are channels with completely unique structures, different approaches to gene isolation must be undertaken. The expression cloning of minK (I_{SK}), the cDNA thought to encode I_{Ks},[25,26] and that of inward rectifiers[27-29] are examples of how an alternative approach may yield channels with very little structural similarity to "traditional" sodium, calcium, or potassium channel genes.

The molecular approach to the question of correlating currents in native myocytes with ion channel genes has taken a "reductionist" strategy. That is, it is now possible to express individual ion channel products in heterologous expression systems (such as *Xenopus* oocytes or mouse fibroblasts) that have few, if any, native currents. Thus, the behavior of a protein encoded by a specific cDNA can be studied in isolation. However, this approach is but a first step to understanding the reconstituted behavior of native currents. For example, Po et al[30] showed that coexpression of two different potassium channel cDNAs results in behavior typical of neither alone. As Whalley and Grant point out, it is likely that potassium channel proteins are made up by assembly of four subunits. The most attractive interpretation of the data of Po et al is that potassium channel gene products can assemble as heterotetrameric channels (ie, different subunits) in native myocytes. Given the multiplicity of cardiac potassium channel genes already isolated, this "mix and match" approach[31] to the genesis of functional channels could certainly account for some of the heterogeneity of cardiac potassium currents in native myocytes. Similarly, we now recognize that the reconstitution of certain sodium current behaviors is more likely if small protein subunits are coexpressed. Thus, the challenge of understanding how ion channel genes encode ion currents will require studies using both the electrophysiological and molecular biological approaches.

Whalley and Grant point out the major mechanisms thought to underlie the arrhythmia-suppressing and the proarrhythmic effects of drugs currently used for the management of cardiac arrhythmias. A number of issues they raise deserve further discussion.

On and Off Rates in Cloned Channels

The availability of ion channel clones in heterologous expression systems has provided new information on the molecular determinants of drug binding. For example, Snyders et al[32,33] showed that both quinidine and quinine are open-channel blockers of the potassium channel clone referred to as Kv1.5. Interestingly, both agents appear to bind at the same position within the ion channel pore and with the same on-rates. However, the affinity of the channel for quinidine is substantially greater than that for quinine, a difference attributable exclusively to differences in off-rates (greater for quinine). It is likely that the two agents share a common binding site within the ion channel pore but that the extent to which the drug side chain interacts with adjacent regions on the ion channel molecule to stabilize or destabilize drug binding accounts for this difference. Thus, at least in this case, we have an example of compounds with similar physicochemical characteristics whose on-rates of block are similar but whose off-rates are different. Further understanding of the molecular determinants of these drug-channel interactions may lead to the development of compounds with target on- and off-rates sufficient to develop rate-dependent antiarrhythmic effects and to avoid rate-dependent proarrhythmic effects. Whalley and Grant point out the structural similarities among potassium, calcium, and sodium channels cloned to date and suggest that this similarity has translated into relative nonspecificity of currently available blocking agents. However, with further information on the molecular determinants of drug block, it may be possible to develop compounds specifically targeted at specific regions or at specific channels.

Reverse Use Dependence and I_{Kr} Block

The concept of "reverse use dependence" as an impediment to the use of many action-prolonging agents is a useful one in the sense that it emphasizes that QT prolongation is exaggerated at slow rates and is undesirable because it may predispose to torsade de pointes.[34] Considerable evidence, however, suggests that such drugs may not completely "lose" efficacy at fast rates. For example, action-prolonging compounds are very effective in animal models of ventricular fibrillation,[35-37] and limited clinical data suggest that faster tachycardias may be more readily suppressed by action potential–prolonging drugs than slower ones.[38] It is possible that these antifibrillatory effects reflect primarily events at the initiation of a tachycardia. Thus, further studies of rate dependence should include evaluation of the action potential during abrupt changes in stimulation rate. Limited data, for example, suggest that dofetilide retains substantial action potential–prolonging characteristics at rapid rates when assessed in this fashion.[39] Hondeghem and Snyders[34] proposed that open-channel blockers of cardiac potassium currents would be less likely to produce reverse use dependence than would closed-state blockers. However, emerging data suggest that many action potential–prolonging agents are indeed blockers of open potassium channels.[10] Further studies of the detailed mechanisms of block may help define characteristics associated with greater or lesser proarrhythmic potential.

It now seems probable that the phenomenon of reverse use dependence with specific blockers of I_{Kr} is determined at least in part by the presence of multiple repolarizing currents in the heart.[40] Even in the absence of drug, cardiac action potentials are shorter at rapid stimulation rates than they are at slow stimulation rates, reflecting increased sodium-potassium ATPase activity as well as incomplete deactivation I_{Ks} (at least in preparations in which I_{Ks} is important). Thus, when I_{Kr} is blocked, only a modest effect is observed at fast rates, because these other phenomena control action potential duration. However, at slower rates, when I_{Ks} deactivation is more complete and sodium-potassium ATPase less active, I_{Kr} block assumes a greater role, and action potentials do become prolonged. Whether other mechanisms of action potential prolongation, such as I_{Ks} or I_{to} block, are associated with reverse use dependence and bradycardia-dependent drug toxicity remains to be determined.

Even though clinical experience with specific I_{Kr} blockers is limited, it is already apparent that each of them has the potential to produce torsade de pointes.[13] This proarrhythmic effect is actually not completely simple to explain. I_{Kr} activates only at potentials ≥ -30 mV and displays strong inward rectification. That is, the channel is open between -30 and $+30$ mV and is maximal around 0 mV. Thus, block of I_{Kr} would be predicted to produce action potential prolongation at the plateau and not substantially affect the trajectory of the terminal portion of the action potential. In fact, in guinea pig myocytes, exactly this effect is observed.[11,40] However, early afterdepolarizations, which are thought to contribute to the genesis of torsade de pointes,[41,42] usually arise at membrane potentials more negative than -30 mV, implying that "specific" I_{Kr} blockers must also affect terminal repolarization, at least in some preparations. Several explanations for this discrepancy are possible. First, a large I_{Ks} in guinea pig myocytes (which now appears atypical for many other species) may account for drug effects in that preparation. Second, it is possible that the "specific" I_{Kr} blockers actually block other channels that contribute to terminal repolarization. Third, I_{Kr} may activate and rectify over a different range of potentials in other species. Fourth, the time course of onset of and recovery from voltage-dependent block of I_{Kr} may be sufficiently different in other species to allow terminal repolarization changes. Finally, it is possible that the currents contributing to early afterdepolarizations, possibly through calcium channels[43] or via sodium-calcium exchange,[44] are more readily elicited in other preparations but not in guinea pig myocytes. If I_{Kr}-blocking antiarrhythmics are to be further developed and widely used, a greater understanding of these subtle details among preparations is desirable.

Amiodarone

When antiarrhythmic drugs are discussed, amiodarone is often presented as an exception to many generalizations. It is highly non-specific in the sense that it blocks many different types of ion channels, and what data are available indicate that it does not display marked reverse use dependence.[45] However, the mechanism underlying amiodarone's antiarrhythmic effect has not been identified with any certainty. Block of various ion channels can be demonstrated acutely in vitro,[18,46,47] but it is recognized that the drug may take weeks to months before an optimal antiarrhythmic effect is observed. It seems possible that the ion channel blocking properties of amiodarone may contribute only in part to its long-term antiarrhythmic effects; conceivably, its uptake into the lipid membrane environment[48,49] in which ion channels exist may account for its effects. Gillis et al[50] reported that changes in dietary lipid resulted in altered propafenone block of cardiac sodium channels, implying that the lipid milieu in which channels exist may be modifiable and thus, perhaps, a target for antiarrhythmic drugs. Given the increasing use of amiodarone, studies of its mechanism of action during chronic treatment seem desirable.

Drug Action in a Syncytium?

Whalley and Grant rightly point out that a clear understanding of antiarrhythmic drug action requires a consideration of drug effects not only at the ion channel level but also in the integrated syncytium. A good example is sodium channel block, which can produce both antiarrhythmic and proarrhythmic effects. In the simplest of all reentrant circuits, such as a jellyfish ring, an intervention that only slows conduction cannot be antiarrhythmic. However, we recognize that sodium channel blockers can suppress reentrant arrhythmias. Some of this effect may reflect changes in refractoriness consequent to the complex relationship between repolarization and recovery from sodium channel inactivation outlined by Whalley and Grant. Alternatively, conduction slowing in a circuit with nonuniform characteristics may eventually lead to block of propagation and extinction of reentry. Moreover, it should be emphasized that the drugs we use as sodium channel blockers may have important potassium channel blocking effects (the example of flecainide in the atria is a good one[51]) and may be potent suppressors of nonreentrant arrhythmogenic mechanisms. The increasing recognition that tachycardias have different underlying pathophysiological characteristics (excitable gap vs no excitable gap, reentrant vs nonreentrant, etc) reinforces the concept that understanding of antiarrhythmic drug action in an arrhythmogenic syncytium is an important requirement to improve antiarrhythmic therapy.[52] Moreover, it is increasingly recognized that the electrophysiological substrate targeted by drugs is dynamic: factors such as ischemia, neurohormones, or myocardial stretch can alter ion channel function in a single cardiac cycle and cause arrhythmias. In addition, slower alteration in channel number or function as a consequence of disease[5,6,53] or even drug therapy[54] is a potentially important area of investigation that is only now evolving.

Targets for Antiarrhythmic Drug Action

The treatment of cardiac arrhythmias with drugs has traditionally relied on ion channel blockers. However, the one class of antiarrhythmic drugs that indisputably prolong life are β-blockers, which are not thought to act directly by blocking ion channels. One hope of new molecular and cellular knowledge is that completely new targets for antiarrhythmic drug action may be identified: these might include mechanisms of channel and/or subunit assembly, mechanisms that phosphorylate or dephosphorylate these proteins to alter their function, mechanisms controlling cell-cell communication, the lipid environment, the cytoskeleton to which channels are anchored, or the mechanisms controlling expression of the genes themselves. Appropriate drug development will also recognize that drugs should maintain this efficacy (and minimize their toxicity) in the face of a dynamic external milieu. The view that antiarrhythmic drug therapy is "doomed" to nonspecificity should be tempered by an open mind about what are appropriate targets for drug treatment of arrhythmias.

The best of the science of medicine has always been based on the premise that improvement in understanding of underlying mechanisms will necessarily lead to safer and more effective forms of pharmacological and nonpharmacological therapy of disease. Scientists involved in the care of patients with cardiac arrhythmias have been at the forefront of applying this principal. The availability of the very new technologies of molecular cloning and of single-cell and single-channel electrophysiology now offers us opportunities for increasing our understanding of basic mechanisms underlying normal and abnormal cardiac electrogenesis and thus improving patient care.

References

1. Whalley D, Grant AO. Role of sodium and potassium channels in atrial electrogenesis and their blockade by antiarrhythmic drugs. This volume.
2. Antzelevitch C, Sicouri S, Litovsky SH, Lukas A, Krishnan SC, Di Diego JM, Gintant GA, Liu DW. Heterogeneity within the ventricular wall: electrophysiology and pharmacology of epicardial, endocardial, and M cells. *Circ Res.* 1991;69:1427–1449.
3. Furukawa T, Kimura S, Furukawa N, Basset AL, Myerburg RJ. Potassium rectifier currents differ in myocytes of endocardial and epicardial origin. *Circ Res.* 1992;70:91–103.
4. Wang Z, Fermini B, Nattel S. Repolarization differences between guinea pig atrial endocardium and epicardium: evidence of a role of I_{TO}. *Am J Physiol.* 1991;260:H1501–H1506.
5. Lue W, Boyden P. Abnormal electrical properties of myocytes from chronically infarcted canine heart. *Circulation.* 1992;85:1175–1188.
6. Beuckelmann D, Näbauer M, Erdmann E. Alterations of K^+ currents in isolated human ventricular myocytes from patients with terminal heart failure. *Circ Res.* 1993;73:379–385.
7. Follmer CH, Colatsky TJ. Block of delayed rectifier potassium current, I_K, by flecainide and E-4031 in cat ventricular myocytes. *Circulation.* 1990;82:289–293.
8. Yang T, Wathen MS, Field LJ, Tamkun MM, Roden DM, Snyders DJ. I_{Kr}: a major repolarizing current in cultured AT1 cells. Submitted, *American Heart Association 66th Scientific Sessions.* November 1993.
9. Fish F, Selby L, Bhattacharyya M, Roden D. Non-inactivating outward currents in rabbit ventricular myocytes. *Biophys J.* 1992;61:A253. Abstract.
10. Carmeliet, E. Voltage- and time-dependent block of the delayed K^+ current in cardiac myocytes by dofetilide. *J Pharmacol Exp Ther.* 1993; 262:809–817.
11. Sanguinetti MC, Jurkiewicz NK. Two components of cardiac delayed rectifier K^+ current: differential sensitivity to block by class III antiarrhythmic agents. *J Gen Physiol.* 1990;96:195–215.
12. Balser JR, Bennett PB, Roden DM. Time-dependent outward current in guinea pig myocytes: gating kinetics of the delayed rectifier. *J Gen Physiol.* 1990;96:835–863.
13. Roden DM. Current status of class III antiarrhythmic therapy. *Am J Cardiol.* 1993;72(suppl):44B–49B.
14. Wang Z, Fermini B, Nattel S. Delayed rectifier outward current and repolarization in human atrial myocytes. *Circ Res.* 1993;73:276–285.
15. Tseng GN, Hoffman BF. Two components of transient outward current in canine ventricular myocytes. *Circ Res.* 1989;64:633–647.
16. Zygmunt AC, Gibbons WR. Calcium-activated chloride current in rabbit ventricular mycytes. *Circ Res.* 1991;68:424–437.
17. Roden DM, Bennett PB, Snyders DJ, Balser JR, Hondeghem LM. Quinidine delays I_K activation in guinea pig myocytes. *Circ Res.* 1988;62: 1055–1058.
18. Balser JR, Bennett PB, Hondeghem LM, Roden DM. Suppression of

time-dependent outward current in guinea pig ventricular myocytes: actions of quinidine and amiodarone. *Circ Res.* 1991;69:519–529.

19. Bean BP. Two kinds of calcium channels in canine atrial cells. *J Gen Physiol.* 1985;86:1–30.

20. Rogart RB, Cribbs LL, Muglia LK, Kephart DD, Kaiser MW. Molecular cloning of a putative tetrodotoxin-resistant rat heart Na^+ channel isoform. *Proc Natl Acad Sci U S A.* 1989;86:8170–8174.

21. Gellens ME, George AL, Chen L, Chahine M, Horn R, Barchi RL, Kallen RG. Primary structure and functional expression of the human cardiac tetrodotoxin-insensitive voltage-dependent sodium channel. *Proc Natl Acad Sci U S A.* 1992;89:554–558.

22. George AL, Knittle TJ, Tamkun MM. Molecular cloning of an atypical voltage-gated sodium channel expressed in human heart and uterus: evidence for a distinct gene family. *Proc Natl Acad Sci U S A.* 1992;89: 4893–4897.

23. Papazian DM, Schwarz TL, Tempel BL, Jan YN, Jan LY. Cloning of genomic and complementary DNA from *Shaker*, a putative potassium channel gene from *Drosophila*. *Science*. 1987;237:749–753.

24. Roberds SL, Knoth KM, Po S, Blair TA, Bennett PB, Hartshorne RP, Snyders DJ, Tamkun MM. Molecular biology of the voltage-gated potassium channels of the cardiovascular system. *J Cardiac Electrophysiol.* 1993;4:68–80.

25. Takumi T, Ohkubo H, Nakanishi S. Cloning of a membrane protein that induces a slow voltage-gated potassium current. *Science*. 1988;242: 1042–1045.

26. Folander K, Smith JS, Antanavage J, Bennett C, Stein RB, Swanson R. Cloning and expression of the delayed rectifier IsK channel from neonatal rat heart and diethylstilbestrol-primed rat uterus. *Proc Natl Acad Sci U S A.* 1990;87:2975–2979.

27. Ho K, Nichols CG, Lederer WJ, Lytton J, Vassilev PM, Kanazirska MV, Hebert SC. Cloning and expression of an inwardly rectifying ATP-regulated potassium channel. *Nature*. 1993;362:31–38.

28. Kubo Y, Baldwin TJ, Jan YN, Jan LY. Primary structure and functional expression of a mouse inward rectifier potassium channel. *Nature*. 1993;362:127–133.

29. Kubo Y, Reuveny E, Slesinger P, Jan YN, Jan LY. Primary structure and functional expression of a rat G-protein-coupled muscarinic potassium channel. *Nature*. 1993;364:802–806.

30. Po S, Roberds S, Snyders DJ, Tamkun MM, Bennett PB. Heteromultimeric assembly of human potassium channels. *Circ Res.* 1993;72:1326–1336.

31. Stühmer W, Ruppersberg JP, Schröter KH, Sakmann B, Stocker M, Giese KP, Perschke A, Baumann A, Pongs O. Molecular basis of functional diversity of voltage-gated potassium channels in mammalian brain. *EMBO J.* 1989;8:3235–3244.

32. Snyders DJ, Knoth KM, Roberds SL, Tamkun MM. Time-, voltage-, and state-dependent block by quinidine of a cloned human cardiac potassium channel. *Mol Pharmacol.* 1992;41:322–330.

33. Snyders D, Tamkun M, Bennett P. Stereoselective block of a cloned

human cardiac K⁺ channel by quinidine isomers. *Circulation.* 1992;86 (suppl I):I–77. Abstract.

34. Hondeghem LM, Snyders DJ. Class III antiarrhythmic agents have a lot of potential, but a long way to go: reduced effectiveness and dangers of reverse use-dependence. *Circulation.* 1990;81:686–690.

35. Bacaner MB, Clay JR, Shrier A, Brochu RM. Potassium channel blockade: a mechanism for suppressing ventricular fibrillation. *Proc Natl Acad Sci U S A.* 1985;83:2223–2227.

36. Chi L, Mu D, Driscoll EM, Lucchesi BR. Antiarrhythmic and electrophysiologic actions of CK-3579 and sematilide in a conscious canine model of sudden coronary death. *J Cardiovasc Pharmacol.* 1990;16:312–324.

37. Lynch JJ Jr, Heaney LA, Wallace AA, Gehret JR, Selnick HG, Stein RB. Suppression of lethal ischemic ventricular arrhythmias by the class III agent E4031 in a canine model of previous myocardial infarction. *J Cardiovasc Pharmacol.* 1990;15:764–775.

38. Kuchar DL, Garan H, Venditti FJ, Finkelstein D, Rottman JN, McComb J, McVoern BA, Ruskin JN. Usefulness of sotalol in suppressing ventricular tachycardia or ventricular fibrillation in patients with healed myocardial infarcts. *Am J Cardiol.* 1989;64:33–36.

39. Knilans T, Lathrop DA, Nanasi PB, et al. Rate and concentration-dependent effects of UK-68, 798, a potent new Class III antiarrhythmic agent, on canine Purkinje fibre action potential duration and Vmax. *Br J Pharmacol.* 1991;103:1568–1572.

40. Jurkiewicz NK, Sanguinetti MC. Rate-dependent prolongation of cardiac action potentials by a methanesulfonamide class III antiarrhythmic agent: specific block of rapidly activating delayed rectifier K⁺ current by dofetilide. *Circ Res.* 1993;72:75–83.

41. Roden DM. Early afterdepolarizations and torsade de pointes: implications for the control of cardiac arrhythmias by controlling repolarization. *Eur Heart J.* In press.

42. Jackman WM, Friday KJ, Anderson JL, Aliot EM, Clark M, Lazzara R. The long QT syndromes: A critical review, new clinical observations and a unifying hypothesis. *Prog Cardiovasc Dis.* 1988;31:115–172.

43. January CT, Riddle JM. Early afterdepolarizations: mechanism of induction and block: a role for L-type Ca²⁺ current. *Circ Res.* 1989;64:977.

44. Szabo B, Rajagopalan CV, Lazzara R. The role of Na⁺:Ca²⁺ exchange in the genesis of early afterdepolarizations in cardiac action potentials. *FASEB J.* 1992;A1164. Abstract.

45. Anderson KP, Walker R, Dustman T, et al. Rate-related electrophysiological effects of long-term administration of amiodarone on canine ventricular myocardium *in vivo. Circulation.* 1989;79:948–953.

46. Mason JW, Hondeghem LM, Katzung BG. Block of inactivated sodium channels and of depolarization-induced automaticity in guinea pig papillary muscle by amiodarone. *Circ Res.* 1984;55:277–285.

47. Nishimura M, Follmer C, Singer D. Amiodarone blocks calcium current in single guinea pig ventricular myocytes. *J Pharmacol Exp Ther.* 1989;251:650–659.

48. Chatelain P. Effects of amiodarone and related drugs on membrane fluidity and enzymatic properties. *Drug and Anesthetic Effects on Membrane Structure and Function.* 1991:183–202.
49. Chester DW, Herbette LG. Membrane pathway for drug binding to protein receptors. In: Hondeghem L, ed. *Molecular and Cellular Mechanisms of Antiarrhythmic Agents.* Mount Kisco, NY: Futura Publishing Co Inc; 1989:241–268.
50. Gillis AM, Keashly R, Watson PA, Mathison HJ, Parsons HG. Influence of dietary fat on the pharmacodynamics of propafenone in isolated, perfused rabbit hearts. *Circulation.* 1992;85:1501–1509.
51. Wang Z, Pagé P, Nattel S. Mechanism of flecainide's antiarrhythmic action in experimental atrial fibrillation. *Circ Res.* 1992;71:271–287.
52. Task Force of the Working Group on Arrhythmias of the European Society of Cardiology. The Sicilian Gambit: a new approach to the classification of antiarrhythmic drugs based on their actions on arrhythmogenic mechanisms. *Circulation.* 1991;84:1831–1851. *Eur Heart J.* 1991;12:1112–1131.
53. Bandyopadhyay S, Mashburn C, Tamkun M, Roden D. Modulation of cardiac K+ channel mRNA transcript level and electrocardiographic effect by hypertension. *Circulation.* 1992;86(suppl I):I–77. Abstract.
54. Taouis M, Sheldon RS, Duff HJ. Upregulation of the rat cardiac sodium channel by *in vivo* treatment with a class I antiarrhythmic drug. *J Clin Invest.* 1991;88:375–378.

Chapter 9

Animal Models of Atrial Arrhythmias

Albert L. Waldo, MD

The Early Work: Mayer, Mines, Lewis, and Garrey

The overriding message in this brief review is that models of cardiac arrhythmias, in this case atrial arrhythmias, are invaluable for gaining insights into the nature, mechanism, and treatment of arrhythmias, with ultimate application to the care of patients. Perhaps the most powerful support of that statement comes from the fact that, as emphasized by Cranefield,[1] on the basis of studies in the subumbrella of the jellyfish (Fig 1), ray and dogfish auricles, and turtle heart by Mayer[2,3] and Mines,[4,5] the basic principles of reentry were understood by 1914. Thus, the need for a substrate (pathway) with a central obstacle around which a reentrant wave front could circulate, the critical need for unidirectional block in that substrate, and the need to have the wave length of excitation shorter than the path length were already understood from some basic experiments in simple animal models. Mines even recognized the necessary presence of what we now call dual atrioventricular (AV) nodal pathways to explain "return extrasystoles," ie, echo beats following a premature ventricular beat.[4] As remarkable as these early studies were, a rereading of them at this time demonstrates that Mayer apparently missed an opportunity to identify the importance of anisotropic

Supported in part by grant RO1-HL38408 from the National Institutes of Health, National Heart, Lung, and Blood Institute, Bethesda, Md; a Research Initiative Award from the Northeast Ohio Affiliate of the American Heart Association, Cleveland, Ohio; and a grant from the Wuliger Foundation, Cleveland, Ohio.

From DiMarco JP, Prystowsky EN (eds): *Atrial Arrhythmias: State of the Art*. Armonk, NY, Futura Publishing Company, Inc., © 1995.

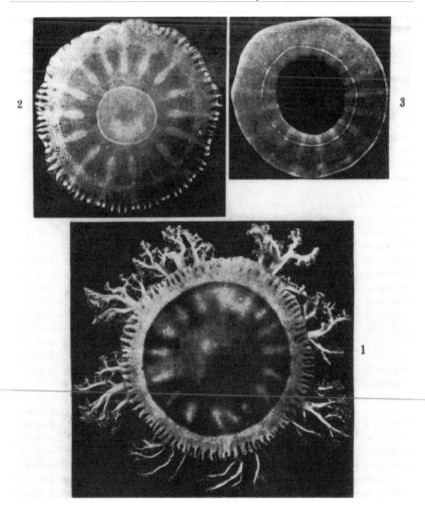

FIGURE 1. *Three views of* Cassiopea xamachana *as published by A.G. Mayer. 1: An aboral view; 2: an oral view of the subumbrella with stomach and mouth-arms removed; and 3: a ring of subumbrella tissue made by cutting off the marginal sense organs and removing the center of the disk. Reproduced with permission from Reference 13.*

conduction, presently a major consideration in understanding reentry. It appears that Mayer was puzzled by an experiment in which he made an incision in the jellyfish ring such that he doubled its length (Fig 2). He assumed that conduction time around the rings also would double. However, what he observed was that conduction

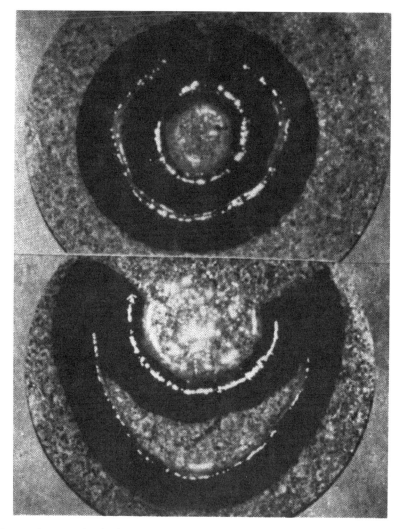

FIGURE 2.   *Method of A.G. Mayer for doubling the length of the pathway of the entrapped circuit wave in* Cassiopea xamachana. *The diameter of the underlying cork platter on which the* Cassiopea xamachana *rests is 20 cm. Reproduced with permission from Reference 13.*

time actually more than doubled. In retrospect, it is clear from examining the study and the nature of the incision in the ring that when the reentrant wave front passed from one ring to the other (as occurred because of the incision), the circulating impulse had to cross perpendicular to the longitudinal orientation of the muscle fibers of the ring. This almost surely caused slowing of conduction. Some nine decades later, we now recognize this as anisotropic conduction.[6]

The major points of this early work on reentry were well understood by Sir Thomas Lewis and his laboratory. In fact, they published simple diagrams illustrating the principles of reentry using a ring model (Fig 3A and 3B).[7] Importantly, this understanding also produced an unspoken assumption that the center of the reentrant circuit was an anatomic obstacle. This apparently influenced Lewis and others for a long time. Although the work on reentry due to reflection by Schmitt and Erlanger[8] could be interpreted otherwise, it does not seem that any investigators considered that the central area of block in the reentrant circuit could, in whole or in part, be functional. Thus, in studies in the canine heart in which atrial flutter was initiated by faradic stimulation of the atria and sequential site activation mapping from remarkably few atrial sites (usually 7 to 15) was performed, Lewis and colleagues concluded that atrial flutter was due to reentrant excitation around the superior and inferior venae cavae, two naturally occurring obstacles (Fig 4).[9] Implicit in this conclusion was the fact that there must be an area of functional block between the superior and inferior venae cavae, but that was not discussed by these authors. The assumption that an anatomic obstacle was required for reentry can be also seen in the interpretation of one canine study in which Lewis and colleagues concluded, again on the basis of recording from relatively few sites on both atria, that the reentrant circuit ". . . would appear to circulate, not around the cavae, but in some other ring of muscle such as that surrounding the mitral orifice" (Fig 5). In fact, this conclusion may have been prescient, in that we now are aware from the studies of Frame et al[10,11] that at least one model of atrial flutter is due to reentrant excitation around the muscular ring of the tricuspid valve orifice.

Nevertheless, it should be emphasized that it was really quite difficult for these early investigators to develop animal models of atrial arrhythmias. It is noteworthy to quote a paragraph in this regard from the work of Lewis et al[9] on atrial flutter:

> A chief difficulty is in obtaining flutter, or fibrillation when it is desired, of sufficient duration. The observations are to be made during the after-effect when stimulation has been withdrawn. In mapping out the auricle, during the progress of the flutter after-effect, an after-effect of considerable duration is essential.

An after-effect lasting 20, 30 or more minutes is usually necessary. We know of no sure method by which these long after-effects are to be obtained, and this lack of knowledge adds much to the difficulty of the work. It is impossible to say at the moment stimulation is withdrawn how long the after-effect will last. It is even impossible to say with certainty that an after-

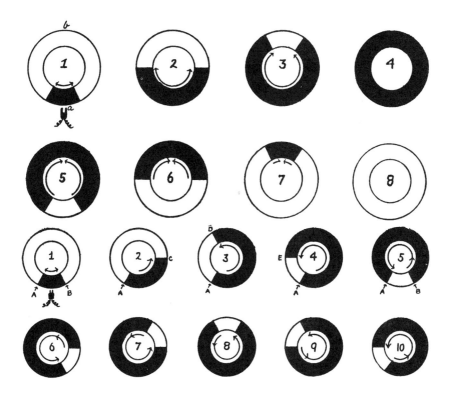

FIGURE 3. Diagram illustrating the progress of a single wave passing through a ring of muscle as a result of stimulation at site a. The black portion of the ring represents the refractory state, and the figure shows its progress through the ring until it involves the whole (4); later the figure shows its subsidence. B: Diagram to illustrating the establishment of a circus movement in a ring of muscle. The ring is stimulated in its lower quadrant, and the wave spreads to A and to B. At A it is blocked, but from B it continues around the ring. When it arrives at E (4), the refractory state at 4 is passing, and so the wave continues to travel around the circle (5 to 10). Reproduced with permission from Reference 7.

effect will be obtained. On many occasions, there will be no after-effect, on very many other occasions there will be a short after-effect, lasting a few seconds or perhaps a minute; on rare occasions an after-effect of many minutes' duration, very rarely of 30 or 60 minutes' duration, will be seen. It is upon these long after-effects that our observations have been undertaken. It will be apparent that there are many disappointments; some auricles will be stimulated repeatedly and only fleeting after-effects

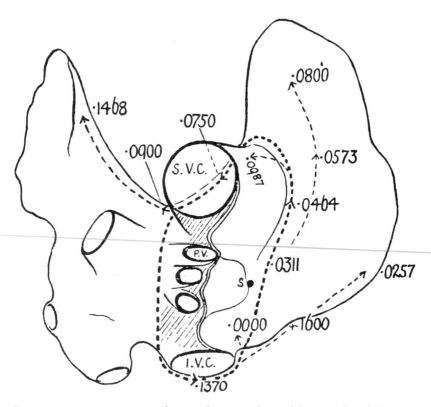

FIGURE 4.   *An accurate and natural-size outline of the auricle of dog KQ showing the readings obtained during the period of flutter. These have been reduced to a new common zero. The broken arrows represent the path pursued by the excitation wave, as ascertained from the direction of the deflections in direct leads and from the surface recordings; the former and latter evidences were entirely confirmatory of each other. An area is shaded to display the pericardial reflection more prominently. S.V.C. = superior and I.V.C = inferior vena cava; P.V. = right pulmonary veins. S marks the point stimulated. Reproduced with permission from Reference 9.*

will be obtained; in others longer after-effects will be obtained, but these will cease spontaneously before the mapping out is complete; in yet others the after-effect will be of sufficient duration, but more often than not it will consist of fibrillation or impure flutter, to which the method of mapping out is unsuited.

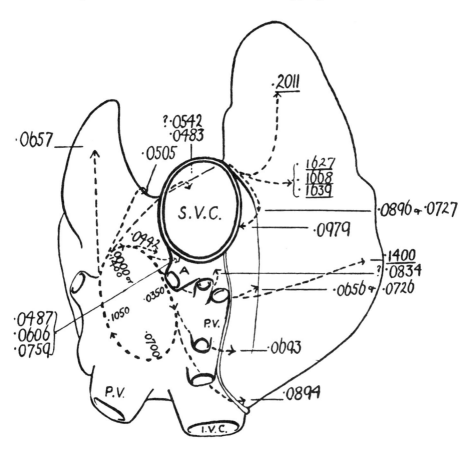

FIGURE 5.   *An accurate outline of the auricle of dog KD, reproduced at natural size. The readings have been reduced to a new common zero. The heavy broken circle represents the supposed track of the circus movement around the left auriculoventricular orifice. The readings inside this cycle are hypothetical. The arrows are drawn in directions compatible with the path of the excitation wave, as ascertained by the directions of the deflections in direct leads, and with the readings obtained from the surface of the heart. S.V.C. = superior and I.V.C. = inferior vena cava; P.V. = left and right pulmonary veins. A = azygous vein. Reproduced with permission from Reference 9.*

Clearly, both the value of and the need for animal models of stable atrial arrhythmias was understood by Lewis and his laboratory. At this point, the work of Walter E. Garrey[12] should be mentioned. As emphasized by Rytand,[13] in a single study published some 80 years ago and remarkable for the fact that it presented only descriptions of what the author had observed in a dying heart rather than any electrophysiological or even mechanical records, Garrey contributed very importantly to a fundamental concept; namely, that a critical mass of tissue is necessary to sustain fibrillation of any sort (atrial or ventricular). Thus, he induced atrial fibrillation by faradic stimulation from the top of one of the atrial appendages. He then separated the tip from the fibrillating atria and found that "as a result of this procedure the appendage came to rest, but the auricles invariably continued their delirium unaltered." Simple but fundamental studies such as these permitted Garrey to conclude that "any small auricular piece will cease fibrillating even though the excised pieces retained their normal properties."

Development of Models of Atrial Tachyarrhythmias: Reentry vs a Single Focus Firing Rapidly

The assumption about anatomic obstacles serving as the center of reentrant circuits is again seen in the important theoretical work of Wiener and Rosenblueth in Mexico City. In the mid 1940s, Wiener and Rosenblueth[14] calculated theoretically that certain anatomic orifices were too small to sustain reentrant excitation. On the basis of estimates of the velocity of the potential circulating reentrant wave front, they calculated that the orifice of the inferior vena cava might be large enough to serve as a possible obstacle for reentrant atrial flutter. They also inferred that the smaller orifice of the superior vena cava would serve for atrial fibrillation. Furthermore, they mentioned without any discussion "the possibility that the pulmonary veins, singly or jointly, may provide effective obstacles for flutter or fibrillation" but indicated that further investigation was necessary. Implicit in this work were two other important principles. First, not only was atrial flutter due to a single reentrant circuit, but atrial fibrillation also could be. The latter is still not proven, but from recent studies in animal models from several laboratories,[15-17] it appears more and more viable that atrial fibrillation may be due to a single focus (in this case, a reentrant circuit) generating a rapid rhythm that the remainder of the atria cannot follow 1:1. Second was the apparent absence of consideration of functional or anatomical areas of slow conduction in the reentrant circuit. The latter, in fact, does not seem to have been part of the consideration of many investigators, although again, the presence of such an area or areas is clear from the work of Schmitt and Erlanger in the late 1920s.[8] Thus, it seems that most investigators assumed constant conduction velocity in the reentrant circuit, something we now know is unusual.

The work of Lewis and colleagues and the work of Wiener and Rosenblueth were instrumental in the development of the Rosenblueth–Garcia Ramos[18] model of atrial flutter. The latter team, also from Mexico City, reasoned that to place a crush lesion between the superior and inferior venae cavae would enlarge the anatomic obstacle sufficiently to permit induction of a stable reentrant circuit. In their experiments, later repeated by Kimura and colleagues[19] (Fig 6A), to ensure stable atrial flutter, they crushed the right atrial tissue between the superior vena cava and the inferior vena cava. Atrial flutter was then initiated by rapid atrial pacing. Using sequential site mapping from relatively few sites, they concluded that circus movement around this anatomic obstacle was either clockwise or counterclockwise. Then, Rosenblueth and Garcia Ramos found that an appropriately placed lesion in the right atrium terminated the atrial flutter, fulfilling the criterion or, in fact, the admonition of Mines[5] that "the test for a circulating excitation is to cut through the ring at one point thereby terminating the flutter." As shown in Fig 6B, Kimura et al[19] repeated this portion of the study as well. Their initial lesion did not terminate the atrial flutter; it simply prolonged the atrial flutter cycle length. They thought the latter was because the lesion made the reentrant circuit longer. Interestingly enough, Rosenblueth and Garcia Ramos in their studies also made a Y-like lesion that they also noted prolonged the atrial flutter cycle length. Neither group considered that the lesion might have fundamentally changed the location of the reentrant pathway. The latter could have been possible, according to the tricuspid ring reentry model.[10,11] In any event, to interrupt the atrial flutter, the lesion had to be extended completely to the AV boundary in this model (Fig 6B).

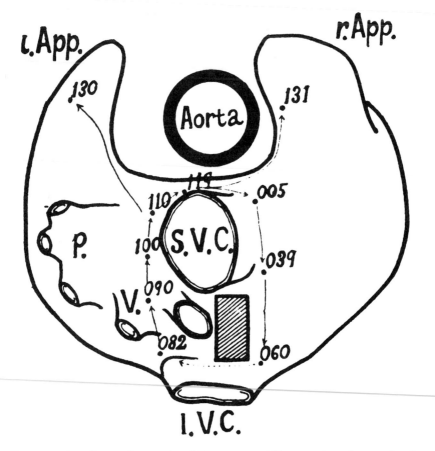

FIGURE 6.A: *From the work of Kimura et al,[19] repeating the work of Rosenblueth and Garcia Ramos. A: Outline of the cephalic surface of a dog's auricle, showing the reading for the arrival of the excitation wave. The obliquely hatched area was injured by Pean's forceps.*

During this period came the important work from Scherf and colleagues,[20-22] also repeated by Kimura et al.[19] They demonstrated that both atrial flutter and atrial fibrillation could be generated from a single focus firing rapidly. This was accomplished by placing aconitine on the heart. As shown in Fig 7, placing aconitine on the atrial appendage caused very rapid activation of the rest of the atria from that site, as evident from the nature of the relative sequence of

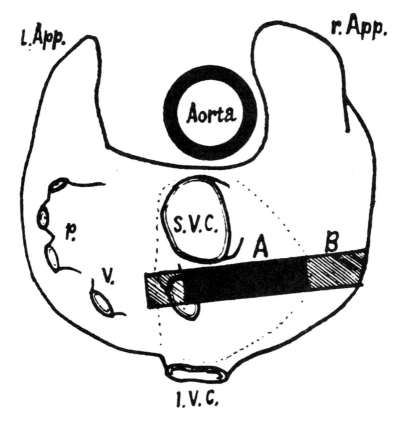

FIGURE 6.B: *Diagram showing enlargement of the blocked area. The flutter persists by the blocking of the area A alone, while it returns instantly to sinus rhythm when the blocked area is widened to the area plotted by oblique lines (B). l.App. = left atrial appendage; r.App. = right atrial appendages; S.V.C. = superior vena cava; I.V.C. = inferior vena cava; P.V. = pulmonary veins. Reproduced with permission from Reference 13.*

atrial activation demonstrated by the sequential site mapping. When the site of aconitine application was excluded, the tachycardia was terminated. Additionally, it seemed that it was the degree of rapidity of firing at the aconitine site that determined whether the rhythm generated was atrial flutter or atrial fibrillation. As summarized recently, we now know that aconitine causes early afterdepo-

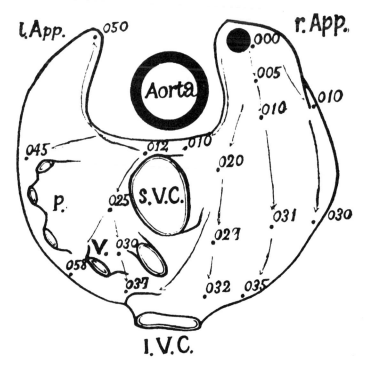

Figure 7. *From work by Kimura et al.[19] Outline of the cephalic surface of a dog's auricle, showing the reading for the arrival of the excitation wave. Aconitine solution was injected at the black shaded portion. Note that the activation sequence is consistent with activation from the site of the placement of the aconitine in the right atrial appendage. Note also the brevity of the duration of the activation sequence. l.App.=left atrial appendage; r.App=right atrial appendage; S.V.C.=superior vena cava; I.V.C.=inferior vena cava; P.V.=pulmonary veins. Reproduced with permission from Reference 13.*

larizations in Purkinje fibers and ventricular muscle.[23] Although it is probably reasonable to assume that it does the same in atrial tissue, repolarization in the latter is sufficiently different from that in ventricular tissue that this assumption must be tested. As summarized recently,[23] the few studies that have been done in rabbit atrial fibers ". . . found an increase in rate, flutter, and even fibrillation in the absence of early afterdepolarizations. In such preparations, it may be that the increase in background inward current caused by aconitine was sufficient to cause a marked increase in the rate of phase 4 depolarization." In any event, while there clearly is no clinical counterpart to aconitine-induced atrial flutter or atrial fibrillation in patients, these findings do indicate that a single focus firing rapidly (whatever the cause) is capable of producing both atrial flutter and atrial fibrillation. In the latter instance, as suggested above, it is assumed that the impulses generated from the site are too rapid for the rest of the atria to following in a 1:1 fashion. The result is atrial fibrillation. As we begin to understand some of the more contemporary models of atrial flutter and atrial fibrillation, this concept is again quite relevant. That this is possible in patients is clearly demonstrated by the continuous rapid atrial pacing studies to precipitate and sustain atrial fibrillation deliberately as a therapeutic maneuver.[24,25]

In 1964, Moe and colleagues[26] developed a computer model of both atrial fibrillation and atrial flutter. It is in part from these studies that the multiple, simultaneously circulating reentrant wavelet hypothesis evolved for the mechanism of atrial fibrillation. In addition, in this computer model, Moe and colleagues[26] showed that atrial flutter developed only when obstacles that were sufficiently long were placed in the model and atrial fibrillation was first precipitated. The latter concept is a continuing theme, present in the original as well as the more recent models, namely, that in virtually all studies, atrial flutter is not initiated de novo. Rather, a transitional rhythm with all the earmarks of atrial fibrillation precedes the development of atrial flutter. The recent work of Shimizu et al[27] indicates that it is during the transitional rhythm that the requisites for the initiation of a stable reentrant circuit develop.

A Functional Model of Reentry: Allessie and Colleagues

As indicated earlier, the importance of the presence of an anatomic obstacle for the evolution of reentrant excitation was either explicit or implicit until Allessie and colleagues[28-30] in the 1970s demonstrated in the isolated left atrium of the rabbit heart that reentrant excitation could occur in which the reentrant circuit was totally functionally determined. The requisite unidirectional block in response to a premature beat results from inhomogeneities of refractoriness. The center of the reentrant circuit around which reentrant excitation travels is functionally determined and is created by centripetal wavelets coming from the reentrant mother wave. These centripetal wavelets continuously bombard the center of the reentrant circuit, thereby maintaining a central area of functional block. This was called leading circle reentry (Fig 8).[30] Thus, Allessie showed for the first time that the center of a reentrant circuit need not be an anatomic obstacle but rather could be functionally determined. This marked an important advance in our understanding of reentry. Also, it provided a new focus on the nature of the excitable gap in the reentrant circuit. In this model, the excitable gap is small and not fully excitable,ie, the excitable gap is such that

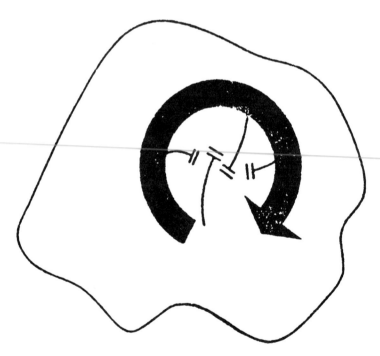

FIGURE 8.   *Diagram of leading circle–type reentry showing a circuit consisting of a reentrant wave front (black arrow) circulating around a functionally refractory center produced by converging wavelets that block in the center. Block is indicated by double bars. Reproduced with permission from Reference 30.*

the head of excitability bites the tail of refractoriness. Thus, the excitable gap consists of tissue in the relative refractory period. Still, the presence of functional areas of slow conduction in the reentrant circuit was not greatly appreciated.

Stable Models of Atrial Flutter and Atrial Fibrillation: The Era of Simultaneous Multisite Mapping Techniques

The next advance in animal models of atrial arrhythmias was the studies by Boineau and colleagues[31] of a dog with spontaneous atrial flutter. Using simultaneous multisite mapping (56 electrodes) of the atria, Boineau and colleagues showed that the reentrant circuit during atrial flutter was in the right free wall. In this model, we see for the first time the presence of crowding of atrial activation isochrones in the reentrant circuit, indicating the presence of areas of functionally slow conduction. They also repeated the studies of Rosenblueth and Garcia Ramos, and on the basis of those studies as well as the studies of the spontaneous atrial flutter in the canine heart, they emphasized the importance of the architecture in the right atrium in contributing to the reentrant substrate. These observations can be considered a prelude to the very important subsequent work on anisotropy by Spach and colleagues.[6]

At about the same time, Allessie and colleagues[32–34] developed a Langendorff-perfused canine atrial model of both atrial fibrillation and atrial flutter. In this model, rapid atrial pacing was initiated during infusion of acetylcholine. Then, after cessation of rapid atrial pacing, either atrial fibrillation or atrial flutter evolved. By recording simultaneously from 192 electrodes from specially designed electrode arrays inserted through the tricuspid and mitral valve orifices to record endocardially from either or both atria, Allessie and colleagues were able to map the sequence of endocardial atrial activation during whichever arrhythmia developed, atrial fibrillation or atrial flutter. Mapping during atrial fibrillation clearly demonstrated the presence of multiple, simultaneously circulating reentrant wave fronts of the random reentry type (Fig 9). This was the first demonstration in an animal model that the multiple reentrant wave front theory of Moe and colleagues[26] was, in fact, operative. Mapping during atrial flutter in this model showed a leading

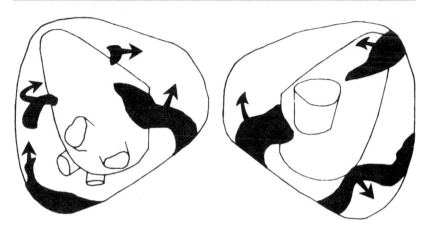

FIGURE 9.   *Multiple propagating wavelets in canine atria encountered at an arbitrary moment during self-sustained atrial fibrillation. A total of 7 wavelets were present, 3 in the right and 4 in the left atrium. The crest of the depolarization waves is indicated by arrows, which point to the general direction in which the wavelets propagate. Reproduced with permission from Reference 34.*

circle–type reentrant circuit that could occur almost anywhere in either atrium (Fig 10). No anatomic orifices functioned as the center of the reentrant circuit in this model. However, the cycle lengths of the induced atrial flutter were so short (<100 msec) that Wells et al[35] suggested this might represent a type II atrial flutter.

Three other atrial flutter models were developed in the 1980s. One by Boyden and Hoffman[36] was created in a canine heart by banding of a pulmonary artery and creation of tricuspid regurgitation. The animal was then allowed to recover, and over time, right atrial enlargement developed. After a period of about 3 months, rapid atrial pacing then always initiated sustained atrial flutter. Importantly, simultaneous multisite endocardial mapping during atrial flutter demonstrated the reentrant circuit to be functionally determined and to be present in the right atrial free wall.[37] Furthermore, standard intracellular microelectrode studies of tissue from this model failed to show any electrophysiological abnormalities.[36] The latter particularly emphasized the importance of functional aspects of reentry in this model.

At the same time, the sterile pericarditis model of atrial flutter

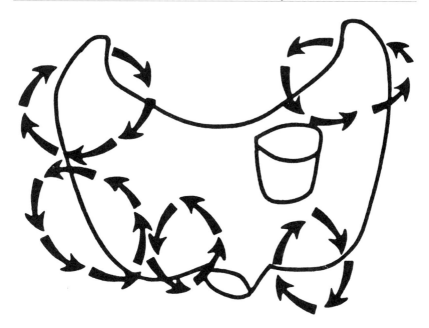

FIGURE 10.   *Demonstration of the location and direction of circus movement in six different examples of atrial flutter induced by Allessie and colleagues in a canine acetylcholine infusion model of atrial flutter. Reproduced with permission from Reference 33.*

was developed by our laboratory.[38] This model was suggested by the observation that atrial flutter is a very common tachyarrhythmia in patients after open heart surgery even though most patients who develop this rhythm after surgery never had it before surgery. Furthermore, the spontaneous occurrence of this arrhythmia seemed to follow the time course of the sterile pericarditis that virtually all patients get after open heart surgery. Thus, when the pericarditis subsided, this arrhythmia spontaneously disappeared and, in most instances, was no longer a clinical problem. Using a sterile pericarditis canine model, we could induce stable atrial flutter and show that it is due to a functionally determined reentrant circuit in the right atrium.[27,39–41] Moreover, the reentrant circuit seems to be of the anisotropic reentrant type.[42]

Simultaneous multisite (190 electrodes on the right atrial free wall) mapping studies from the sterile canine pericarditis atrial flutter model provided new insights into the evolution and maintenance of functionally determined reentrant circuits. Of particular note, the onset of atrial flutter was shown to first require a transitional rhythm (atrial fibrillation) during which the requisites for reentry develop, namely, unidirectional block and a functional center around which reentrant wave front can circulate (Fig 11A and

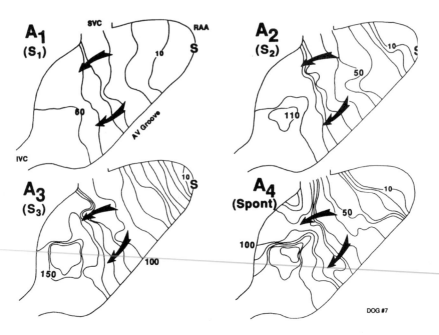

FIGURE 11. A: *Isochronous maps during the onset of atrial flutter in the canine pericarditis model induced by an eight-beat drive train (S_1) followed by two premature beats (S_2 and S_3, respectively) (300/130/80 msec) delivered from the right atrial appendage (RAA) at site S. Isochrones are displayed at 10-msec intervals. Arrows indicate the direction of the main activation wave front. Beats A_1, A_2, and A_3 represent isochronous maps corresponding to S_1, S_2, and S_3, respectively. Beat A_1 (S_1) was the last driven beat at a cycle length of 300 mesc. Beat A_2 (S_2) was the first premature beat. Beat A_3 (S_3) was the second premature beat. In beats A_2 and A_3, radial activation preceded from the pacing site, and crowding of 10-msec isochrones developed in some areas. In beat A_4, the first spontaneous (Spont) beat, the earliest activated area was close to the pacing site. SVC = superior vena cava; IVC = inferior vena cava; AV = atrioventricular.*

11B).[27] This model has also served to demonstrate the importance of functional areas of slow conduction in the reentrant circuit, particularly at pivot points. These areas of slow conduction seem to be the Achilles' heel of these reentrant circuits, since intervention, such as drug therapy or pacing, that causes termination of the atrial flutter reentrant circuit results in its termination in an area of slow con-

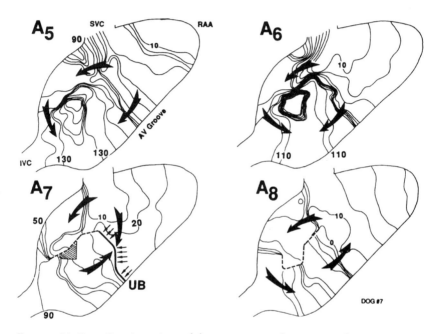

FIGURE 11. B: *Continuation of the sequence of activation from Fig 11A. Beats A_5 to A_8 represent subsequent spontaneous beats. Beats A_5 and A_6 showed development of the areas of slow conduction along the sulcus terminalis and in the pectinate muscle region. With beat A_7, unidirectional block (UB) (solid thick black line) of the inferior wave front occurred at the pectinate muscle region in the area of slow conduction. Then, the nonblocked superior activation wave front conducted around a line of functional block (dashed lines) and through an area of slow conduction close to the inferior vena cava to conduct through the areas of unidirectional block from the opposite direction. The shaded area represents an area of localized block. Beat A_8 was the first spontaneous atrial flutter beat, which traveled counterclockwise around an area of functional block (dashed line) at a cycle length of 152 msec. Reproduced with permission from Reference 27.*

duction.[40,41,43,44] Furthermore, when this rhythm stops spontaneously, it also results from block of the circulating reentrant wave front in an area of slow conduction.[45] Principles of entrainment have also been demonstrated in this model.[40]

Another important atrial flutter model, referred to earlier, is the tricuspid ring reentry model developed by Frame et al.[10,11] In this model, these workers used the intercaval lesion of Rosenblueth and

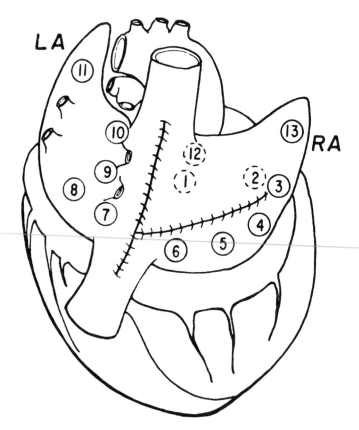

FIGURE 12. A: *This diagram of the heart viewed from the right posterior oblique projection shows the location of the Y-shaped lesion to create the model of Frame et al.[10,11] The intercaval lesion extends from the superior vena cava to the inferior vena cava, and another lesion extends from the intercaval lesion across the right atrium toward the right atrial appendage. Each number indicates the position of a bipolar pair of electrodes. LA = left atrial appendage; RA = right atrial appendage.*

Garcia Ramos but made a second lesion that extended from the intercaval region toward the right atrial appendage. Thus, a Y-type lesion was created surgically in the right atrial free wall (Fig 12A). Then, with rapid atrial stimulation, sustained atrial flutter developed. The reentrant wave front during this rhythm was shown to be due to either clockwise or counterclockwise circus movement around the tricuspid valve ring (Fig 12B).[10,11] This model has been helpful in understanding the importance of boundaries for the development and maintenance of reentrant excitation, to help understand drug actions in interruption of reentrant excitation, and also to help understand entrainment.[46-48] It should be noted that the significance of boundaries was, in part, appreciated by Mayer[2,3] and Mines.[4,5] They indicated in their work that the central obstacle

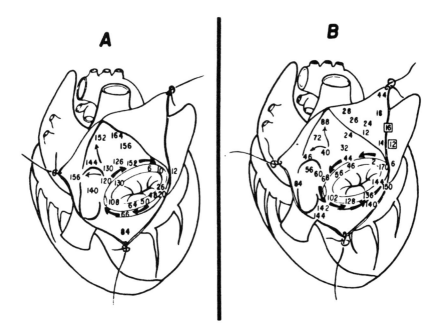

FIGURE 12. B: *Endocardial activation times recorded at the right atrium during atrial flutter while the heart is on total cardiopulmonary bypass. Panel A shows a clockwise activation sequence around the ring of the tricuspid valve orifice. Panel B shows a counterclockwise activation sequence around the ring of the tricuspid valve orifice. Reproduced with permission from Reference 10.*

around which the reentrant wave front circulated was important because short-circuiting of the central obstacle would result in premature arrival of the activation wave front at the site of unidirectional block. If it arrived before that site had time to repolarize, the reentrant excitation would cease because the tissue simply could not depolarize again. Frame et al[10,11] and Boyden and Graziano[47] extended the appreciation of the importance of boundaries in development and maintenance of reentrant arrhythmia to include the importance of the lateral boundaries of the reentrant circuit. Finally, regarding the tricuspid ring reentry model, as summarized recently,[49] it should be noted that this rhythm probably has a clinical counterpart in the appearance of atrial flutter in patients after various surgical procedures such as the Mustard, the Senning, and the Fontan procedures used to repair congenital heart lesions.

Other models of atrial flutter have also been used recently to understand the nature of circus movement and to discover the effects of various interventions (drugs, pacing, etc) on these circuits. This includes the crush lesion model of Feld and Shahandeh-Rad[50] and Yamashita and colleagues.[51] Our laboratory also developed a cryolesion model of atrial flutter.[52] These and the above models also provided insights into the nature of recordings from the reentrant circuit.[41,50] The latter have important implications for interpreting data from clinical studies in which the mapping techniques are far more difficult and, to date, less sophisticated than in animal models. Extrapolation from these data has already been used by Feld and colleagues,[53] Saoudi and colleagues,[54] and Cosio and colleagues[55] in their use of ablative techniques to cure atrial flutter in patients.

Most recently, several new models of atrial fibrillation have been described. Most are still being characterized but clearly are of interest and already have demonstrated usefulness. The first is an in vitro canine right atrial model of Schuessler et al,[16] in which a figure-8 reentrant circuit of very short cycle length was induced during acetylcholine infusion. This reentrant circuit was shown to generate an atrial fibrillation rhythm in the remainder of the preparation. The second model is produced in sheep simply by pacing the atria rapidly for a brief period.[56] After this pacing, the atrial fibrillation persists for relatively long periods. This model remains to be more fully characterized but has already been used to study atrial defibrillation.[56]

The third model of atrial fibrillation is the canine sterile pericarditis model.[57] It is produced the same way as the canine sterile pericarditis model of atrial flutter. The difference is that stable atrial fibrillation rather than atrial flutter is induced when the pacing induction protocol is initiated during days 1 and 2 after surgery. On days 3 and 4 after surgery, the inducibility of atrial fibrillation decreases. Furthermore, the sterile pericarditis atrial fibrillation model appears to be a model of paroxysmal atrial fibrillation, since the duration of induced atrial fibrillation rarely exceeds 60 to 70 minutes. This model already has been used to study atrial defibrillation.[58]

The fourth model of atrial fibrillation is also in the canine heart; it is a continuous vagal stimulation model in which atrial fibrillation is initially induced by a burst of rapid atrial pacing.[59,60] Although not fully characterized, it is thought to resemble the model described by Allessie et al[32,34] in the isolated Langendorff preparation and has been used to study antiarrhythmic drug action. The fifth model, just presented by Allessie's group (Wijffels et al[61]) and currently being characterized, is the goat model of atrial fibrillation. This model, produced by recurrent rapid pacing to precipitate and sustain atrial fibrillation, has already provided new and important data regarding changes in atrial refractoriness following prolonged periods of atrial fibrillation. In sum, all these models provide new and important opportunities to understand better the nature and treatment of atrial fibrillation.

Concept of Functionally Slow Conduction

During this time, the significant work of Spach and colleagues[6,62,63] demonstrating the presence of the anisotropy and its value in understanding normal and abnormal cardiac conduction evolved. These studies emphasized the importance of the direction of the wave front relative to fiber orientation, both for refractoriness and conduction velocity and for the safety factor for conduction. Thus, in terms of conduction velocity, when an impulse crosses perpendicular to the longitudinal orientation of the cardiac muscle fibers, a marked decrease in conduction velocity will occur. These concepts were soon shown to be very important in the reentrant ventricular tachycardia model of Wit, Dillon, et al.[42,64] In this model, ventricular tachycardia can be induced in a thin rim of surviving myocardial tissue following a Harris two-stage procedure to occlude the left anterior descending coronary artery to produce an infarct. In fact, Wit and colleagues[42,64] described anisotropic reentry in this model. In this type of reentry, direction of the activation wave front relative to fiber orientation is a critical factor in the initiation and maintenance of reentrant excitation. Relative to atrial arrhythmias, it is thought that anisotropic conduction is important in the sterile pericarditis atrial flutter model, in which functional areas of slow conduction, principally at the pivot points of the reentrant circuit, are uniformly present.[27,39–41,43–45]

Summary

Thus, it is clear that animal models already have provided significant insights into the nature and mechanism of atrial arrhythmias. Undoubtedly, further studies and development of additional models will continue to provide valuable new insights and should continue to have important implications for patient care. Of course, the ultimate animal model to study is the human being. Such studies have already begun during open heart surgery[65] and hold promise that with the new techniques of simultaneous multisite mapping and other technologies, we will indeed continue to gain the requisite insights and understanding of these arrhythmias to advance patient care.

References

1. Cranefield PF. *The Conduction of the Cardiac Impulse.* Mt Kisco, NY: Futura Publishing Co; 1975:153–197.
2. Mayer AG. Rhythmical pulsation in scyphomedusae. Washington, DC: Carnegie Institution of Washington. Publication 47;1906:1–62.
3. Mayer AG: Rhythmical pulsation in scyphomedusae. II. In: *Papers from the Tortugas Laboratory of the Carnegie Institution of Washington.* 1908;1:113–131.
4. Mines GR: On dynamic equilibrium in the heart. *J Physiol (Lond).* 1913;46:349–383.
5. Mines GR: On circulating excitation in heart muscles and their possible relations to tachycardia and fibrillation. *Trans R Soc Can.* 1914;43: 8–52.
6. Spach MS, Miller WT III, Dolber PC, Kootsey JM, Sommer JK, Mosher CE Sr. The functional role of structural complexities in the propagation

of the polarization in the atrium of the dog: cardiac conduction disturbances due to discontinuities of effective axial resistivity. *Circ Res.*
1982;50:175–191.

7. Lewis T. Observations upon flutter and fibrillation, IV: impure flutter;
theory of circus movement. *Heart.* 1920;7:293–345.

8. Schmitt FO, Erlanger J. Directional differences in the conduction of the
impulse through heart muscle and their possible relation to extrasys-
tolic and fibrillary contractions. *Am J Physiol.* 1928–29;87:326–347.

9. Lewis T, Feil HS, Stroud WD. Observations upon flutter and fibrillation, II: the nature of auricular flutter. *Heart.* 1920;7:191–245.

10. Frame LH, Page RL, Hoffman BF. Atrial reentry around an anatomic
barrier with a partially refractory excitable gap: a canine model of atrial
flutter. *Circ Res.* 1986;58:495–511.

11. Frame LH, Page RL, Boyden PA, Fenoglio JJ Jr, Hoffman BF. Circus
movement in the canine atrium around the tricuspid ring during experimental atrial flutter and during reentry in vivo. *Circulation.* 1987;76:
1155–1175.

12. Garrey W. The nature of fibrillary contraction of the heart: its relation
to tissue mass and form. *Am J Physiol.* 1914;33:397–414.

13. Rytand DA. The circus movement (entrapped circuit wave) hypothesis
of atrial flutter. *Arch Intern Med.* 1966;65:125–159.

14. Wiener N, Rosenblueth A. The mathematical formulation of the problem of conduction of impulses in a network of connected excitable elements, specifically in cardiac muscle. *Arch Inst Cardiol Mex.* 1946;16:
205–265.

15. Pertsov AM, Davidenko JM, Salomonsz R, Baxter WT, Jalife J. Spiral
waves of excitation underlie reentrant activity in isolated cardiac muscle. *Circ Res.* 1993;72:631–650.

16. Schuessler RB, Grayson TM, Bromberg BI, Cox JL, Boineau JP. Cholinergically mediated tachyarrhythmias induced by a single extrastimulus
in the isolated canine right atrium. *Circ Res.* 1992;71:1254–1276.

17. Ortiz J, Niwano S, Abe H, Gonzalez HX, Rudy Y, Johnson NJ, Waldo
AL. Mapping the conversion of atrial flutters to atrial fibrillation and
atrial fibrillation to atrial flutter: insights into mechanism. *Circ Res.*
Submitted.

18. Rosenblueth A, Garcia Ramos J. Studies on flutter and fibrillation, II:
the influence of artificial obstacles on experimental auricular flutter.
Am Heart J. 1947;33:677–684.

19. Kimura E, Kato K, Murao S, Ajisaka H, Koyama S, Omiya Z. Experimental studies on the mechanism of auricular flutter. *Tohoku J Exp
Med.* 1954;60:197–207.

20. Scherf D. Studies on auricular tachycardia caused by aconitine administration. *Proc Exp Biol Med.* 1947;64:233–239.

21. Scherf D, Romano FJ, Terranova R. Experimental studies on auricular
flutter and auricular fibrillation. *Am Heart J.* 1958;36:241–251.

22. Scherf D, Terranova R. Mechanism of auricular flutter and fibrillation.
Am J Physiol. 1949;159:137–142.

23. Cranefield PF, Aronson RS. *Cardiac Arrhythmias: The Role of Triggered
Activity and Other Mechanisms.* Mt Kisco, NY: Futura Publishing Co,
Inc; 1988:426–465.

24. Waldo AL, MacLean WAH, Karp RB, Kouchoukos NT, James TN. Continuous rapid atrial pacing to control recurrent or sustained supraventricular tachycardias following open heart surgery. *Circulation.* 1976; 54:245–250.
25. Moreira DAR, Shepard RB, Waldo AL. Chronic rapid atrial pacing to maintain atrial fibrillation: use to permit control of ventricular rate in order to treat tachycardia induced cardiomyopathy. *PACE Pacing Clin Electrophysiol.* 1989;12:761–775.
26. Moe GK, Rheinboldt WC, Abildskov JA. A computer model of atrial fibrillation. *Am Heart J.* 1964;67:200–220.
27. Shimizu A, Nozaki A, Rudy Y, Waldo AL. Onset of induced atrial flutter in the canine pericarditis model. *J Am Coll Cardiol.* 1991;17:1223–1234.
28. Allessie MA, Bonke FIM, Schopman FJG. Circus movement in rabbit atrial muscle as a mechanism of tachycardia. *Circ Res.* 1973;33:54–62.
29. Allessie MA, Bonke FIM, Schopman FJG. Circus movement in rabbit atrial muscle as a mechanism of tachycardia; II: the role of nonuniform recovery of excitability in the occurrence of unidirectional block as studied with multiple microelectrodes. *Circ Res.* 1976;39:168–177.
30. Allessie MA, Bonke FIM, Schopman FJG. Circus movement in rabbit atrial muscle as a mechanism of tachycardia, III: the "leading circle" concept: a new model of circus movement in cardiac tissue without the involvement of an anatomic obstacle. *Circ Res.* 1977;41:9–18.
31. Boineau JP, Schuessler RB, Mooney CR, Miller CB, Wylds AC, Hudson RD, Borremans JM, Brockus CW. Natural and evoked atrial flutter due to circus movement in dogs. *Am J Cardiol.* 1980;45:1167–1181.
32. Allessie M, Lammers W, Smeets J, Bonke F, Hollen J. Total mapping of atrial excitation during acetylcholine-induced atrial flutter and fibrillation in the isolated canine heart. In: Kulbertus HE, Olsson SB, Schlepper M, eds. *Atrial Fibrillation.* Molndal, Sweden: A.B. Hassle; 1982:44–59.
33. Allessie MA, Lammers WJEP, Bonke FIM, Hollen J. Intraatrial reentry as a mechanism for atrial flutter induced by acetylcholine in rapid pacing in the dog. *Circulation.* 1984;70:123–135.
34. Allessie M, Lammers WJEP, Bonke FI, Hollen J. Experimental evaluation of Moe's multiple wavelet hypothesis of atrial fibrillation. In: Zipes DP, Jalife J, eds. *Cardiac Electrophysiology and Arrhythmias.* New York, NY: Grune & Stratton; 1985:265–275.
35. Wells JL Jr, MacLean WAH, James TN, Waldo AL. Characterization of atrial flutter: studies in man after open heart surgery using fixed atrial electrodes. *Circulation.* 1979;60:665–673.
36. Boyden PA, Hoffman BF. The effects on atrial electrophysiology and structure of surgically induced right atrial enlargement in dogs. *Circ Res.* 1981;49:1319–1331.
37. Boyden PA. Activation sequence during atrial flutter in dogs with surgically induced right atrial enlargement; I: observations during sustained rhythms. *Circ Res.* 1988;62:596–608.
38. Pagé P, Plumb VJ, Okumura K, Waldo AL. A new model of atrial flutter. *J Am Coll Cardiol.* 1986;8:872–879.

39. Okumura K, Plumb VJ, Pagé PL, Waldo AL. Atrial activation sequence during atrial flutter in the canine pericarditis model and its effects on the polarity of the flutter wave in the electrocardiogram. *J Am Coll Cardiol.* 1991;17:509–518.
40. Shimizu A, Nozaki A, Rudy Y, Waldo AL. Multiplexing studies of effects of rapid atrial pacing on the area of slow conduction during atrial flutter in canine pericarditis model. *Circulation.* 1991;83:983–994.
41. Shimizu A, Nozaki A, Rudy Y, Waldo AL. Characterization of double potentials in a functionally determined reentrant circuit: multiplexing studies during interruption of atrial flutter in the canine pericarditis model. *J Am Coll Cardiol.* 1993;22:2022–2032.
42. Dillon SM, Allessie MA, Ursell PC, Wit AL. Influence of anisotropic tissue structure on reentrant circuits in the epicardial border zone of subacute canine infarcts. *Circ Res.* 1988;63:182–206.
43. Schoels W, Yang H, Gough WB, El-Sherif N. Circus movement atrial flutter in the canine sterile pericarditis model: differential effects of procainamide on the components of the reentrant pathway. *Circ Res.* 1991;68:1117–1126.
44. Ortiz J, Nozaki A, Shimizu A, Khrestian C, Rudy Y, Waldo AL. Mechanism of interruption of atrial flutter by moricizine: electrophysiologic and multiplexing studies in the canine sterile pericarditis model of atrial flutter. *Circulation.* Submitted.
45. Ortiz J, Igarashi M, Gonzalez HX, Laurita K, Rudy Y, Waldo AL. Mechanism of spontaneous termination of stable atrial flutter in the canine sterile pericarditis model. *Circulation.* 1993;88:1866–1877.
46. Spinelli W, Hoffman BF. Mechanisms of termination of reentrant atrial arrhythmias by class I and class III antiarrhythmic agents. *Circ Res.* 1989;1565–1579.
47. Boyden PA, Graziano JN. Activation mapping of reentry around an anatomical barrier in the canine atrium: observations during the action of class III agent d-sotalol. *J Cardiovasc Electrophysiol.* 1993;4:266–279.
48. Boyden PA, Frame LH, Hoffman BF. Activation mapping of reentry around an anatomic barrier in the canine atrium: observations during entrainment and termination. *Circulation.* 1989;79:406–416.
49. Waldo AL. Mechanisms of atrial fibrillation, atrial flutter, and ectopic atrial tachycardia: a brief review. *Circulation.* 1987;75(suppl III):III–37–III–40.
50. Feld GK, Shahandeh-Rad F. Mechanism of double potentials recorded during sustained atrial flutter in the canine right atrial crush-injury model. *Circulation.* 1992;86:628–641.
51. Yamashita T, Inoue H, Nozaki A, Sugimoto T. Role of anatomic architecture in sustained atrial reentry and double potentials. *Am Heart J.* 1992;124:938–946.
52. Shimizu A, Igarashi M, Rudy Y, Waldo AL. Insights into atrial flutter from experimental models. *PACE Pacing Clin Electrophysiol.* 1991;14:627. Abstract.
53. Feld GK, Fleck P, Cheng P-S, Boyce K, Bahnson TD, Stein JB, Calisi CM, Ibarra M. Radiofrequency catheter ablation for the treatment of human type I atrial flutter: identification of a critical zone in the reen-

trant circuit by endocardial mapping techniques. *Circulation.* 1992;86: 1233–1240.
54. Saoudi N, Atallah G, Kirkorian G, Touboul P. Catheter ablation of the atrial myocardium in human type I atrial flutter. *Circulation.* 1990;81: 762–771.
55. Cosio FG, Lopez-Gil M, Giocolea A, Arribas F, Barroso JL. Radiofrequency ablation of the inferior vena cava-tricuspid valve isthmus in common atrial flutter. *Am J Cardiol.* 1993;71:705–709.
56. Powell AC, Garan H, McGovern BA, Fallon JT, Krishnan S, Ruskin JN. Low energy conversion of atrial fibrillation in sheep. *J Am Coll Cardiol.* 1992;20:707–711.
57. Ortiz J, Igarashi M, Gonzalez X, Johnson NJ, Waldo AL. A new, reliable atrial fibrillation model with a clinical counterpart. *J Am Coll Cardiol.* 1993;21:183A. Abstract.
58. Ortiz J, Sokoloski MC, Niwano S, Abe H, Gonzalez X, Ayers GM, Alferness CA, Waldo AL. Successful atrial defibrillation using temporary pericardial electrodes. *J Am Coll Cardiol.* 1994;23:125A. Abstract.
59. Wang Z, Pagé P, Nattel S. Mechanism of flecainide's antiarrhythmic action in experimental atrial fibrillation. *Circ Res.* 1992;71:271–287.
60. Wang J, Bourne GW, Wang Z, Villemaire C, Talajic M, Nattel S. Comparative mechanisms of antiarrhythmic drug action in experimental atrial fibrillation: importance of use-dependent effects on refractoriness. *Circulation.* 1993;88:1030–1044.
61. Wijffels M, Kirchhof C, Fredericks J, Boersma L, Allessie M. Atrial fibrillation begets atrial fibrillation. *Circulation.* 1993;88(suppl I):I–18. Abstract.
62. Spach MS, Dolber PC. The relation between discontinous propagation in anisotropic cardiac muscle and the "vulnerable period of reentry." In: Zipes DP, Jalife J, eds. *Cardiac Electrophysiology and Arrhythmias.* New York, NY: Grune & Stratton; 1985:241–252.
63. Spach MS, Dolber PC, Heidlage JF. Resolution of discontinuous versus continuous propagation: microscopic mapping of the derivatives of extracellular potential wave forms. In: Zipes DP, Jalife J, eds. *Cardiac Electrophysiology. From Cell to Bedside.* Philadelphia, Pa: WB Saunders Co; 1990:139–148.
64. Wit AL, Dillon SM. Anisotropic reentry. In: Shenasa M, Borggrefe M, Breithardt G, eds. *Cardiac Mapping.* Mt Kisco, NY: Futura Publishing Co, Inc; 1993:127–154.
65. Cox JL, Canaven TE, Schuessler RB, Cain ME, Lindsay BD, Stone C, Smith PK, Corr PB, Boineau JP. The surgical treatment of atrial fibrillation, II: intraoperative electrophysiologic mapping and description of the electrophysiologic basis of atrial flutter and atrial fibrillation. *J Thorac Cardiovasc Surg.* 1991;101:406–426.

Chapter 9

Editorial Comments

Penelope A. Boyden, PhD

Animal models of atrial arrhythmias have been in use for at least 100 years. From an animal model, one can provide an essential link needed to answer mechanistically driven questions. An investigator would venture into developing an animal model of an arrhythmia for the following reasons. First, the arrhythmia can be studied in the chronically instrumented, conscious animal. This is an advantage because with the proper placement of pacing electrodes, changes in the electrocardiogram can be monitored during overdrive protocols and the arrhythmia. Furthermore, after the arrhythmia is studied in the animal in the conscious state, the arrhythmic heart can be isolated or the chest opened and studied by multisite mapping techniques. The arrhythmic heart may also be removed and portions of the endocardial/epicardial tissues mapped in vitro by use of fine-tipped microelectrodes. In this way, the cellular electrical basis of the arrhythmia may be determined. Finally, the arrhythmic heart of the animal can provide tissues that can be used for correlative myocyte electrophysiological experiments (ie, voltage clamp experiments) and/or pathological studies.

In the past 5 years, several of these approaches using existing animal models of atrial arrhythmias have provided new information concerning the several subtypes of reentrant rhythms that give rise to atrial tachycardias, as well as the meaning of changes in the electrocardiogram observed during specific pacing protocols.

For instance, the use of an animal model of an atrial arrhythmia has provided us with new information about the mechanism of entrainment of a reentrant atrial rhythm. The concept of entrainment originated in work by Waldo et al[1,2] during a series of pacing

From DiMarco JP, Prystowsky EN (eds): *Atrial Arrhythmias: State of the Art*. Armonk, NY, Futura Publishing Company, Inc., © 1995.

This work was supported by funds from the National Heart, Lung, and Blood Institute (HL-30557).

studies in patients with atrial tachycardias. In these studies, Waldo et al suggested the patterns of activation and the four electrocardiogram-based criteria that had to be satisfied to demonstrate that an arrhythmia was due to reentry. However, a more precise understanding of the way in which paced stimuli actually influence patterns of activation during reentry around a functional barrier has now arisen from the recent multisite mapping study using the canine sterile pericarditis model of atrial flutter.[3] Results from this experimental study confirmed the third criterion of entrainment proposed by Waldo et al in their patient studies (Fig 1).

The use of an animal model of atrial flutter has also allowed us

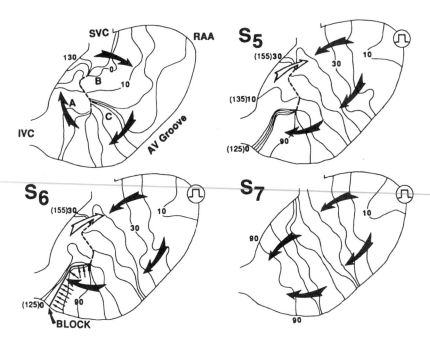

FIGURE 1. *Schematics of 10-msec isochrone maps during pacing interruption of atrial flutter in canine sterile pericarditis model. Numbers in each map show activation time for isochrone. Arrows depict main direction of wave front. Upper left is flutter during control (142-msec cycle length). Upper right, lower left, and lower right schematics show maps for fifth (S_5), sixth (S_6), and seventh (S_7) paced beats during rapid pacing at a cycle length of 125 msec. S_7 map shows interruption of flutter. See Reference 3 for more detail. RAA = right atrial appendage; SVC = superior vena cava; IVC = inferior vena cava; AV = atrioventricular.*

to probe the mechanism of action of a specific pharmacological agent, in particular, the action of the class III agent d-sotalol. In an earlier study using the chronically instrumented conscious animal in which a Y-shaped surgical lesion had been placed in the right atrium, Spinelli and Hoffman[4] showed that d-sotalol was quite effective in terminating sustained atrial flutters. This was not at all surprising, since it had been shown previously that in this canine model of flutter, the circus path is provided by the supravalvular tissues of the tricuspid ring.[5] Therefore, in this particular subtype of reentry around an anatomic barrier, it was hypothesized that a drug-induced increase in atrial refractoriness would increase the wavelength of the reentering impulse, reduce the excitable gap within the reentrant circuit, and cause termination of the reentry. However, Spinelli and Hoffman found that the affect of d-sotalol to terminate the reentrant flutter rhythm was not always consistent with a large drug-induced increase in the wavelength of the impulse. Careful examination of the few electrograms recorded in the chronically instrumented conscious animal at the time of d-sotatol–induced termination showed that while a modest prolongation of flutter cycle length occurred, termination was immediately preceded by one or two short flutter cycle lengths (Fig 2). Therefore, what was predicted to occur in this anatomic reentrant circuit with a class III agent did not always happen.

The effects of d-sotalol on atrial flutter in this animal model have now been mapped.[6] An example of a sequence of flutter beats during this particular type or mode of termination with this agent is illustrated in Fig 3. The changes in flutter cycle length preceding the drug-induced termination in the conscious dog also occurred during the drug-induced termination in the mapping studies in the isolated heart (Fig 4). The results of this study illustrate that the marked oscillations in cycle length that immediately preceded termination were secondary to failure of a lateral boundary of the circuit. This resulted in the entry of a broad excitatory impulse into the circuit. This wave front reset the flutter for one beat (Fig 3E), and then, presumably because of its prematurity, terminated the flutter in the next (Fig 3F). Our ability to map changes in activation patterns in the heart of an animal with an experimental atrial reentrant rhythm has enabled us to add to our knowledge about how drugs might terminate atrial reentry. For instance, we know now that drugs can affect reentrant rhythms not only by altering the electrical properties of fibers within the primary reentrant circuit but also by altering properties of fibers far from but contiguous with the tis-

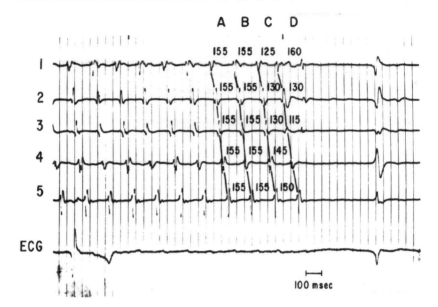

FIGURE 2. *Electrograms (1–5) and electrocardiogram (ECG) showing termination of flutter by d-sotalol in dog in which a Y-shaped lesion had been placed in right atrium. Note the change in flutter cycle length immediately preceding drug induced termination. See Reference 4 for more detail.*

sues of the primary circuit. By virtue of their complex three-dimensional nature, the atrial chambers have numerous ways by which an extra impulse could arise and subsequently impact on the electrical activity of the primary circuit. Our findings with a d-sotalol[6] emphasize further our need to consider not only the nature of the central barrier of the atrial reentrant circuit but also the nature of the lateral boundaries. In particular, we must consider the importance of the lateral boundaries in the initiation of atrial rhythms (in that they can provide stabilization of a rhythm [for discussion see Frame et al[5]]) as well as in their termination. In reference to the latter, we must become more knowledgeable about the role of "failure of lateral boundaries" in the mechanism of spontaneous and drug-induced terminations of reentrant rhythms.

With all that we have gained with our use of existing animal models of atrial arrhythmias, there is still much that we need to know that we may never achieve with models that exist today. First, for the models described above, as well as those described by Waldo

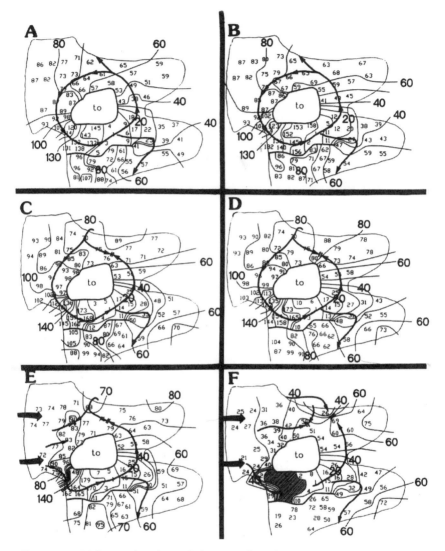

FIGURE 3. *Right atrial endocardial maps of one beat of control flutter in dog in which a Y-shaped lesion had been placed in the right atrium (flutter due to anatomic reentry) (panel A). Panel B depicts one beat of flutter after d-sotalol had increased the flutter cycle length. Panels C through F depict the patterns of activation during the last four consecutive beats of flutter during the action of d-sotalol to terminate this flutter. Note the different path of the circulating impulse (compare panels B and C). Large broad arrows in panels E and F depict the location of the large broad excitatory wavefront that resets (panel E) and then terminates the reentry (panel F).*

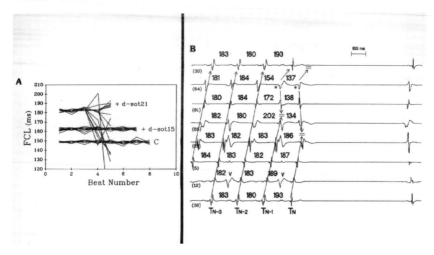

FIGURE 4. *Patterns of flutter cycle length (FCL) oscillations (panel A) and electrograms recorded from several sites (panel B) during* d-sotalol–*induced termination depicted in maps of Fig 3. For this episode, CL variability is depicted for the control (C) flutter, for the fluter after* d-sotalol *(+d-sot15), and for the last consecutive beats at the time of termination (+d-sot21). Note the short CLs at the time of termination.This is similar to what occurred in the chronically instrumented dog with* d-sotalol *(see Fig 2). The asterisk corresponds to activation by a broad excitatory wave front in the intercaval region (see panels E and F in Fig 3). See Reference 21 for more details.*

in the previous chapter, the rhythms are initiated by electrical stimulation of the atria. No animal model available today has reproducible naturally occurring initiating events. Even the most recent animal models of atrial fibrillation (see preceding chapter) need repeated electrical stimulation for initiation of the fibrillation. Second, although several models of atrial arrhythmias have been developed that may mimic human disease, animal models of arrhythmias that are sustained for long periods of time (ie, years) have yet to be developed. In the sterile pericarditis model,[7] atrial flutter and now atrial fibrillation[8] occur after surgery. However, the mechanisms of these rhythms may not be the same as those chronic atrial tachyarrhythmias that develop in humans over years. In the chronic animal models in which right[9,10] or left[11] atrial enlargement is produced surgically, atrial rhythms result. However, at best, "chronic" in these animals means months and not years. Although these models are perhaps an improvement, we are still far from actually "mimicking" the human arrhythmic condition.

What is needed is models of atrial arrhythmias in animals in which long-standing and naturally occurring heart disease has occurred. There have been only a few scattered reports of such models.

In the report by Boineau et al,[12] two different forms of flutter were accidentally discovered in a dog without apparent heart disease. Epicardial multisite activation maps obtained showed that flutters were due to circus movement of impulses around a functional barrier in the right atrium. Slowed conduction necessary for the stabilization of this type of macroreentry was associated with right atrial hypoplasia.

Dogs can have naturally occurring mitral valvular disease and marked left atrial enlargement secondary to a pressure-volume overload of the chamber. In these animals, atrial fibrillation is persistent, lasting at least 3 years.[13] Careful examination of sections of these enlarged atria isolated and studied in vitro showed that dramatic abnormalities of cellular electrophysiology were not involved in the genesis of fibrillation. More likely, the dramatic alterations in the atrial wall architecture altered the anisotropic properties of the atrial myocardium (see the chapter by Spach in this volume), increasing the possibilities for slowed conduction, conduction block, and reentrant excitation.

Atrial enlargement and persistent atrial arrhythmias are also present in a population of domestic cats with naturally occurring primary myocardial disease.[14] The gross and pathological changes in the hearts that are associated with this feline disease mimic those of human hearts with hypertrophic and congestive cardiomyopathy. In contrast to the findings in dogs with mitral insufficiency and atrial fibrillation, the cell electrophysiology of the enlarged atria of these myopathic cats was abnormal. Often, fibers were inexcitable. Some fibers had action potentials followed by delayed afterdepolarizations or were abnormally automatic.

These studies illustrate that the mechanism of atrial fibrillation may differ depending on the changes in myocyte electrophysiology and/or anatomic structure that accompany the underlying heart disease. This idea is not new, since several studies have illustrated the marked changes in cellular electrophysiology that occur in the fibers in sections of diseased human atria.[15-17] Since our understanding of the impact of changes in atrial chamber macroscopic and microscopic structure on conduction of cardiac impulse was limited at the time of these latter studies, we were unable to distinguish whether the abnormalities in electrophysiology described were secondary to the altered anatomy of the sections of atrium studied in vitro or were due to chronic changes in ion channel function of the myocytes that provide the substrate for these rhythms.

At the time of this writing, no one has yet dispersed myocytes from the persistently fibrillating atria to help us distinguish between these two possibilities. Therefore, once again we are at the brink of a very important step in atrial arrhythmogenesis. To take this step, we must take full advantage of the animal models of atrial arrhythmias. It is clear that by dispersing the myocytes from persistently fibrillating atria, we can determine whether certain ion channels that we know to function in normal myocytes also exist in the myocytes of the long-term fibrillating atria. Such studies would certainly contribute to a more complete understanding of the relationship between chronic (up to years) changes in ion channel function and pharmacological and nonpharmacological approaches to atrial arrhythmias.

But this task could be enormous. Although atrial myocyte preparations have been routine for several years, only lately have we begun to appreciate that the heterogeneity in the voltage profiles of atrial myocytes appears to be related to differences in the densities of specific ion channels. In a recent report using human atrial myocytes,[18] the variability in the transmembrane action potentials of normal atrial myocytes was secondary to a difference in the relative magnitudes of the time-dependent outward currents (Fig 5). Furthermore, an earlier report suggested that long-term treatment with cardiac drugs could by itself alter the atrial electrophysiology of human myocytes[19] (Fig 6). Therefore, depicting changes in ion channel function in myocytes from fibrillating human tissue could be very difficult if controls for heterogeneity and drug-free conditions are not rigorous. Again, studies could be more easily completed using tissues obtained from an animal model of a long-standing atrial arrhythmia.

A change in ion channel function in a myocyte dispersed from the fibrillating atria could be a consequence of the atrial pathology, such as cardiomyopathy or cardiac hypertrophy. However, it is also not difficult to imagine that just the presence of a persistent tachyarrhythmia (or rapid stimulation) could by itself alter ion channel function. Allessie and colleagues (this volume) showed that persistent stimulation of goat atria increases the duration of the fibrillation episode. This may be due to a change in the atrial wall archi-

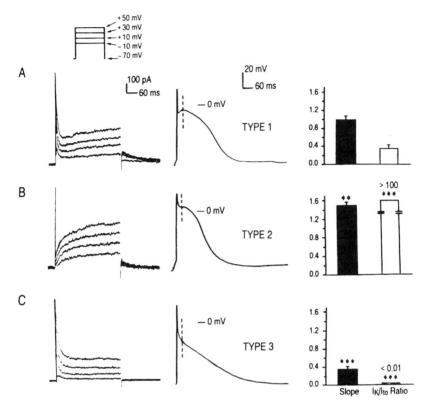

FIGURE 5. *Characterization of three different outward current patterns (types 1 to 3) observed in normal human atrial myocytes. I_k=delayed rectifier current; I_{to}=transient outward current. Shown on the left of each panel are ionic currents elicited by 300-msec depolarizing steps to -10, +10, +30, and +50 mV from a holding potential of=-70 mV. Shown in the middle of each panel are action potentials recorded from the same cells. Shown on the right are average slopes of phase 3 repolarization and the I_k/I_{to} ratio. See Reference 18 for more details.*

tecture and/or ion channel function caused by the rapid stimulation. Studies in an animal model of seizures suggested that after a brief period of drug-induced generalized seizure activity, the levels of mRNA corresponding to two potassium channel clones (delayed rectifier currents of 1.2 and 4.2 kV) were repressed by 90 minutes after the seizure, remained maximally repressed between 3 and 6

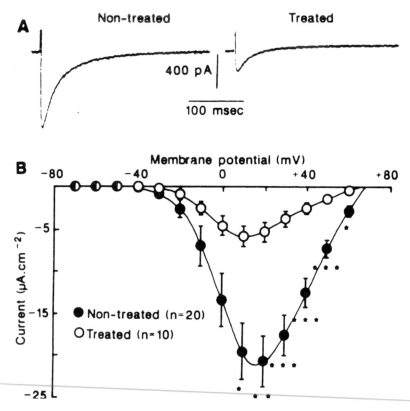

FIGURE 6. *Panel A shows calcium current tracings recorded in response to 350-msec depolarizing pulses from a holding potential of -80 to +10 mV in myocytes from the nontreated patient group and the treated patient group. Panel B depicts the current density–voltage relationships for calcium currents recorded in these human myocytes. Treated means patients were treated with nifedipine, nicardipine, or diltiazem before myocyte dispersion. See Reference 19 for more details.*

hours, and returned to normal by 12 hours.[20] These data suggest that specific neuronal K+ channels can be regulated by rapid repetitive activity at the transcriptional level. At this time, it is not clear how rapid stimulation affects K+ channel message and/or function in the atrial myocardium. This is certainly a question that can be answered by use of an appropriate animal model of an arrhythmia.

References

1. Waldo AL, Plumb VJ, Arciniegas JG, et al. Transient entrainment and interruption of the atrioventricular bypass pathway type of paroxysmal atrial tachycardia: a model for understanding and identifying reentrant arrhythmias. *Circulation*. 1983;67:73–83.
2. Waldo AL, MacLean WAH, Karp RB, Kouchoukos NT, James TN. Entrainment and interruption of atrial flutter with atrial pacing: studies in man following open heart surgery. *Circulation*. 1977;56:737–745.
3. Shimizu A, Nozaki A, Rudy Y, Waldo AL. Multiplexing studies of effects of rapid atrial pacing on the area of slow conduction during atrial flutter in canine pericarditis model. *Circulation*. 1991;83:983–994.
4. Spinelli W, Hoffman BF. Mechanisms of termination of reentrant atrial arrhythmias by class I and class III antiarrhythmic agents. *Circ Res.* 1989;65:1565–1579.
5. Frame LH, Page RL, Boyden PA, Fenoglio JJ Jr, Hoffman BF. Circus movement in the canine atrium around the tricuspid ring during experimental atrial flutter and during reentry in vitro. *Circulation*. 1987; 76:1155–1175.
6. Boyden PA, Graziano JN. Activation mapping of reentry around an anatomic barrier in the canine atrium: observations during the action of the class III agent, d-sotalol. *J Cardiovasc Electrophysiol.* 1993;4:266–279.
7. Okumura K, Plumb VJ, Page PL, Waldo AL. Atrial activation sequences during atrial flutter in the canine pericarditis model and its effects on the polarity of the flutter wave in the electrocardiogram. *J Am Coll Cardiol.* 1991;17:509–518.
8. Ortiz J, Niwano S, Abe H, Gonzalez X, Johnson NJ, Waldo AL. Mapping the conversion of atrial flutter to atrial fibrillation and vice versa: insights into mechanism. *PACE Pacing Clin Electrophysiol.* 1993;16:890.
9. Boyden PA, Hoffman BF. The effects on atrial electrophysiology and structure of surgically induced right atrial enlargement in dogs. *Circ Res.* 1981;49:1319–1331.
10. Boyden PA. Activation sequence during atrial flutter in dogs with surgically induced right atrial enlargement, I: observations during sustained rhythms. *Circ Res.* 1988;62:596–608.
11. Cox JL, Schuessler RB, D'Agostino HJ, et al. The surgical treatment of atrial fibrillation, III: Development of a definitive surgical procedure. *J Thorac Cardiovasc Surg.* 1991;101:569–583.
12. Boineau JP, Schuessler RB, Mooney CR, et al. Natural and evoked atrial flutter due to circus movement in dogs: role of abnormal atrial pathways, slow conduction, nonuniform refractory period distribution and premature beats. *Am J Cardiol.* 1980;45:1167–1181.
13. Boyden PA, Tilley LP, Pham Tuan Duc, Liu Si-kwang, Fenoglio JJ Jr, Wit AL. Effects of left atrial enlargement on atrial transmembrane potentials and structure in dogs with mitral valve fibrosis. *Am J Cardiol.* 1982;49:1896–1908.
14. Boyden PA, Tilley LP, Albala A, Liu SK, Fenoglio JJ Jr. Wit AL. Mechanisms for atrial arrhythmias associated with cardiomyopathy: a study

of feline hearts with primary myocardial disease. *Circulation.* 1984;69: 1036–1047.

15. Hordof AJ, Edie R, Malm JR, Hoffman BF, Rosen MR. Electrophysiologic properties and response to pharmacologic agents of fibers from diseased human atria. *Circulation.* 1976;54:774–779.

16. Mary-Rabine L, Hordof AJ, Danilo P Jr, Malm JR, Rosen MR. Mechanisms for impulse initiation in isolated human atrial fibers. *Circ Res.* 1980;47:267–277.

17. Ten Eick RE, Baumgarten CM, Singer DH. Ventricular dysrhythmia: membrane basis or of currents, channels, gates, and cables. *Prog Cardiovasc Dis.* 1981;24:157–188.

18. Wang Z, Fermini B, Nattel S. Delayed rectifier outward current and repolarization in human atrial myocytes. *Circ Res.* 1993;73:276–285.

19. LeGrand B, Hatem S, Deroubaix E, Couetil JP, Coraboeuf E. Calcium current depression in isolated human atrial myocytes after cessation of chronic treatment with calcium antagonists. *Circ Res.* 1991;69:292–300.

20. Tsaur M, Sheng M, Lowenstein DH, Jan YN, Jan LY. Differential expression of K channel mRNAs in the rat brain and down regulation in the hippocampus following seizures. *Neuron.* 1992;8:1055–1067.

21. Boyden PA, Graziano JN. Multiple modes of termination of reentrant excitation around an anatomic barrier in the canine atrium during the action of *d*-sotalol. *Eur Heart J.* 1993;14(Suppl H):41–49.

Chapter 10

Maintenance of Sinus Rhythm In Patients at Risk of Atrial Fibrillation

*Francis D. Murgatroyd, MRCP; and
A. John Camm, MD, FRCP, FACC, FESC*

Introduction

Why Try to Restore and Maintain Sinus Rhythm?

Atrial fibrillation (AF) has traditionally been regarded as a benign arrhythmia. However, there is growing evidence that its adverse consequences are not limited to the symptoms of palpitations and dyspnea: AF may trigger ventricular arrhythmias in susceptible individuals; it may cause left ventricular dysfunction; and it is a major cause of preventable stroke.

In AF, the loss of atrial transport, combined with an irregular and poorly controlled ventricular rate, causes a largely unpredictable reduction in cardiac output: this is a particular problem in those with reduced ventricular compliance or contractility. In addition to causing irregular palpitations, AF may therefore give rise to symptoms of dyspnea and dizziness and may precipitate angina and cardiac failure in susceptible individuals. It has long been known that AF associated with rheumatic valvular disease carries a very high risk of stroke (approximately 17% per annum),[1] but the SPAF and other trials conducted recently have demonstrated that there is also a significant thromboembolic risk in patients with non-rheumatic AF.[2–6]

From DiMarco JP, Prystowsky EN (eds): *Atrial Arrhythmias: State of the Art*. Armonk, NY, Futura Publishing Company, Inc., © 1995.

Recent work in an animal model has found that artificially maintained AF causes changes to the electrophysiological substrate of the atrium (principally shortening of the atrial refractory period) that tend to facilitate AF induction and maintenance—in other words, AF "begets" further AF.[7] Most importantly, this process of electrical remodeling appears to be reversible. These findings, if applicable to humans, have several important ramifications. They may explain the fact that the duration of AF is a primary determinant of successful cardioversion and the subsequent maintenance of sinus rhythm.[8] They may account for the special value of drugs that prolong the atrial refractory period in terminating sustained AF. Furthermore, they would suggest that an aggressive initial approach to the maintenance of sinus rhythm may allow the atrium to normalize electrically, so that it becomes less susceptible to arrhythmia recurrence in the longer term.

Thus, far from being benign, AF has adverse symptomatic and hemodynamic consequences and in many instances is associated with an increased risk of stroke and an adverse prognosis. It is a substantial cause of cardiovascular morbidity and mortality and in the United States accounts for more days spent in hospital than any other arrhythmia.[9] The suppression of AF results in an increased cardiac output and exercise capacity[10,11] and a decrease in arrhythmic symptoms. It also appears that the left ventricular dysfunction sometimes seen in sustained AF due to consistently high rates (so-called "tachycardia-cardiomyopathy") is largely reversible.[12] AF is self-perpetuating, so that termination of a prolonged episode may reduce the risk of the next. If initial treatment is successful, sinus rhythm (in the absence of worsening underlying heart disease) should become progressively easier to maintain. The alternative approach, of accepting AF and attempting to control the ventricular rate and reduce the thromboembolic risk with drugs, is suboptimal.

Types of AF

In addition to the possible causes of AF, the temporal pattern of the arrhythmia in each patient can be characterized and has an important bearing on the goals and choice of treatment. The role of antiarrhythmic therapy for the prevention of AF has been studied in three very different groups of patients. First, patients in whom sinus rhythm has been restored electrically, pharmacologically, or spontaneously have a high risk of AF recurrence, which generally declines with time. Second, treatment may be considered for those patients in whom AF may never have occurred but in whom there is a known risk of the arrhythmia over a specific period of time, such as following acute myocardial infarction and cardiac surgery. Finally, the largest group is of patients with recurrent spontaneous episodes of AF: while usually self-terminating, these may cause symptoms of sufficient severity to warrant antiarrhythmic treatment. This group is highly diverse in terms of the frequency, duration, and severity of symptoms and the pattern of onset of arrhythmia: each of these features has a bearing on the choice of treatment.

Restoration of Sinus Rhythm

Transthoracic DC shocks have been used to restore sinus rhythm for three decades, with reported success rates of between 70% and 95%.[8,13] In 246 patients undergoing attempted cardioversion for AF and atrial flutter (AFL), multivariate analysis identified short arrhythmia duration ($P<.01$), low age ($P<.05$) and AFL ($P<.02$) as independent predictors of success.[8] Surprisingly, other features in the clinical history and the left atrial diameter were not independent predictors: a finding borne out elsewhere.[14,15] Antiarrhythmic drugs can also be given to terminate AF (Fig 1), although their efficacy is limited to arrhythmia of short duration and is significantly lower in AFL. Drugs in Vaughan Williams classes IA and IC are most commonly used, but amiodarone is also highly effective,[16] and some of the newer class III drugs currently under investigation may be effective in terminating both sustained AF and AFL. For example, in a dose-ranging study of intravenous dofetilide, 10 of 19 patients with AF and 4 of 5 with AFL were converted to sinus rhythm.[17] Ibutilide has shown 100% efficacy in terminating both AF and AFL in acute canine models.[18,19] Established antiarrhythmic drugs are generally ineffective in AFL: the apparent efficacy of these new agents underlines the power of class III drugs in reentrant arrhythmias.

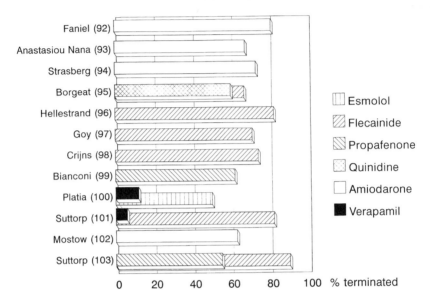

FIGURE 1.   *Acute termination of AF: studies of antiarrhythmic drug effi-cacy. That of esmolol, an ultrashort-acting β-blocker, is unusual, since this group of drugs is generally thought to be as ineffective as digitalis and the calcium channel antagonists. References are given in parenthesis.*

Maintenance of Sinus Rhythm by Use of Antiarrhythmic Drugs

Maintenance of Sinus Rhythm After Cardioversion

AF recurs in approximately two thirds of patients within 1 year after cardioversion: this is more likely in patients with AF of long dura-tion, rheumatic origin, and heart failure with high New York Heart Association functional class.[8,15] In such patients and in those with recurrent AF following previous cardioversion, antiarrhythmic ther-apy may be given to maintain sinus rhythm. Quinidine is the most common agent used for this purpose in the United States, and several controlled trials indicate that it reduces the recurrence rate by approx-imately 50%.[20–24] The other class IA drugs, such as disopyramide and procainamide, are equally effective,[25-27] as is flecainide.[28] Amiodarone has a higher efficacy than quinidine[29] and is also useful in cases refractory to other drugs.[30] Its use is generally avoided in the United States because of its many side effects. However, these are far less common with the low doses (100 to 200 mg/d) commonly used in Europe, which are still highly effective.[31] The degree of success that can be achieved with an aggressive antiarrhythmic strategy is illustrated by a recent study of serial antiarrhythmic therapy for maintaining sinus rhythm after cardioversion.[32] One hundred twenty-seven patients were given flecainide after a first successful cardioversion: in the event of recurrence, repeat cardioversion was given and sotalol substituted (39 patients), or quinidine if sotalol was not tolerated (14 patients). Amiodarone was used following cardioversion if these treatments failed (34 patients). This strategy required 1.8 ± 0.8 cardioversions per patient: actuarially, two thirds of patients eventually achieved a 2-year period free of recurrent AF.

Prevention of AF After Cardiac Surgery

AF complicates up to 28.4% of coronary artery bypass graft operations and an even higher proportion of valvular procedures; it is especially common in elderly patients.[33] Most episodes occur 2 to 4 days after surgery, and this timing closely reflects a peak in circulating catecholamines, which are higher in patients who develop AF than in those who do not.[34] The prophylactic value of β-adrenergic blocking agents also supports an adrenergic mechanism, but both pericarditis and atrial infarction have also been suggested as causes, and it is likely that the pathogenesis is multifactorial. The effects of digitalis on the incidence of AF following cardiac surgery are unclear. Preoperative loading with digoxin was found to halve the incidence of postoperative AF in at least one randomized study[35] but to increase it in another.[36] This paradox may be accounted for by the different loading regimens used and serum levels achieved. Postoperative digitalization does not appear to reduce the incidence of AF,[37] nor does digoxin given to treat AF affect the rate of conversion to sinus rhythm.[38] Prophylactic verapamil does not affect the incidence of AF following cardiac surgery, and it increases the likelihood of hypotension.[39] However, a large number of trials of a variety of β-blockers have demonstrated their efficacy while failing to show significant adverse effects.[40] In a randomized comparison of propranolol, digoxin, and no treatment, the β-blocker was found to halve the incidence of AF, whereas digoxin had no effect.[41] Therefore, if a policy of routine antiarrhythmic prophylaxis for cardiac surgery is to be implemented, a β-blocker is the obvious choice. Amiodarone is an alternative, attractive in view of its minimal negative inotropic and proarrhythmic effects, and has been shown to suppress both atrial and ventricular arrhythmias in a placebo-controlled study.[42] However, since postoperative AF is usually self-terminating and tolerated hemodynamically, the need for such a policy is uncertain.

Prevention of AF After Myocardial Infarction

AF follows about 1 in 10 acute myocardial infarctions and indicates a relative risk of death between 1.28 and 1.7. However, the arrhythmia appears to be a marker of adverse prognosis reflecting infarct severity rather than an independent risk factor.[43,44] AF may become a less common complication of myocardial infarction in the era of routine β-blockade, thrombolysis, and anticoagulant/antiplatelet drugs, but the true effect of these treatments on its incidence is unclear, an unfortunate result of the limited end points of the "megatrials" that established their benefit. Unlike ventricular arrhythmias, AF complicating myocardial infarction is not perceived as a sufficient problem to warrant the consideration of routine antiarrhythmic prophylaxis. Furthermore, pharmacological issues should not be allowed to eclipse the importance of general measures such as hemodynamic optimization and the maintenance of a high serum potassium level. Nevertheless, the occurrence of AF in patients with substantial infarcts may be poorly tolerated and precipitate hemodynamic deterioration and further ischemia. In this situation, the use of most antiarrhythmic drugs carries a substantial risk because of their negative inotropy and potential for proarrhythmia: these patients are already compromised hemodynamically and have highly unpredictable electrophysiology. Unfortunately, DC cardioversion is of limited use because of the high rate of early recurrence, and sometimes drug therapy is necessary. The clinician usually has to choose between the goals of ventricular rate control and the abolition of AF: the former is usual, since most patients eventually spontaneously revert to sinus rhythm. Of the antiarrhythmic agents currently available, only amiodarone and racemic sotalol combine the ability to slow atrioventricular conduction with an antifibrillatory action. Digitalis, which is traditionally given to slow the ventricular rate, may be ineffective because of its slow onset of action and antagonism by high sympathetic tone. β-Blockers and calcium antagonists do not have these limitations but may be contraindicated because of impaired ventricular function.

These considerations are well illustrated in a study by Cowan et al,[45] in which 34 patients with AF complicating acute myocardial infarction were randomized to receive digoxin or amiodarone intravenously. After 24 hours, a similar proportion of each group had reverted to sinus rhythm, and the ventricular rates were similar. However, there was a marked tendency to earlier reversion in the group receiving amiodarone (Fig 2); furthermore, the ventricular rate fell significantly earlier in this group. The adverse prognosis associated with AF following myocardial infarction is illustrated by the fact that 25% of patients in both groups died before hospital dis-

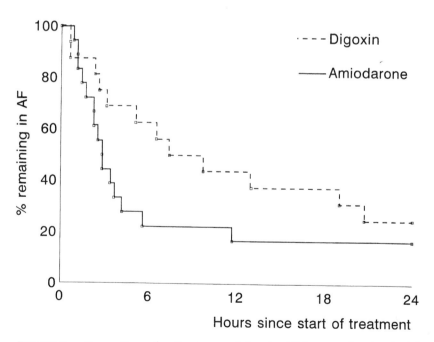

FIGURE 2.   *Proportion of patients remaining in AF in a randomized trial of intravenous amiodarone and intravenous digoxin for AF complicating acute myocardial infarction (intention-to-treat analysis).[45]*

charge. Although it is not licensed for this indication in the United States, amiodarone is frequently used in Europe for the treatment of arrhythmias complicating myocardial infarction. In addition to its relative lack of negative inotropy, it appears to have a remarkably low incidence of proarrhythmia even in these high-risk patients. Several multicenter studies of prophylactic amiodarone in high-risk myocardial infarction patients are in progress, and it is hoped that these will shed light on the drug's effects on atrial as well as ventricular arrhythmias and its safety in this group of patients.

Prevention of Paroxysmal AF

The term "paroxysmal AF" is generally applied to patients with recurrent self-terminating arrhythmic episodes, but this is a heterogeneous group. Both the need for treatment and the choice of therapy are determined by three considerations: the presence and nature of any underlying disease, the symptoms and potential complications caused by AF episodes, and the temporal pattern of attacks.

Underlying Disease

The enumeration of the many illnesses that can give rise to paroxysms of AF is not within the scope of this discussion. However, it is self-evident that such causative factors are of primary importance and that their successful treatment, where possible, is preferable to long-term antiarrhythmic therapy. Although for the most part paroxysmal AF is considered benign, its potential risks include the provocation of ventricular arrhythmias, hemodynamic deterioration, and thromboembolism. These risks are determined to a large extent by the nature of any coexisting cardiac pathological conditions, as is the safe selection of antiarrhythmic therapy. Therefore, while the majority of patients with paroxysmal AF do not have significant underlying disease,[46] it is important to actively investigate this possibility.

Symptoms

The choice of therapy is also affected by the degree and nature of any symptoms caused, which vary greatly between patients.

Symptoms of sufficient severity to warrant prophylaxis may be related to the sensation of cardiac irregularity, the lack of atrial transport, or simply to a rapid ventricular rate. Accordingly, a drug may be selected for its effect on the atrioventricular node rather than an antifibrillatory action, although there is no evidence to support this strategy.

Patterns of AF

One approach to treatment is based on the hypothesis that, particularly in patients with idiopathic AF, paroxysms may be triggered by autonomic factors. In the "vagotonic" group (typically men, with episodes starting in their fourth decade), attacks occur when parasympathetic tone is high, especially during the evening and night and after exercise.[47] Conversely, patients in the "adrenergic" group (often middle-aged and of either sex) suffer episodes of AF related to elevated sympathetic tone. In animal models, both vagal and adrenergic stimulation affect atrial electrophysiology in ways that facilitate AF; however, this mechanism has not been demonstrated in humans. Nevertheless, patients with vagotonic AF often respond to strongly anticholinergic antiarrhythmic drugs, such as disopyramide, while those with adrenergic AF may improve with intense β-blockade, even when other drugs have failed.[48]

Antiarrhythmic Drug Trials in Paroxysmal AF

The evaluation of antiarrhythmic therapy in patients with paroxysmal AF is considerably more difficult than in the categories described earlier. Trial designs must take account of patients with a variety of arrhythmia frequencies and drug dose requirements, but the most serious challenge is the documentation of infrequent, brief arrhythmic episodes, for which hospital electrocardiography (ECG) and ambulatory monitoring are inadequate. For these reasons, there was no evidence for the efficacy of any antiarrhythmic drug in this specific group of patients until recently.

These methodological problems were first adequately addressed by Anderson et al,[49] who concentrated on symptomatic attacks of AF in the evaluation of flecainide in what came to be a benchmark for studies of supraventricular arrhythmias. Arrhythmia documentation was achieved using patient-activated ECG monitors with telephone transmission of recordings. Only patients who transmitted AF during screening and who tolerated antiarrhythmic treatment were eligible for randomization to the double-blind treatment phase. The principal end point was the interval between documented attacks of AF, rather than the number of episodes in a given time. This approach allowed patients with frequent symptoms to finish treatment early, while those with infrequent arrhythmia were monitored for correspondingly longer. A crossover design allowed each patient to act as his/her own control, and thus considerable statistical power was achieved in a relatively small study. The study showed a highly significant reduction in the frequency of symptomatic episodes of AF: the median time to the first attack was increased from 3 days on placebo to 14.5 days on flecainide, and the median interval between attacks rose from 6.2 to 27 days ($P<.001$ for both end points). Using a similar crossover design, Pietersen and Hellemann[50] again found that flecainide was effective compared with placebo. Clementy et al[51] reported on a large series in which 944 patients were started on flecainide for paroxysmal AF and followed up for 9 months with periodic Holter monitoring. Of those patients remaining on treatment for the entire 9 months, 65% appeared to remain free of arrhythmia. This is an overestimate of the true efficacy of the drug, since inclusion criteria were wide, 382 patients were lost to follow-up or discontinued therapy, and Holter monitoring has a low probability of detecting rare arrhythmia recurrences. In all of these studies, a high incidence of side effects was found, but these rarely required discontinuation of therapy.

Propafenone, another class IC agent, has also been found to be effective in treating symptomatic paroxysmal AF, although in fewer and smaller studies. Connolly and Hoffert[52] studied 18 patients in whom active and placebo treatments were alternated monthly for 4 months, during which arrhythmias were documented by transtelephonic monitoring. Seven patients withdrew during dose ranging because of adverse effects, poor compliance, or lack of efficacy. In those patients entering the efficacy phase, the percentage of days with an attack of AF was reduced from 51% to 27% ($P<.01$). Pritchett et al[53] found that the rate of recurrence of supraventricular arrhythmias in 33 patients (17 with paroxysmal AF and 16 with supraventricular tachycardia) was reduced by propafenone to one fifth of that during placebo treatment (P=.004).

Both propafenone and sotalol have been examined in two interesting trials of patients refractory to other drugs. Antman et al[54] reported on 109 patients with AF (paroxysmal in 51%) resistant to drugs in 1 to 5 previous antiarrhythmic drug trials. Patients were initially treated with propafenone and transferred to sotalol if arrhythmia recurred. Thirty-nine percent of patients were free of symptomatic arrhythmia after 6 months of propafenone and 50% after 6 months of sotalol. Cumulatively, 55% were free of recurrence after 6 months on one or both drugs. Reimold et al[55] randomized 100 patients with AF (both paroxysmal and chronic) to treatment with propafenone or sotalol. A mean of 1.9 ± 1.0 class IA antiarrhythmic drugs had previously been unsuccessful. Over a 1-year follow-up, both drugs were found to be equally effective in maintaining sinus rhythm, and the effects were not found to be dependent on arrhythmia pattern or left atrial size.

The efficacy of sotalol is probably attributable to its class III effects, since β-adrenergic blockade alone seldom seems to be of value in paroxysmal AF. The class III effect makes other drugs in this group likely to suppress AF, and amiodarone is in widespread use in Europe, where experience suggests that it is highly effective and well tolerated in doses of 100 to 200 mg/d, with serious complications rare. Unfortunately, its long half-life makes amiodarone unsuitable for crossover comparisons with placebo or other drugs. For this reason, when amiodarone has been included in clinical trials for the prevention of AF, it has usually been reserved for patients who have failed to respond to other treatments. There is a clear need for prospective, placebo-controlled studies of amiodarone as the first treatment in maintaining sinus rhythm after cardioversion and in the prophylaxis of paroxysmal AF.[56] d-Sotalol, dofetilide, and sematilide are all currently undergoing clinical trials in paroxysmal AF. In view of the potential market and the perceived lack of satisfactory treatments, other new class 3 drugs will probably also be clinically evaluated in the near future for this indication. The future of each is likely to be determined by its tendency for proarrhythmia, the most common type being torsade de pointes; this is very low with amiodarone but unknown for the other agents.[57]

Digoxin is very commonly given to patients with paroxysmal AF, despite the absence of any evidence of benefit. The effect of digitalis is controversial: theoretically, its vagotonic action would be expected to slow atrial conduction and reduce the effective refractory period, increasing susceptibility to AF.[58] Rawles et al[59] examined 139 episodes of AF in ambulatory ECG recordings from 72 patients and found that episodes lasting for more than 30 minutes occurred more commonly in patients taking digoxin: no difference was found in either the frequency of episodes or the mean ventricular rate during AF between patients taking digoxin and others. Similarly, Galun et al[60] found no difference between the ventricular rate during AF in 13 patients who were taking long-term digoxin and 14 patients who were not. It can be argued that these retrospective studies might be biased against the drug, since patients with more frequent or rapid episodes of AF are more likely to be treated. The CRAFT-1 trial, recently reported,[61] prospectively evaluated digoxin in a placebo-controlled crossover study whose primary end point was the time between episodes of AF documented by transtelephonic monitoring. The drug was found to cause a modest reduction in the frequency of symptomatic attacks, possibly related to a lower ventricular rate during recorded AF.[61] Comparison of single ambulatory ECG recordings made during active and placebo treatment failed to show any difference in either the number or duration of AF episodes for each patient.[62] It can be concluded that digoxin, in conventional doses, probably has very little true effect on susceptibility to AF but may marginally reduce symptoms. There is little to be gained by instituting digoxin for this indication, but treatment need not be ceased when it is indicated for other reasons.

Thus, the efficacy of class IC drugs in paroxysmal AF is established, and the actions of digitalis and class III agents are becoming clearer. There is little evidence to support the use of class IA drugs for this specific indication, although they are the most commonly used in the United States and the worldwide. Similarly, the affects of β-adrenergic blocking agents in this group of patients are unknown, although they are frequently given either for exercise-induced attacks or with the aim of reducing the ventricular rate during AF. The ongoing CRAFT-2 study is comparing disopyramide, atenolol, and placebo in a double-blind crossover trial in patients with symptomatic AF: in addition to evaluating the overall efficacy of these drugs, it will be possible to determine whether the "vagal" and "adrenergic" patterns of onset of AF predict the response to a particular class of agent.

In the absence of trials supporting the use of the commonest antiarrhythmic drugs for paroxysmal AF, current treatment recommendations are based largely on extrapolation and clinical experience. A "stepped care" approach, such as the algorithm illustrated in Table 1, is finding increasing favor. If antiarrhythmic therapy is deemed necessary, an attempt is made is individualize therapy according to the pattern of onset of episodes, using an anticholnergic class IA drug for "vagotonic" patients and a β-blocker for "adrenergic" AF. Newer antiarrhythmic drugs from classes IC and III are tried in sequence if this approach fails: in younger patients with normal hearts, flecainide and propafenone are usually safe and highly effective, whereas sotalol may cause unacceptable side effects. Conversely, in older patients with hypertensive or ischemic heart disease, sotalol seems to be better tolerated, and its β-blocking effects may actually be an advantage. Amiodarone may also be considered at this stage and may be particularly suited to patients with heart failure, in whom AF is poorly tolerated yet other antiarrhythmic drugs cannot be given because of the risk of negative inotropy and proarrhythmia. We generally reserve intervention approaches (see below) for patients in whom this "stepped care" approach has been exhausted.

TABLE 1.   A Stepped-Care Approach to the Management of Paroxysmal Atrial Fibrillation

1. Is antiarrhythmic treatment necessary?
   Consider severity of symptoms
   Consider risks of treatment versus no treatment
2. Therapy guided by arrhythmia pattern
   "Vagotonic": anticholinergic antiarrhythmic drugs, eg, disopyramide
   "Adrenergic": β-blockers
3. Sequential trials of
   Class IC Drug (flecainide or propafenone)
   Sotalol
4. Consider
   Low-dose amiodarone
   Combined class IC+III therapy
   AF surgery ("maze," "corridor")
   AV nodal ablation + permanent pacemaker implantation

Limitations of Drug-Based Strategies to Prevent AF: Failure, Intolerance, Proarrhythmia

Current pharmacological treatments for the prevention of AF have several shortcomings. While the studies above have shown the superiority of certain drugs to placebo in specific circumstances, complete suppression of AF is rarely possible. The meta-analysis by Coplen et al[63] showed that quinidine reduced the rate of recurrence of AF after cardioversion by about 50%; nevertheless, half of the patients on active treatment were back in AF within 1 year. Again, in the study by Anderson et al[49] of flecainide for paroxysmal AF, only 31% of patients remained free of arrhythmia for the entire 8-week period of active treatment: this was a significant improvement over placebo treatment but represented far from complete suppression. These outcomes are demonstrated in Fig 3.

Antiarrhythmic drugs are further limited by their side-effect profiles. In the case of class IA drugs, intolerance is most commonly due to negative inotropy, anticholinergic side effects, or autoantibody formation. Class IC drugs are associated with a variety of less serious side effects but affect contractility even more. Among the class III drugs, sotalol is limited chiefly by intolerance of β-blockade, and amiodarone has numerous side effects that can occasionally be life-threatening.[64] Most of the new antiarrhythmic drugs under development cause little or no reduction in contractility: since they are chemically dissimilar to amiodarone, it is also hoped that they will not share its side-effect profile.

A less frequent but more serious problem is the risk of proarrhythmia. Torsade de pointes due to quinidine given for supraventricular arrhythmias was first described in 1964,[65] but has been highlighted by Coplen et al's[63] meta-analysis: although quinidine was moderately effective, its use was associated with a statistically significant increase in mortality. This controversial study is open to methodological criticism: the trials examined do not reflect modern use of quinidine, and most importantly, they were designed to examine efficacy rather than safety; indeed, few of the deaths in the meta-analysis were known to be arrhythmic. Whatever the shortcomings of this meta-analysis, the use of quinidine for the prevention of atrial fibrillation does seem to carry a small risk of torsade de pointes, even in the absence of structural heart disease, and is therefore difficult to predict. The same probably applies to other class IA drugs

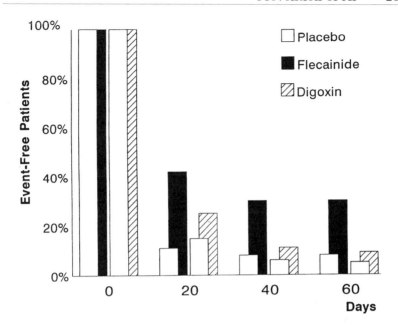

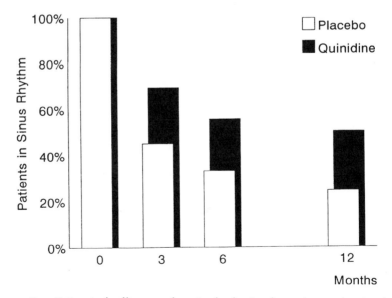

FIGURE 3.   *Estimated efficacy of antiarrhythmic drugs in randomized, placebo-controlled trials for the prevention of AF. Top, Flecainide and digoxin for the prevention of symptomatic paroxysmal AF.[49,61] Bottom, Quinidine for the prevention of AF recurrence after cardioversion.[63]*

that have not been studied in as much detail, and torsade is known to occur in at least 2% of patients taking sotalol.[66] Torsade is unusual with the class IC drugs, but concern over their proarrhythmic potential has arisen from the CAST study, in which flecainide and encainide were associated with an increased mortality in patients with ventricular arrhythmias following myocardial infarction.[67] Although there have been reports of ventricular arrhythmias arising from the use of class IC drugs for atrial fibrillation,[68] this risk seems to be limited largely to patients with significant structural cardiac disease, especially active ischemia. Comparison between 579 patients receiving flecainide or encainide for supraventricular arrhythmias and 154 similar patients treated otherwise found no increase in mortality in the former group; indeed, the trend was for decreased mortality, with survival similar to that predicted for a closely matched population without arrhythmia.[69] The relative safety of antiarrhythmic drug treatment in patients with good ventricular function was supported by a retrospective analysis of participants in the Stroke Prevention in AF study. This showed that the use of antiarrhythmic medication (principally class I) was associated with an increased mortality but that this increase was seen entirely in the patients with heart failure.[70] Nevertheless, the widespread perception that antiarrhythmic drug therapy for the prevention of AF is not particularly effective, well tolerated, or safe has prompted the search for alternative approaches.

Nonpharmaceutical Approaches

Retrospective studies such as that of Rosenqvist et al[71] indicate that in patients paced for sinus node disease, the incidence of AF is lower among those receiving atrial pacemakers than those receiving ventricular devices; these findings have recently been confirmed by the preliminary results of a large randomized study in Denmark.[72] Therefore, while it is clear that the choice of pacing mode can substantially influence the risk of subsequent AF, at present AF is not itself an indication for pacemaker implantation.

Experimentally, a combination of slow intra-atrial conduction and a short atrial effective refractory period is necessary for the atria to be able to sustain the multiple coexisting wavelets that constitute AF.[73] Studies in patients have demonstrated inhomogeneously slowed conduction, fractionated electrograms, and refractoriness that is shortened or adapts poorly with rate.[74-76] These factors may be exaggerated by bradycardia and atrial ectopic beats, which may explain the increased tendency of patients with sinus node disease to develop AF. In acute studies, pacing at a higher rate reduces the dispersion of conduction and may restore homogeneity of refractoriness, as well a suppressing ectopic activity. Indeed, temporary overdrive pacing is commonly used in the acute setting to prevent atrial and ventricular arrhythmias.[77] Permanent atrial pacing for bradycardia often appears to reduce the frequency of AF episodes in patients with the sick sinus syndrome, and occasionally the arrhythmia is entirely abolished. Attuel et al[78] reported a series of 10 patients in whom electrophysiological studies were performed before the implantation of dual chamber pacemakers for the "brady-tachy" syndrome. Seven patients showed intra-atrial conduction delay that paradoxically disappeared at higher rates: in these patients, long-term suppression of AF was obtained by pacing at 90 beats per minute. The same group had earlier reported some clinical improvement by long-term pacing, again at 90 beats per minute, in 6 patients without sinus node disease but with resistant paroxysmal AF of the "vagal" variety.[79] Maintenance of such a high rate on a permanent basis may be poorly tolerated, so it would be ideal to be able to "overdrive" the atrium only when necessary. One possibility is to use the presence of ectopic activity as a marker of vulnerability, and a pacing algorithm has been developed that causes an increase in heart rate with each sensed atrial premature beat, as well as preventing any postextrasytolic pause (Fig 4).[80] A more radical strategy is to attempt to force synchronous activation in an atrium affected by abnormal conduction using triggered (AAT mode) pacing connected to more than one atrial site. Initial experience in patients suggests that atrial vulnerability can be significantly reduced by use of this technique.[81] Such results from individual investigators need to be confirmed in larger, controlled studies, but the possibility that an intervention as simple as atrial pacing could be used to normalize atrial electrophysiology is attractive.

Another possible application for devices has been raised by the demonstration that local capture of AF can obtained at a single site by rapid pacing.[82] This has not yet been reproduced in humans, let alone at multiple sites, but theoretically such a technique could be used to reduce the fibrillating mass to such an extent that AF is extinguished. Another electrical method for terminating AF is the use of biphasic shocks delivered between the coronary sinus and right atrium. This technique has been found to require very low

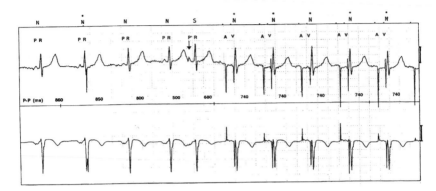

FIGURE 4.   *Ambulatory recording of a pacing algorithm intended to prevent AF by overdrive suppression of atrial premature complexes (APCs). Each time an APC is sensed (arrow), the algorithm causes the pacemaker to increase the heart rate by a small factor. If no more premature beats occur, the pacemaker is allowed to gradually slow down to its normal lower-rate behavior. The algorithm thus seeks a heart rate that suppresses most APCs.*

energies in sheep[83]; its usefulness will depend on whether sufficiently low defibrillation energies can be achieved to make shocks tolerable in conscious humans and whether there is any risk of inducing ventricular arrhythmias. While pacing the heart out of AF remains a distant prospect, the implanted atrial defibrillator is likely to undergo clinical evaluation in the next 2 to 3 years.[84] Such devices, by aborting arrhythmic episodes before they become established, could prevent the structural and electrophysiological changes that accompany established AF.

Modification of Atrioventricular Conduction

A common approach to resistant AF is to "ignore" the arrhythmia and aim for control of the ventricular rate by use of atrioventricular nodal blocking drugs. When these drugs fail, catheter ablation of the atrioventricular node with implantation of a rate-adaptive pacemaker is now routine.[85] Furthermore, because of its simplicity, this technique is increasingly used at an early stage. However, while it has many advantages in poorly controlled chronic AF, especially in the elderly, it is less successful if symptoms are due to a sensation of cardiac irregularity rather than a fast heart rate. Atrioventricular nodal ablation often gives disappointing symptomatic results in patients with paroxysmal AF. Despite the advent of sophisticated mode-switching pacemakers that are able to preserve atrioventricular synchrony during sinus rhythm and switch to adaptive-rate ventricular pacing during AF, patients continue to be aware of the change in rhythm. A possible alternative to the obliteration of atrioventricular conduction is the selective ablation of the slow atrioventricular pathway,[86] which appears to reduce the maximum ventricular rate without affecting normal conduction. In general, it is far from clear that the overall quality of life is improved by ablative procedures. The risk of thromboembolic complications is at best unaffected, and the intervention can be considered a treatment of last resort other than in those patients whose symptoms are entirely due to an uncontrolled ventricular rate.

Surgery

Improved understanding of the pattern of activation of the fibrillating atrium has led to the development of operations designed to abolish the arrhythmia. Biatrial isolation and the "compartment" and "corridor" operations all aim to exclude AF from a strip of tissue maintaining continuity between the sinus and atrioventricular nodes.[87-89] In theory, therefore, these procedures are not expected to stop fibrillation in the entire atrium, and their end result should be akin to that of atrioventricular nodal ablation. In practice, however, the divided atrium often does not fibrillate. Cox et al[90] devised a more a radical procedure in which a series of incisions force atrial activation into channels that are too small to allow fibrillation, yet allow the entire atrium to be depolarized. This "maze" operation has proved successful in maintaining sinus rhythm, even in patients with previous longstanding AF, and restoration of atrial contractility has been reported. However, it is clearly a major procedure— postoperative complications are frequent—and both safety and a substantial improvement in quality of life need to be demonstrated if it is to become a more routine therapy.[91]

Conclusions

AF is the most common sustained arrhythmia and carries a significant morbidity and mortality: whenever possible, sinus rhythm should be restored and maintained. Episodes of AF that do not resolve spontaneously can usually be terminated without difficulty, but recurrence is frequent. Paroxysmal AF is also very common; while it is probably less dangerous, it is often more symptomatic than sustained AF. The efficacy of the drugs most commonly used worldwide to prevent recurrent AF has not been fully established, and no drug is wholly effective, tolerated, and safe. The prevention of AF may one day be an indication for specialized pacemakers and implanted devices, and a variety of surgical procedures have been developed. However, these treatments are likely to be reserved for a minority of cases. The management of an individual patient depends on a detailed knowledge of the clinical features and pattern of AF; these determine the need for treatment and both the efficacy and likely adverse effects of the available therapies.

References

1. Wolf PA, Dawber TR, Thomas HE, Kannel WB. Epidemiologic assessment of chronic atrial fibrillation and risk of stroke: the Framingham study. *Neurology.* 1978;28:973–977.
2. Stroke Prevention in Atrial Fibrillation Study. Final results. *Circulation.* 1991;84:527–539.
3. The effect of low-dose warfarin on the risk of stroke in patients with nonrheumatic atrial fibrillation: the Boston Area Anticoagulation Trial for Atrial Fibrillation Investigators. *N Engl J Med.* 1990;323:1505–1511.
4. Petersen P, Boysen G, Godtfredsen J, Andersen ED, Andersen B. Placebo-controlled, randomised trial of warfarin and aspirin for prevention of thromboembolic complications in chronic atrial fibrillation: the Copenhagen AFASAK study. *Lancet.* 1989;1:175–179.
5. Connolly SJ, Laupacis A, Gent M, Roberts RS, Cairns JA, Joyner C. Canadian Atrial Fibrillation Anticoagulation (CAFA) Study. *J Am Coll Cardiol.* 1991;18:349–355.
6. Ezekowitz MD, Bridgers SL, James KE, et al. Warfarin in the prevention of stroke associated with nonrheumatic atrial fibrillation: Veterans Affairs Stroke Prevention in Nonrheumatic Atrial Fibrillation Investigators [see comments]. *N Engl J Med.* 1992;327:1406–1412.
7. Wijffels MC, Kirchhof C, Frederiks J, Boersma L, Allessie MA. Atrial fib-

rillation begets atrial fibrillation. *Circulation.* 1993;88(suppl I):I–18. Abstract.

8. Van Gelder IC, Crijns HJ, Van Gilst WH, Verwer R, Lie KI. Prediction of uneventful cardioversion and maintenance of sinus rhythm from direct-current electrical cardioversion of chronic atrial fibrillation and flutter. *Am J Cardiol.* 1991;68:41–46.

9. Bialy D, Lehmann MH, Schumacher DN, Steinman RT, Meissner MD. Hospitalization for arrhythmias in the United States: importance of atrial fibrillation. *J Am Coll Cardiol.* 1992;19:41A Abstract.

10. Atwood JE, Myers JN, Sullivan MJ, Forbes SM, Sandhu S, Callaham P, Froelicher VF. The effect of cardioversion on maximal exercise capacity in patients with chronic atrial fibrillation. *Am Heart J.* 1989;118:913–918.

11. Lipkin DP, Frenneaux M, Stewart R, Joshi J, Lowe T, McKenna WJ. Delayed improvement in exercise capacity after cardioversion of atrial fibrillation to sinus rhythm. *Br Heart J.* 1988;59:572–577.

12. Grogan M, Smith HC, Gersh BJ, Wood DL. Left ventricular dysfunction due to atrial fibrillation in patients intially believed to have idiopathic dilated cardiomyopathy. *Am J Cardiol.* 1992;69:1570–1573.

13. Lown R, Amarasingham R, Neuman J. New method for terminating cardiac arrhythmias: use of synchronized capacitor discharge. *JAMA.* 1962;182:548–555.

14. Dalzell GW, Anderson J, Adgey AA. Factors determining success and energy requirements for cardioversion of atrial fibrillation. *Q J Med.* 1990;76:903–913.

15. Dittrich HC, Erickson JS, Schneiderman T, Blacky AR, Savides T, Nicod PH. Echocardiographic and clinical predictors for outcome of elective cardioversion of atrial fibrillation. *Am J Cardiol.* 1989;63:193–197.

16. Blevins RD, Kerin NZ, Benaderet D, Frumin H, Faitel K, Jarandilla R, Rubenfire M. Amiodarone in the management of refractory atrial fibrillation. *Arch Intern Med.* 1987;147:1401–1404.

17. Suttorp MJ, Polak PE, van't Hof A, Rasmussen HS, Dunselman PH, Kingma JH. Efficacy and safety of a new selective class III antiarrhythmic agent dofetilide in paroxysmal atrial fibrillation or atrial flutter. *Am J Cardiol.* 1992;69:417–419.

18. Nabih M, Prcevski P, Fromm B, Lavine S, Elnabtity M, Munir A, Steinman R, Meissner M, Lehmann M. Ibutilide, a new class III agent, rapidly terminates sustained atrial fibrillation (AF) in a canine model of acute left ventricular (LV) dysfunction. *PACE Pacing Clin Electrophysiol.* 1992;15:517. Abstract.

19. Gibson JK, Buchanan LV, Kabell GG. Ibutilide, a class III antiarrhythmic agent, rapidly terminates sustained atrial flutter in a canine model. *Pharmacologist.* 1992;34:168. Abstract.

20. Boissel JP, Wolf E, Gillet J, Soubrane A, Cavallaro A, Mazoyer G, Delahaye JP. Controlled trial of a long-acting quinidine for maintenace of sinus rhythm after conversion of sustained atrial fibrillation. *Eur Heart J.* 1981;2:49–55.

21. Sodermark T, Jonsson B, Olsson A, Oro L, Wallin H, Edhag O, Sjogren A, Danielsson M, Rosenhamer G. Effect of quinidine on maintaining sinus rhythm after conversion of atrial fibrillation or flutter: a multicentre study from Stockholm. *Br Heart J.* 1975;37:486–492.
22. Byrne Quinn E, Wing AJ. Maintenance of sinus rhythm after DC reversion of atrial fibrillation: a double-blind controlled trial of long-acting quinidine bisulphate. *Br Heart J.* 1970;32:370–376.
23. Hillestad L, Bjerkelund C, Dale J, Maltau J, Storstein O. Quinidine in maintenance of sinus rhythm after electroconversion of chronic atrial fibrillation: a controlled clinical study. *Br Heart J.* 1971;33:518–521.
24. Hartel G, Louhija A, Konttinen A, Halonen PI. Value of quinidine in maintenance of sinus rhythm after electric conversion of atrial fibrillation. *Br Heart J.* 1970;32:57–60.
25. Karlson BW, Torstensson I, Abjorn C, Jansson SO, Peterson LE. Disopyramide in the maintenance of sinus rhythm after electroconversion of atrial fibrillation: a placebo-controlled one-year follow-up study. *Eur Heart J.* 1988;9:284–290.
26. Hartel G, Louhija A, Konttinen A. Disopyramide in the prevention of recurrence of atrial fibrillation after electroconversion. *Clin Pharmacol Ther.* 1974;15:551–555.
27. Szekely P, Sideris DA, Batson GA. Maintenance of sinus rhythm after atrial defibrillation. *Br Heart J.* 1970;32:741–746.
28. Van Gelder IC, Crijns HJ, Van Gilst WH, Van Wijk LM, Hamer HP, Lie KI. Effcacy and safety of flecainide acetate in the maintenance of sinus rhythm after electrical cardioversion of chronic atrial fibrillation or atrial flutter. *Am J Cardiol.* 1989;64:1317–1321.
29. Vitolo E, Tronci M, Larovere MT, Rumolo R, Morabito A. Amiodarone versus quinidine in the prophylaxis of atrial fibrillation. *Acta Cardiol.* 1981;36:431–444.
30. Graboys TB, Podrid PJ, Lown B. Efficacy of amiodarone for refractory supraventricular tachyarrhythmias. *Am Heart J.* 1983;106:870–876.
31. Gosselink AT, Crijns HJ, Van Gelder IC, Hillige H, Wiesfeld AC, Lie KI. Low-dose amiodarone for maintenance of sinus rhythm after cardioversion of atrial fibrillation or flutter. *JAMA.* 1992;267:3289–3293.
32. Crijns HJ, Van Gelder IC, Van Gilst, WH, Hillege H, Gosselink AM, Lie KI. Serial antiarrhythmic drug treatment to maintain sinus rhythm after electrical cardioversion for chronic atrial fibrillation or atrial flutter. *Am J Cardiol.* 1991;68:335–341.
33. Fuller JA, Adams GG, Buxton B. Atrial fibrillation after coronary artery bypass grafting: is it a disorder of the elderly? *J Thorac Cardiovasc Surg.* 1989;97:821–825.
34. Kalman J, Howes L, Louis W, Munawar M, Yapanis A, Tonkin A. Atrial fibrillation following cardiac surgery: a manifestation of increased sympathetic activity. *PACE Pacing Clin Electrophysiol.* 1992;15:519. Abstract.
35. Johnson LW, Dickstein RA, Fruehan CT, Kane P, Potts JL, Smulyan H, Webb WR, Eich RH. Prophylactic digitalization for coronary artery bypass surgery. *Circulation.* 1976;53:819–822.

36. Tyras DH, Stothert JCJ, Kaiser GC, Barner HB, Codd JE, Willman VL. Supraventricular tachyarrhythmias after myocardial revascularization: a randomized trial of prophylactic digitalization. *J Thorac Cardiovasc Surg.* 1979;77:310–314.

37. Weiner B, Rheinlander HF, Decker EL, Cleveland RJ. Digoxin prophylaxis following coronary artery bypass surgery. *Clin Pharmacol.* 1986;5: 55–58.

38. Falk RH, Knowlton AA, Bernard SA, Gotlieb NE, Battinelli NJ. Digoxin for converting recent-onset atrial fibrillation to sinus rhythm: a randomized, double-blinded trial. *Ann Intern Med.* 1987;106:503–506.

39. Davison R, Hartz R, Kaplan K, Parker M, Feiereisel P, Michaelis L. Prophylaxis of supraventricular tachyarrhythmia after coronary bypass surgery with oral verapamil: a randomized, double-blind trial. *Ann Thorac Surg.* 1985;39:336–339.

40. Lauer MS, Eagle KA. Atrial fibrillation following cardiac surgery. In: Falk RH, Podrid PJ, eds. *Atrial Fibrillation: Mechanisms and Management.* New York, NY: Raven Press; 1992:127–143.

41. Rubin DA, Nieminski KE, Reed GE, Herman MV. Predictors, prevention, and long-term prognosis of atrial fibrillation after coronary artery bypass graft operations. *J Thorac Cardiovasc Surg.* 1987;94:331–335.

42. Hohnloser SH, Meinertz T, Dammbacher T, Steiert K, Jahnchen E, Zehender M, Fraedrich G, Just H. Elecrocardiographic and antiarrhythmic effects of intravenous amiodarone: results of a prospective, placebo-controlled study. *Am Heart J.* 1991;121:89–95.

43. Behar S, Zahavi Z, Goldbourt U, Reicher Reiss H. Long-term prognosis of patients with paroxysmal atrial fibrillation complicating acute myocardial infarction: SPRINT Study Group. *Eur Heart J.* 1992;13:45–50.

44. Goldberg RJ, Seeley D, Becker RC, Brady P, Chen ZY, Osganian V, Gore JM, Alpert JS, Dalen JE. Impact of atrial fibrillation on the in-hospital and long-term survival of patients with acute myocardial infarction: a community-wide perspective. *Am Heart J.* 1990;119:996–1001.

45. Cowan JC, Gardiner P, Reid DS, Newell DJ, Campbell RW. A comparison of amiodarone and digoxin in the treatment of atrial fibrillation complicating suspected acute myocardial infarction. *J Cardiovasc Pharmacol.* 1986;8:252–256.

46. Murgatroyd FD, Curzen NP, Aldergather J, Ward DE, Damm AJ. Clinical features and drug therapy in patients with paroxysmal atrial fibrillation: results of the CRAFT multi-center database. *J Am Coll Cardiol.* 1993;21:380A. Abstract.

47. Coumel P, Attuel P, Lavellée JP, Flammang D, Leclercq JF, Slama R. Syndrome d'arythmie auriculaire d'origine vagale. *Arch Mal Coeur.* 1978;71:645–656.

48. Coumel P, Escoubet B, Attuel P. Beta-blocking therapy in atrial and ventricular tachyarrhythmias: experience with nadolol. *Am Heart J.* 1984;108:1098–1108.

49. Anderson JL, Gilbert EM, Alpert BL, Henthorn RW, Waldo AL, Bhandari AK, Hawkinson RW, Pritchett ELC. Prevention of symptomatic

recurrences of paroxysmal atrial fibrillation in patients initially tolerating antiarrhythmic therapy: a multicenter, double-blind, crossover study of flecainide and placebo with transtelephonic monitoring: Flecainide Supraventricular Tachycardia Study Group. *Circulation.* 1989; 80:1557–1570.

50. Pietersen AH, Hellemann H. Usefulness of flecainide for prevention of paroxysmal atrial fibrillation and flutter: Danish-Norwegian Flecainide Multicenter Study Group. *Am J Cardiol.* 1991;67:713–717.

51. Clementy J, Dulhoste MN, Laiter C, Denjoy I, Dos Santos P. Flecainide acetate in the prevention of paroxysmal atrial fibrillation: a nine-month follow-up of more than 500 patients. *Am J Cardiol.* 1992;70:44A–49A.

52. Connolly SJ, Hoffert DL. Usefulness of propafenone for recurrent paroxysmal atrial fibrillation. *Am J Cardiol.* 1989;63:817–819.

53. Pritchett ELC, McCarthy EA, Wilkinson WE. Propafenone treatment of symptomatic paroxysmal supraventricular arrhythmias: a randomized, placebo-controlled, crossover trial in patients tolerating oral therapy. *Ann Intern Med.* 1991;114:539–544.

54. Antman EM, Beamer AD, Cantillon C, McGowan N, Friedman PL. Therapy of refractory symptomatic atrial fibrillation and atrial flutter: a staged care approach with new antiarrhythmic drugs. *J Am Coll Cardiol.* 1990;15:698–707.

55. Reimold SC, Cantillon CO, Friedman PL, Antman EM. Propafenone versus sotalol for suppression of recurrent symptomatic atrial fibrillation. *Am J Cardiol.* 1993;71:558–563.

56. Middlekauff HR, Wiener I, Saxon LA, Stevenson WG. Low-dose amiodarone for atrial fibrillation: time for a prospective study? *Ann Intern Med.* 1992;116:1017–1020.

57. Katritsis D, Camm AJ. New class III antiarrhythmic drugs. *Eur Heart J.* 1993;14(H):93–99.

58. Coumel P, Leclercq JF, Attuel P. Paroxysmal atrial fibrillation. In: Kulbertus HE, Olsson SB, Schlepper M, eds. *Atrial Fibrillation.* Mölndal, Sweden: AB Hässle; 1982:158–175.

59. Rawles JM, Metcalfe MJ, Jennings K. Time of occurrence, duration, and ventricular rate of paroxysmal atrial fibrillation: the effect of digoxin. *Br Heart J.* 1990;63:225–227.

60. Galun E, Flugelman MY, Glickson M, Eliakim M. Failure of long-term digitalization to prevent rapid ventricular response in patients with paroxysmal atrial fibrillation. *Chest.* 1991;99:1038–1040.

61. Murgatroyd FD, O'Nunain S, Gibson SM, Ward DE, Camm AJ, CRAFT Investigators. The results of CRAFT-1: a multi-center, double-blind, placebo-controlled crossover study of digoxin in symptomatic paroxysmal atrial fibrillation. *J Am Coll Cardiol.* 1993;21:478A. Abstract.

62. Murgatroyd FD, Xie B, Ward DE, Malik M, Camm AJ. Effects of digoxin in patients with paroxysmal atrial fibrillation: analysis of Holter data. *Br Heart J.* 1993; 69:P66. Abstract.

63. Coplen SE, Antman EM, Berlin JA, Hewitt P, Chalmers TC. Efficacy and safety of quinidine therapy for maintenance of sinus rhythm after cardioversion: a meta-analysis of randomized control trials. *Circulation.* 1990;82:1106–1116.

64. Vrobel TR, Miller PE, Mostow ND, Rakita L. A general overview of amiodarone toxicity: its prevention, detection, and management. *Prog Cardiovasc Dis.* 1989;31:393–426.
65. Selzer A, Wray HW. Quinidine syncope: paroxysmal ventricular fibrillation occurring during treatment of chronic atrial arrhythmias. *Circulation.* 1964;30:17–26.
66. Soyka LF, Wirtz C, Spangenberg RB. Clinical safety profile of sotalol in patients with arrhythmias. *Am J Cardiol.* 1990;65:74A–81A.
67. The Cardiac Arrhythmia Suppression Trial (CAST) Investigators. Preliminary report: effect of encainide and flecainide on mortality in a randomized trial of arrhythmia suppression after myocardial infarction. *N Engl J Med.* 1989;321:406–412.
68. Falk RH. Flecainide-induced ventricular tachycardia and fibrillation in patients treated for atrial fibrillation. *Ann Intern Med.* 1989;111:107–111.
69. Pritchett ELC, Wilkinson WE. Mortality in patients treated with flecainide and encainide for supraventricular arrhythmias. *Am J Cardiol.* 1991;67:976–980.
70. Flaker GC, Blackshear JL, McBride R, Kronmal RA, Halperin JL, Hart RG. Antiarrhythmic drug therapy and cardiac mortality in atrial fibrillation. *J Am Coll Cardiol.* 1992;20:527–532.
71. Rosenqvist M, Brandt J, Schuller H. Long-term pacing in sinus node disease: effects of stimulation mode on cardiovascular morbidity and mortality. *Am Heart J.* 1988;116:16–22.
72. Andersen HR, Thuesen L, Bagger JP, Vesterlund T, Bloch Thomsen PE. Atrial versus ventricular pacing in sick sinus syndrome: a prospective randomized trial in 225 consecutive patients. *Eur Heart J.* 1993;14:252. Abstract.
73. Allessie MA, Rensma PL, Brugada J, Smeets JLRM, Penn O, Kirchhof CJHJ. Pathophysiology of atrial fibrillation. In: Zipes DP, Jalife J eds. *Cardiac Electrophysiology: From Cell to Bedside.* Philadelphia, Pa: WB Saunders; 1990:548–559.
74. Tanigawa M, Fukatani M, Konoe A, Isomoto S, Kadena M, Hashiba K. Prolonged and fractionated right atrial electrograms during sinus rhythm in patients with paroxysmal atrial fibrillation and sick sinus node syndrome. *J Am Coll Cardiol.* 1991;17:403–408.
75. Ohe T, Matsuhisa M, Kamakura S, Yamada J, Sato I, Nakajima K, Shimomura K. Relation between the widening of the fragmented atrial activity zone and atrial fibrillation. *Am J Cardiol.* 1983;53:1219–1222.
76. Kumagai K, Akimitsu S, Kawahira K, Kawanami F, Yamanouchi Y, Hiroki T, Arakawa K. Electrophysiological properties in chronic lone atrial fibrillation. *Circulation.* 1991;84:1662–1668.
77. Fisher JD. Control of atrial tachyarrhythmias using cardiac pacemakers. In: Touboul P, Waldo AL, eds. *Atrial Arrhythmias: Current Concepts and Management.* St Louis, Mo: Mosby Year Book; 1990:400–410.
78. Attuel P, Pellerin D, Mugica J, Coumel P. DDD pacing: an effective treatment modality for recurrent atrial arrhythmias. *PACE Pacing Clin Electrophysiol.* 1988;11:1647–1654.
79. Coumel P, Friocourt P, Mugica J, Attuel P, Leclercq JF. Long-term prevention of vagal atrial arrhythmias by atrial pacing at 90/minute:

experience with 6 cases. *PACE Pacing Clin Elecrophysiol.* 1983; 6:552–560.
80. Murgatroyd FD, Slade AKB, Nitzsche R, Camm AJ, Ritter P. A new pacing algorithm for the suppression of atrial fibrillation. *PACE Pacing Clin Electrophysiol.* Abstract. In press.
81. Daubert C, Mabo P, Berder V, Le Breton H, Leclerq C, Gras D. Permanent dual atrium pacing in major interatrial conduction blocks: a four years experience. *PACE Pacing Clin Electrophysiol.* 1993;16:885. Abstract.
82. Allessie MA, Kirchhof CJ, Scheffer GJ, Chorro FJ, Brugada J. Regional control of atrial fibrillation by rapid pacing in conscious dogs. *Circulation.* 1991;84:1689–1697.
83. Cooper RA, Alferness CA, Smith WM, Ideker RE. Internal cardioversion of atrial fibrillation in sheep [see comments]. *Circulation.* 1993;87: 1673–1686.
84. Levy S, Camm AJ. An implantable atrial defibrillator: an impossible dream? *Circulation.* 1993;87:1769–1772.
85. Scheinman MM, Morady F, Hess DS, Gonzalez R. Catheter induced ablation of the atrioventricular junction to control refractory supraventricular arrhythmias. *JAMA.* 1982;248:851–855.
86. Fleck RP, Chen PS, Boyce K, Ross R, Dittrich HC, Feld GK. Radiofrequency modification of atrioventricular conduction by selective ablation of the low posterior septal right atrium in a patient with atrial fibrillation and a rapid ventricular response. *PACE Pacing Clin Electrophysiol.* 1993;16:377–381.
87. Williams JM, Ungerleider RM, Lofland GK, Cox JL. Left atrial isolation: a new technique for the treatment of supraventricular arrhythmias. *J Thorac Cardiovasc Surg.* 1980;80:373–380.
88. Harada A, D'Agostino HJJ, Schuessler RB, Boineau JP, Cox JL. Biatrial isolation with preservation of normal sinus node function and sino-ventricular conduction: a surgical treatment for supraventricular tachycardias. *J Am Coll Cardiol.* 1987;9:100. Abstract.
89. Defauw JJ, Guiraudon GM, van Hemel NM, Vermeulen FE, Kingma JH, de Bakker JM. Surgical therapy of paroxysmal atrial fibrillation with the "corridor" operation. *Ann Thorac Surg.* 1992;53:564–570.
90. Cox JL, Schuessler RB, D'Agostino HJJ, Stone CM, Chang BC, Cain ME, Corr PB, Boineau JP. The surgical treatment of atrial fibrillation, III: development of a definitive surgical procedure. *J Thorac Cardiovasc Surg.* 1991;101:569–583.
91. McCarthy PM, Castle LW, Maloney JD, Trohman RG, Simmons TW, White RD, Klein AL, Cosgrove DM. Initial experience with the maze procedure for atrial fibrillation. *J Thorac Cardiovasc Surg.* 1993;105: 1077–1087.
92. Faniel R, Schoenfeld P. Efficacy of i.v. amiodarone in converting rapid atrial fibrillation and flutter to sinus rhythm in intensive care patients. *Eur Heart J.* 1983;4:180–185.
93. Anastasiou Nana MI, Levis GM, Moulopoulos SD. Amiodarone: application and clinical pharmacology in atrial fibrillation and other arrhythmias. *Int J Clin Pharmacol Ther Toxicol.* 1984;22:229–235.

94. Strasberg B, Arditti A, Sclarovsky S, Lewin RF, Buimovici B, Agmon J. Efficacy of intravenous amiodarone in the management of paroxysmal or new atrial fibrillation with fast ventricular response. *Int J Cardiol.* 1985;7:47–58.

95. Borgeat A, Goy JJ, Maendly R, Kaufmann U, Grbic M, Sigwart U. Flecainide versus quinidine for conversion of atrial fibrillation to sinus rhythm. *Am J Cardiol.* 1986;58:496–498.

96. Hellestrand KJ. Intravenous flecainide acetate for supraventricular tachycardias. *Am J Cardiol.* 1988;62:16D–22D.

97. Goy JJ, Kaufmann U, Kappenberger LJ, Sigwart U. Restoration of sinus rhythm with flecainide in patients with atrial fibrillation. *Am J Cardiol.* 1988;62:38D–40D.

98. Crijns HJ, Van Wijk LM, Van Gilst WH, Kingma JH, Van Gelder IC, Lie KI. Acute conversion of atrial fibrillation to sinus rhythm: clinical efficacy of flecainide acetate: comparison of two regimens. *Eur Heart J.* 1988;9;634–638.

99. Bianconi L, Boccadamo R, Pappalardo A, Gentili C, Pistolese M. Effectiveness of intravenous propafenone for conversion of atrial fibrillation and flutter of recent onset. *Am J Cardiol.* 1989;64:335–338.

100. Platia EV, Michelson EL, Porterfield JK, Das G. Esmolol versus verapamil in the acute treatment of atrial fibrillation or atrial flutter. *Am J Cardiol.* 1989;63:925–929.

101. Suttorp MJ, Kingma JH, Lie AH, Mast EG. Intravenous flecainide versus verapamil for acute conversion of paroxysmal atrial fibrillation or flutter to sinus rhythm. *Am J Cardiol.* 1989;63:693–696.

102. Mostow ND, Vrobel TR, Noon D, Rakita L. Rapid control of refractory atrial tachycarrhythmias with high-dose oral amiodarone. *Am Heart J.* 1990;120:1356–1363.

103. Suttorp MJ, Kingma JH, Jessurun ER, Lie AH, van Hemel NM, Lie KI. The value of class IC antiarrhythmic drugs for acute conversion of paroxysmal atrial fibrillation or flutter to sinus rhythm. *J Am Coll Cardiol.* 1990;16:1722–1727.

Chapter 10

Editorial Comments

Douglas L. Packer, MD

Over the past three decades, extraordinary amounts of time, energy, and resources have been expended toward the pharmacological maintenance of normal sinus rhythm in patients with atrial fibrillation. While many patients have been successfully managed, clinicians caring for patients with atrial fibrillation are all too familiar with the failure of the largely empirical drug therapy used for this problem.

Still, the accompanying risk of untoward sequelae of chronic atrial fibrillation, including stroke and peripheral embolic events, provides strong incentive for maintaining normal rhythm. In this regard, it has been a widespread clinical perception that maintenance of normal sinus rhythm decreases this risk in patients with underlying heart disease. Maintaining sinus rhythm is also expected to improve a patient's hemodynamic status, diminish symptoms due to rapid ventricular response rates or tachycardia-induced ventricular dysfunction, and thereby improve the patient's quality of life. Furthermore, experimental evidence now suggests that atrial fibrillation may be self-perpetuating through progressive alteration of the electrophysiological substrate.[1] This suggests that aggressive attempts at maintaining normal sinus rhythm may reverse such changes and make it progressively easier to prevent atrial fibrillation.

While these observations provide appropriate rationale for attempting normal sinus rhythm maintenance, actual reduction of risk of stroke, peripheral embolism and death with antiarrhythmic therapy in patients with atrial fibrillation has never been conclusively demonstrated. Although improvement in an individual patient's hemodynamic status and symptoms have been well-documented, additional studies will be required to support the expendi-

From DiMarco JP, Prystowsky EN (eds): *Atrial Arrhythmias: State of the Art.* Armonk, NY, Futura Publishing Company, Inc., © 1995.

ture of health care dollars on sinus rhythm maintenance to prolong life.

Regardless of the extent to which pharmacological therapy alters untoward sequelae–related morbidity or mortality, the drugs usually used for maintaining sinus rhythm have not been uniformly effective. Most studies, regardless of drug type, show high atrial fibrillation recurrence rates over the first 30 to 60 days of therapy, followed by a plateau in actuarial recurrence curves at the 50% to 60% recurrence level over 6 to 12 months of therapy. The actual failure rates might be even higher, were it possible to document the recurrence of asymptomatic paroxysmal atrial fibrillation episodes.[2] The exception to this 50% to 60% benchmark is seen with amiodarone therapy, which is effective in maintaining normal sinus rhythm in a higher proportion of patients. An additional 10% to 30% of patients enjoy a salutary effect of antiarrhythmic therapy if one accepts a decrease in the frequency of atrial fibrillation or an increase in the time of recurrence as reasonable end points of therapy. Although imperfect, these outcomes of antiarrhythmia therapy are still an improvement over the 20% to 30% sinus rhythm maintenance rate observed in untreated or placebo groups of prior trials.

Pharmacological therapy is also limited by a variety of nuisance side effects and end-organ toxicity. The risk of proarrhythmic events described by Murgatroyd and Camm[3] continues to confound the initiation and long-term usage of antiarrhythmic agents. Because of the potential unfavorable balance between benefits and side effects, it is not surprising that many clinicians view the prevention of recurrent atrial fibrillation as an unrealistic goal for many patients. Similarly, these issues make the avoidance of membrane-active antiarrhythmic therapy very attractive for patients with reversible contributors to atrial fibrillation or infrequent episodes occurring in the absence of other organic heart disease.

Despite these concerns, it may be possible to tip this unfavorable balance between the benefits and side effects of drug therapy in a more positive direction. This, however, will require substantive inroads into better understanding of the pathophysiology of atrial fibrillation, the role of atrial underlying substrate in its development, and the mechanism of action of antiarrhythmic therapy. For example, it is possible that the variable response to antiarrhythmic therapy in attempted maintenance of sinus rhythm may be a function of differences in underlying substrate in nonresponders versus responders. Clarification of this possibility may lead to improved results in appropriate patients. Over the past 10 years, a variety of studies have demonstrated that patients with normal ejection fractions and no underlying heart disease are more likely to respond satisfactorily to antiarrhythmic therapy for ventricular arrhythmias than those with marked ventricular dysfunction. This has raised the question of whether those who respond to drug therapy do so because of efficacy of the drug or the inherent properties of the underlying cardiac substrate.

Unlike the case of ventricular arrhythmia, however, little is known about the impact of abnormalities of atrial substrate on the response to drug therapy. Clarification of this issue is confounded by the absence of methods of characterizing atrial function. Still, the higher atrial fibrillation recurrence rates in patients with underlying heart disease[4] underscores a probable analogous relationship between structural abnormalities and drug response, as observed in patients with ventricular tachycardia. If there is an atrial function/structural equivalence, it may be possible to identify clinical predictors of a favorable drug response in hopes of allowing early focusing of therapeutic efforts and resources on potential responders. In contrast, those who are unlikely to respond to therapy could be more quickly triaged to alternative treatment strategies.

A better elucidation of the mechanisms of atrial fibrillation initiation and the beneficial countering antiarrhythmic drug effects is also needed. Detailed mapping examination of the onset of spontaneously occurring atrial fibrillation is not currently available. Certainly, membrane-active agents decrease APC triggers, although the recurrence of atrial fibrillation indicates that this alone is insufficient for preserving normal rhythm. Unfortunately, the action of drugs on the "substrate" response to those triggers in the atrial fibrillation initiation sequence is unclear. It is conceivable that conventional therapy fails to adequately target the circuit components of the reentrant circuits required for the initiation or early perpetuation of atrial fibrillation.

In contrast, investigations over the past 20 years have elucidated much of the mechanism of sustained atrial fibrillation and its termination by antiarrhythmic agents. The presence of multiple reentrant wavelets around functional areas of block that migrate in time and space has been well defined.[5] In addition, the termination of atrial fibrillation or flutter by (1) the drug-induced development of a critical area of block within a reentrant circuit, (2) collapse of the lateral boundaries of the circuit, (3) slowing of conduction allowing recovery of tissue ahead of the advancing wave front, with subsequent symmetrical activation from a single region, and (4) marked depression of conduction leading to failure of impulse propagation has been documented. Unfortunately, these findings were derived in specific models of established atrial fibrillation or flutter (ie, arrhythmia related to fixed anatomic barriers, vagal stimulation, rapid pacing, or induced pericarditis) and cannot be easily generalized to accommodate the conditions present at the time of spontaneously occurring atrial fibrillation. We hope that, through careful clinical studies or with the development of more representative models of atrial fibrillation, future assessments of the mechanism of initiation of this arrhythmia will be possible and the explanation of the effect of antiarrhythmic therapy in altering that process will be forthcoming. Furthermore, the role of autonomic influences in the initiation and maintenance of atrial fibrillation will be assessable and the role of antiadrenergic or vagolytic agents may be clarified.

It is also possible that subsequent investigations will lead to more focused "clinical" therapy. The recent findings of increased densities of certain ion currents in atrial tissue[6] suggest that drug targeting of strategic "atrium-specific" ion channels might lead to more effective treatment of atrial fibrillation. An increased abundance of several K^+ currents, including I_{to} and I_{KAch}, in atrial tissue has been documented. In addition, a human K^+ channel, H_{K2} with a marked predilection for atrial tissue has been identified and its response to antiarrhythmic agents examined.[7] Based on differences in the prevalence of these channels in atrial tissue, there is reason to believe that more selective block of these K^+ channels might be an important venue of atrial fibrillation–preventing antiarrhythmic agents. Such targeting, if effective, might lead to more marked increases in atrial refractoriness, leading to wavelength alteration and, therefore, prevention of atrial fibrillation or its annihilation after several initial beats. In this regard, the possibility that the newer class III antiarrhythmic agents may more selectively target relevant K^+ channels[8] mandates further clinical trials in patients with atrial fibrillation. Furthermore, effective block of atrium-specific channels could be achieved with less accompanying ventricular proarrhythmia. Obviously, additional studies will be required to determine whether such "poisoning" of specific channels will lead to better atrial fibrillation suppression than available with current antiarrhythmic agents. Furthermore, any potential benefits of atrium-specific therapy must outweigh the problems created by accompanying side effects.

Even with these inroads, the benefit of maintaining sinus rhythm must be weighed against the benefits of alternative therapies. Typically, complete ablation of the AV conduction system is usually viewed as the "court of last resort." Nevertheless, maintaining rate control by ablation of the AV conduction system along with coumarin or aspirin therapy may yield better long-term results than possible with attempted sinus rhythm maintenance. This approach may be less fraught with side effects than membrane-active pharmacological therapy or as effective as drug therapy in decreasing the symptoms related to rapid heart rates and could have an equal benefit of decreasing the risk of peripheral embolic events as documented in recent long-term anticoagulation trials conducted in patients with atrial fibrillation. In contrast, this extreme rate-control approach fails to improve atrial transport, and the risk of bleeding with warfarin (particularly in the elderly) is appreciable. Several questions about the outcome of patients undergoing ablation of the AV conduction system rate-control contrast must be resolved. The long-term consequences of AV conduction modification or ablation are unknown. The quality of life of these patients is unclear. Finally, the effect of ablation on left ventricular function, including exercise tolerance in patients with persistently abnormal atrial transport, has yet to be elucidated.

The requisite comparisons of antiarrhythmic therapy to maintain sinus rhythm vs rate control with anticoagulation are unavailable but will be forthcoming from several ongoing studies. One such trial, the New England Atrial Fibrillation Intervention Trial Pilot Study, is designed to compare the effect of quinidine plus rate control or propafenone plus rate control versus coumarin and rate control alone. End points of this study include recurrent atrial fibrillation, episodic or peripheral embolic events, and death. This and other similar studies should aid in choosing between various treatment options.

An alternative approach to patients with the potential for atrial fibrillation has been suggested by recent pacing studies. A variety of retrospective studies have demonstrated that the propensity for chronic atrial fibrillation appears to be less in patients who have been physiologically paced (DDD or AAI mode) compared with those receiving VVI pacemakers.[9] Several of these studies also suggest a decrease in long-term mortality with physiological pacing.

While these studies are intriguing, several problems remain. First, most of the available studies were retrospective and nonrandomized. Furthermore, the pacing mode selected in these studies may have been biased by clinician preferences. The prevalence of prepacing atrial fibrillation in these studies is also unclear. In most studies, follow-up is incomplete, and the patient cohorts are noncontemporary. Comparison groups were not usually matched, and no untreated control groups were included. Subsequent studies will be required to provide more definitive evidence that physiological pacing prevents atrial fibrillation and that this approach is superior to drug therapy. Such studies may also disclose the relative merits of physiological, dual-site, or premature atrial contraction–responsive pacing and whether antitachycardia pacing will ever become a viable means of terminating atrial fibrillation.

The role of alternative therapy with implanted atrial defibrillators also warrants clarification. With currently available lead arrays, it is difficult to obtain defibrillation thresholds much below 1 or 2 J. Such shocks, however, are poorly tolerated by patients. The cost of initiating treatment is also high, and the propensity for the induction of ventricular tachycardia or fibrillation related to a shock remains a possibility. These limitations must be addressed before this form of therapy will find its niche and become a viable alternative to drug therapy.

Finally, it is unclear whether the results of antiarrhythmic therapy will be superior to those of the surgical "Maze" procedure. Certainly, this approach is highly effective in Dr Cox's hands[10] and is probably as reasonable today as surgical accessory pathway ablation in Wolff-Parkinson-White patients facing lifelong medical therapy was 10 to 15 years ago. As yet, however, no studies have detailed the cost-effectiveness or long-term benefit of such surgery. Furthermore, this approach requires substantial operative expertise and is accompanied by significant morbidity and mortality. Undoubtedly, the attending risks will be greater and the results less favorable in centers with limited experience. As such, the application of this technique should be restricted to centers of excellence, and studies involving cost and efficacy comparisons of this and less invasive approaches would be useful but probably unfeasible.

Thus, many uncertainties remain in the area of long-term therapy for patients with atrial fibrillation. It remains unclear whether the maintenance of sinus rhythm is worth the work, which treatment is best, and at what point a stepped approach to the pharmacological management of patients with atrial fibrillation should be replaced by nonpharmacological measures. These issues will require additional comparative studies to examine the relative benefits, risks, and costs of the various approaches. Undoubtedly, we will learn that no single therapy fits all patients. We can hope that many of the answers to the questions raised here will allow clinicians to eliminate empiricism and lead to an informed selection of more effective mechanism-specific pharmacological or nonpharmacological therapy for an individual patient.

References

1. Wijffels M, Kirchhof C, Fredriks J, Boersma L, Allessie M. Atrial fibrillation begets atrial fibrillation. *Circulation.* 1993;(Suppl 1):I-18, abstract.
2. Page RL, Wilkinson WE, Clair WK, McCarthy EA, Pritchett ELC. Asymptomatic arrhythmias in patients with symptomatic paroxysmal atrial fibrillation and paroxysmal supraventricular tachycardia. *Circulation.* 1994;89:224–227.
3. Murgatroyd FD, Camm AJ. Maintenance of sinus rhythm in patients at risk of atrial fibrillation. This volume.
4. Van Gelder JC, Crijns HJ, Van Gilst WH, Verwer R, Kie KI. Prediction of uneventful cardioversion and maintenance of sinus rhythm from direct-current electrical cardioversion of chronic atrial fibrillation and flutter. *Am J Cardiol.* 1991;68:41–46.
5. Allesie MA, Rensma PL, Brugada J, Smeets JLRM, Penn O, Kirchhof CJHJ. Pathophysiology of atrial fibrillation. In: Zipes DP, Jalife J, eds. *Cardiac Electrophysiology: From Cell to Beside.* Philadelphia, Pa: WB Saunders: 1990:548–559.
6. Giles WR, Imaizumi Y. Comparison of potassium currents in rabbit atrial and ventricular cells. *J Physiol.* 1988;405:123–145.
7. Tamkun MM, Knoth KM, Walbridge JA, Kroemer H, Roden DM, Glover DM. Molecular cloning and characterization of two voltage-gated K^+ channel cDNAS from human ventricle. *FASEB J.* 1991;5:331–337.
8. Colatsky TJ, Follmer CH, Starmer CF. Channel specificity in antiarrhythmic drug action: mechanism of potassium channel block and its role in suppressing and aggravating cardiac arrhythmias. *Circulation.* 1990;82:2235–2242.
9. Lamas GA, Estes NM III, Schneller S, Flaker GC. Does dual chamber of atrial pacing prevent atrial fibrillation? The need for a randomized controlled trial. *PACE Pacing Clin Electrophysiol.* 1992;15:1109–1113.
10. Cox JL, Schuessler RB, D'Agostino HJ, Stone CM, Chang BC, Cain ME, Corr PB, Boineau JP. The surgical treatment of atrial fibrillation, III: development of a definite surgical procedure. *J Thorac Cardiovasc Surg.* 1991;101:569–583.

Chapter 11

Ventricular Rate Control in Atrial Fibrillation

John P. DiMarco, MD, PhD

In patients in sinus rhythm with normal atrioventricular (AV) conduction, the sinus node controls heart rate. The sinus node has extensive neural inputs from the sympathetic and parasympathetic nervous systems and is also responsive to the influence of circulating hormones. In response to any increase in cardiac demand, the sinus rate will increase in a linear fashion. In patients with atrial fibrillation, the sinus node no longer influences heart rate, which is now regulated by the response of the AV node to the fibrillating atrium. In most patients, the resting ventricular rate in the untreated state during atrial fibrillation will be higher than the rate that would be expected were the patient in sinus rhythm. Heart rate responses to physiological stimuli such as exercise or emotion will also be controlled by the AV node. Most patients with atrial fibrillation will require either a pharmacological or a nonpharmacological intervention to control their ventricular rates, but the optimal technique for controlling these rates remains controversial. In clinical practice, attempts to control rate are often ineffective.[1]

Optimal Rate Control

Atrial fibrillation is associated with a number of hemodynamic and electrophysiological consequences that may affect cardiac output.[2] Atrial contractile function and, therefore, the atrial contribution to ventricular filling are absent. This loss may be important in patients with compromised function at rest, in individuals with low

From DiMarco JP, Prystowsky EN (eds): *Atrial Arrhythmias: State of the Art*. Armonk, NY, Futura Publishing Company, Inc., © 1995.

filling pressures, and in those with noncompliant ventricles but is less significant during exercise. RR intervals in atrial fibrillation may be highly variable, so ventricular filling times are unequal. This variation is of particular significance in patients with mitral stenosis, but its significance in other patients is uncertain. At rest, the mean heart rate during atrial fibrillation in untreated individuals is usually >100 beats per minute, but there is wide interindividual variability. Some patients with high levels of vagal tone may actually have lower average heart rates in atrial fibrillation than when they are in sinus rhythm. Patients with paroxysmal atrial fibrillation may have high ventricular rates at the onset of an episode and then stabilize, with rates within a more normal range even without intervention. Exercise heart rates in atrial fibrillation are also highly variable. Only a few patients will manifest a relationship between heart rate and $\dot{V}O_2$ with increasing exercise similar to the linear relationship typically seen in patients with sinus rhythm. Patterns of excess cardioacceleration, persistent bradycardia throughout exercise, and biphasic responses may all be seen[3] (Fig 1). In theory optimal con-

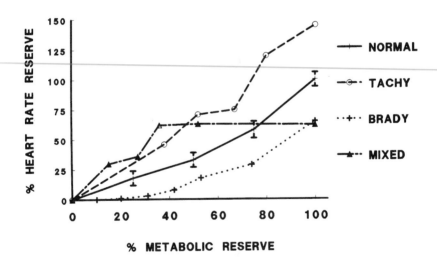

FIGURE 1.   *Patterns of rate response in atrial fibrillation. The relationship between heart rate and metabolic demand in patients in normal sinus rhythm is roughly linear. In patients with atrial fibrillation, patterns of excess tachycardia, inappropriate bradycardia, and mixed patterns can be observed. Based on data in Corbelli et al.[3]*

trol of ventricular rate in atrial fibrillation should mimic the linear response of the sinus node to a full range of physiological stimuli with, perhaps, a small upward shift to counterbalance the adverse effects of absent atrial contraction and the irregularity of ventricular activity.

Role of the AV Node

During atrial fibrillation, atrial activity occurs at rates >400 beats per minute, and this activity may be either fairly regular or totally irregular. The traditional concept of how ventricular response is controlled has been that concealed conduction in the AV node modulates the atrial inputs and controls ventricular response. As described in a classic paper by Langendorf et al,[4] in concealed conduction some of the atrial impulses penetrate into the AV junction but do not reach the ventricle. These "concealed" impulses then affect conduction of the subsequent impulse by "delaying it, blocking it entirely or causing repetitive concealed conduction." Thus, based on these electrocardiographic observations and on later electrophysiological measurements,[5,6] ventricular rates will be determined largely by the effective and functional refractory periods of the AV node. Since the AV node is autonomically sensitive, these properties will change as sympathetic and parasympathetic inputs vary, thus allowing a range of graded responses to physiological stimuli. As recently shown by Chorro et al,[7] the rate and regularity of atrial activity also affect ventricular rates. As atrial rates become faster and/or more irregular with greater impulse-to-impulse variation, more concealed conduction occurs and the overall ventricular rate slows. The converse is true when the rate slows or becomes more regular. This has relevance to potential, unanticipated rate changes during drug therapy that may alter electrical activity in atrial fibrillation without converting the rhythm.

The variable rates at which the AV node conducts can be described in terms of recovery, facilitation, and fatigue.[8,9] Incomplete recovery of calcium channels responsible for conduction produces an abrupt increase in conduction time after a single premature impulse. A second, slower component of adaptation seen with repetitive pacing has been attributed to fatigue. Facilitation describes the effects of one premature impulse on the subsequent impulse. These components, called the "rate-dependent" properties of AV nodal conduction, are subject to mathematical modeling to explain AV nodal behavior, but such modeling of conduction during atrial fibrillation would be very complex.

Recently, an alternative hypothesis concerning the role of the AV node has been proposed by Meijler and colleagues.[10,11] These investigators propose that the AV node functions not to conduct impulses but rather as a pacemaker whose rate is modulated by atrial inputs. As described by Cohen et al,[12] electrotonic modulation of phase 4 depolarization within the AV node by atrial impulses of random strength, duration, and origin could influence the pacemaker function of the AV node and result in the slower and irregular ventricular response observed during atrial fibrillation. In this model, the ventricular rate would be determined by the sum of the effects of atrial electrical activity, electrotonic modulation of the AV nodal pacemaker by atrial activity, the intrinsic properties of the AV node, and the refractory period and threshold of the His-Purkinje system. At present, it is uncertain whether this concept of AV nodal function in atrial fibrillation will prove to be superior to the traditional concepts of concealed conduction of impulses from the atrium described above.

Clinical Scenarios

The approach to rate control in any individual patient must be dictated by several clinical factors. In paroxysmal atrial fibrillation, autonomic tone at the start of the episode will determine the initial ventricular response. This may result in either slower heart rates in vagally mediated atrial fibrillation or accelerated rates when atrial fibrillation occurs with exercise, hyperthyroidism, or illness. The rapid and abrupt change in rate is presumably what produces most of the patient's symptoms. Unfortunately, the magnitude of the rate change during future paroxysmal episodes cannot usually be predicted by the sinus rate prevalent between these episodes. In addition, in some patients with atrial fibrillation, the arrhythmias develop as a result of or in association with sinus node dysfunction. Since agents that slow AV nodal conduction will also usually depress automaticity in the sinus node, it may be difficult to achieve stable rates during both sinus rhythm and fibrillation unless pacing is also prescribed. A second set of problems is presented by patients with chronic atrial fibrillation. In this situation, ventricular rates should ideally remain appropriate through the changes in autonomic tone that occur during normal daily activities and during periods of illness. Finally, the use of drugs for rate control in the acute management of new-onset atrial fibrillation must be considered as a separate problem since, here, the speed at which an agent can safely bring an elevated rate under control will be important.

Cardiac Glycosides

Cardiac glycosides have traditionally been the primary drugs used to control rate in atrial fibrillation. Digitalis works primarily by augmenting parasympathetic tone on the heart, but minor direct effects on the AV node may also occur.[13] Digitalis alone may be used successfully to control rate in some patients with atrial fibrillation, but its efficacy is quite limited in many others. Weiner et al[14] and Falk et al[15] evaluated the onsets of action of intravenous and oral digoxin, respectively. In both studies, the onset of rate slowing was delayed until 4 to 8 hours after initial drug administration. Rawles et al[16] reported on the initial ventricular rate at the onset of episodes in patients with paroxysmal atrial fibrillation and found no difference in initial rate between a group of 41 patients not taking digoxin and a group of 31 patients on the drug (140 ± 25 vs 134 ± 22 beats per minute, respectively). Similar findings were made by Galun et al[17] and by Pritchett.[18] A controlled study of the effects of digoxin on rates in paroxysmal atrial fibrillation (CRAFT-1) is now ongoing. Preliminary data reported to date show an increase in duration between symptomatic attacks and a slight decrease in mean heart rate during arrhythmia among the digoxin-treated patients.[19]

In chronic or established atrial fibrillation, digoxin is often effective in bringing resting heart rates into a more normal range, but rates during exercise are less responsive. Lang et al[20] exercised patients while they were receiving digoxin doses of 0, 0.25, or 0.5 mg/d. Although resting heart rate decreased on both active drug dosages, only at the higher dosage was a small change seen in exercise heart rates. Beasley et al[21] adjusted digoxin doses to achieve either low (0.6 to 1.3 ng/mL) or high (0.8 to 2.9 ng/mL) levels. Mean resting heart rates decreased from 108 to 93 to 83 beats per minute in the three groups as dosage was increased, and mean exercise heart rates at a standard $\dot{V}o_2$ of 20 mL·kg^{-1}·min^{-1} were 191, 182, and 164 beats per minute. Only in the highest-dose group was the difference in exercise heart rate significant. In comparison, the rest and exercise heart rates in a control group of patients in sinus rhythm at the same work level were 72 and 118 beats per minute, respectively. Ahuja et al[22] examined the effects of digoxin on heart rate in 10 patients with mitral stenosis. Again in this study, there was a decrease in resting heart rate from 116 ± 11 to 80 ± 10 beats per minute but no significant change at peak exercise (190 ± 10 vs 182 ± 10 beats per minute) with addition of digoxin. There were, however, moderate increases in time to dyspnea and total work capacity associated with digoxin therapy.

In summary, the widely prevalent clinical practice of relying on digoxin therapy alone to provide adequate rate control in patients with paroxysmal and chronic atrial fibrillation appears to be in need of reexamination. Resting heart rates in sinus rhythm in digitalized patients are of no value for predicting rates during paroxysmal episodes of atrial fibrillation. Resting heart rates during chronic atrial fibrillation in the patient on digoxin may also be misleading and often do not reflect an ability to respond optimally during moderate or vigorous exercise. Although digoxin still has a role in the management of atrial fibrillation, it is certainly not universally effective and no longer should be considered the obvious choice for initial therapy.

Calcium Channel Blockers

The calcium channel blockers verapamil and diltiazem produce frequency-dependent effects on AV nodal refractoriness and enhance the potential for concealed conduction within the AV node.[23,24] Verapamil and diltiazem are available for both intravenous and oral administration. Bolus administration of either drug to hemodynamically stable patients with atrial fibrillation and rapid ventricular rates usually results in a prompt dose-dependent reduction in heart rate. Continuous-infusion regimens using diltiazem (10 to 15 mg/h after initial loading) have been shown to produce stable 30% to 40% increases in heart rate in hospitalized patients with atrial fibrillation.[25–27] Since diltiazem has less negative inotropic potential than verapamil, its use should be preferred in patients with compromised ventricular function.

In chronic atrial fibrillation, both oral verapamil and oral dilti-azem have been shown to be efficacious at controlling ventricular rates. Exercise tolerance and symptoms are improved over the untreated state.[28-30] However, even though average 24-hour heart rates and exercise heart rates are lower during therapy with calcium channel blockers than during therapy with digoxin, improvements in exercise capacity or symptoms have not been consistently noted.

Several cautions concerning the chronic use of calcium chan-nel blockers in patients with atrial fibrillation must be raised. In the Multicenter Diltiazem Post-Infarction Trial,[31] diltiazem was associ-ated with an increased long-term mortality in a subgroup of patients with clinical signs of congestive heart failure. Although the major-ity of the patients were in sinus rhythm, similar deleterious effects would be possible in patients in atrial fibrillation with heart failure.

In patients with paroxysmal atrial fibrillation, the duration of each episode and the frequency of episodes may be as important as rate in determining a patient's symptoms. Two reports have sug-gested that verapamil and diltiazem may produce adverse effects on the electrophysiological properties of the atrium that may prolong individual episodes of arrhythmia. Shenasa et al[32] administered intravenous and oral verapamil and diltiazem to patients undergo-ing electrophysiological study and compared the duration of elec-trically induced atrial fibrillation before and after drug administra-tion. Both drugs prolonged the duration of episodes, with this change being most marked in those patients with a prior history of atrial fibrillation. Kumagai et al[33] examined the effects of intra-venous verapamil on electrophysiological properties of the atrium in 12 patients with paroxysmal atrial fibrillation. They found that verapamil prolonged intra-atrial conduction times and produced increased fragmentation of electrical activity in response to prema-ture stimulation. The clinical relevance of these studies has not been confirmed with long-term monitoring studies in patients with paroxysmal atrial fibrillation, but they should alert us to a possible adverse effect from these drugs.

β-Adrenergic Blocking Drugs

The AV node is heavily influenced by the autonomic nervous system. During periods of increased adrenergic stimulation, AV nodal refractoriness will decrease and ventricular rates during atrial fibrillation will increase. β-Adrenergic blocking agents are, therefore, rational choices for rate control in both acute and chronic settings. The choice of β-blocker is dictated by the desired duration of action, the availability of an intravenous formulation, and the relative cardioselectivity of the compound. The use of agents with intrinsic sympathomimetic activity, such as pindolol or xamoterol, has been advocated to prevent resting bradycardia and may be useful in patients with "brady-tachy" syndromes or autonomic nervous system dysfunction.[34–36]

Although all β-adrenergic blockers control excess heart rates during exercise, studies on their effect on maximal exercise tolerance have yielded inconsistent results. Ahuja et al[22] showed a marked improvement in exercise capacity during β-blocker therapy in patients with mitral stenosis, but patients with this diagnosis may be particularly sensitive to the effects of decreased filling times associated with inappropriately high ventricular rates. Other studies have shown no change or even a decrease in exercise capacity during β-blocker therapy.[37,38] Many patients, however, will report improved symptoms while on a β-blocker, presumably because average cardiac requirements through the day are not accurately reflected by a limitation of peak exercise capacity.

Other Antiarrhythmic Agents

Antiarrhythmic drugs are often used to prevent recurrent episodes of paroxysmal atrial fibrillation or to prevent ventricular arrhythmias in patients with chronic atrial fibrillation. Some of these agents will have effects on ventricular rates should atrial fibrillation occur. Quinidine is frequently described as having vagolytic effects, but these actions are probably of clinical significance only with intravenous administration or during loading. Both flecainide and propafenone slow ventricular rates in paroxysmal atrial fibrillation and may make paroxysmal episodes better tolerated.[18] The intrinsic β-blocking activity of propafenone may be responsible for this rate slowing, but other poorly understood mechanisms are probably also involved. Sotalol and amiodarone cause rate slowing because of their antiadrenergic actions. All of these drugs, however, have more toxicity than agents that work primarily on the AV node, so their use for the sole purpose of rate control should be uncommon.

Nonpharmacological Options

The introduction of catheter techniques for ablation of AV junctional conduction and of rate-adaptive permanent pacemakers has opened new opportunities for reassessment of the effects of rate control on the functional status of patients with atrial fibrillation. This approach allows control of rates both at rest and during periods of increased cardiac demand. Although the various sensors that are used to detect increased demand may produce different rate-response patterns to various physiological stressors, it is generally accepted that these units are superior to fixed-rate ventricular demand pacing. In clinical practice, the sensor-determined rate prescribed will usually be well below that seen in an untreated or digoxin-treated patient with intact AV conduction, suggesting that earlier clinical guidelines for rate control may have overestimated requirements. Several studies have reported rather dramatic increases in left ventricular function, exercise duration, and functional capacity in everyday activities and in psychological well-being in patients after AV junctional ablation.[39,40] However, in these studies, AV junctional ablation was usually performed only after patients had failed vigorous pharmacological attempts at rate control. No trial has randomized patients with either paroxysmal or chronic atrial fibrillation to either drug therapy or ablation-pacemaker therapy as an initial step. However, the observations available in the patients who have undergone AV junctional ablation should cause us to question whether a higher heart rate in atrial fibrillation is required to maintain adequate cardiac output.

Associated Conditions

Rate control during atrial fibrillation may be complicated by the clinical situation in which the arrhythmia occurs. Some of the more commonly encountered clinical problems are listed in Table 1. Patients with severe chronic lung disease and atrial arrhythmias are often poorly responsive to digoxin because of high and unstable levels of adrenergic tone and can rarely tolerate β-adrenergic blockers. When calcium blockers are ineffective or contraindicated in these patients, AV junctional ablation can be of great value. Patients

TABLE 1. Common Settings in Which Rate Control Is Difficult

Chronic obstructive lung disease
"Brady-tachy" syndromes
Vagally mediated atrial fibrillation
Competitive athletes
Hyperthyroidism
After cardiac surgery

with vagally mediated atrial fibrillation or diffuse conduction system disease often do not require drugs for rate control. In these patients, however, pacing may be required to prevent symptomatic bradycardia. At this point, it remains uncertain whether chronic atrial pacing actually prevents the development of atrial fibrillation. Competitive athletes with atrial fibrillation are often particularly difficult to manage because β-blockade may accentuate their physiological resting bradycardia and impair peak performance. In hyperthyroidism, β-blockers are the drugs of choice, but control of thyroid hormone levels is usually required before normal heart rates are restored. Patients who develop atrial arrhythmias after cardiac surgery are poorly responsive to digoxin. Frequently, "cocktails" of several agents are required to control symptoms because of the rapid ventricular rates typically seen in this setting.

Conclusions

It is now appreciated that there are significant limitations in our ability to maintain sinus rhythm in patients with atrial fibrillation. In the absence of any therapy, ventricular rates in most patients with atrial fibrillation will be in excess of an optimal value, and it is generally accepted that attempts at rate control are indicated. In the past, drug therapy has had only a limited ability to produce a smooth rate-response curve in response to normal physiological situations, and the optimal curve, both for the average patient and in any given individual, has been difficult to define. As we move toward a better understanding of the function and pharmacology of the AV node and explore nonpharmacological options that allow more precise titration of ventricular rate, it seems probable that poor rate control alone will no longer compromise patient outcomes.

References

1. Roberts SA, Diaz C, Nolan PE, et al. Effectiveness and costs of digoxin treatment for atrial fibrillation and flutter. *Am J Cardiol.* 1993;72:567.
2. Ueshima K, Myers J, Ribisl PM, et al. Hemodynamic determinants of exercise capacity in chronic atrial fibrillation. *Am Heart J.* 1993; 125: 1301.
3. Corbelli R, Masterson M, Wilkoff BL. Chronotropic response to exercise in patients with atrial fibrillation. *PACE Pacing Clin Electrophysiol.* 1990;13:179.
4. Langendorf R, Pick A, Katz LN. Ventricular response in atrial fibrillation: role of concealed conduction in the AV junction. *Circulation.* 1965; 32:69.
5. Toivonen L, Kadish A, Kou W, et al. Determinants of the ventricular rate during atrial fibrillation. *J Am Coll Cardiol.* 1990;16:1194.
6. Scheinman MM. Atrioventricular nodal conduction and refractoriness. *PACE Pacing Clin Electrophysiol.* 1993;16:592.
7. Chorro FJ, Kirchhof CJHJ, Brugada J, et al. Ventricular response during irregular atrial pacing and atrial fibrillation. *Am J Physiol.* 1990;259 (*Heart Circ Physiol.* 28):H1015.
8. Nayebpour M, Talajic M, Nattel S. Quantitation of dynamic AV nodal properties and application to predict rate-dependent AV conduction. *Am J Physiol.* 1991;261(*Heart Circ Physiol.* 30):H292.
9. Nayebpour M, Talajic, M, Villemaire C, et al. Vagal modulation of the rate-dependent properties of the atrioventricular node. *Circ Res.* 1990; 67:1152.
10. Meijler FL, Fisch C. Does the atrioventricular node conduct? *Br Heart J.* 1989;61:309.
11. Meijler FL, Wittkampf FHM. Role of the atrioventricular node in atrial fibrillation. In: Falk RH, Podrid PJ, eds. *Atrial Fibrillation. Mechanisms and Management.* New York, NY: Raven Press Ltd; 1992:59–100.
12. Cohen RJ, Berger RD, Dushane TE. A quantitative model for the ventricular response during atrial fibrillation. *IEEE Trans Biomed Eng.* 1983;30:769.
13. Klein HO, Kaplinsky E. Digitalis and verapamil in atrial fibrillation and flutter: is verapamil now the preferred agent? *Drugs.* 1986;31:185.
14. Weiner P, Bassan MM, Jarchovsky J, et al. Clinical course of acute atrial fibrillation treated with rapid digitalization. *Am Heart J.* 1983;105:223.
15. Falk RH, Knowlton AA, Bernard SA, et al. Digoxin for converting recent-onset atrial fibrillation to sinus rhythm. *Ann Intern Med.* 1987; 106:503.

16. Rawles JM, Metcalfe MJ, Jennings K. Time of occurrence, duration, and ventricular rate of paroxysmal atrial fibrillation: the effect of digoxin. *Br Heart J.* 1990;63:225.

17. Galun E, Flugelman MY, Glickson M, et al. Failure of long-term digitalization to prevent rapid ventricular response in patients with paroxysmal atrial fibrillation. *Chest.* 1991;99:1038.

18. Pritchett ELC. Management of atrial fibrillation. *N Engl J Med.* 1992; 326:1264.

19. Murgatroyd FD, O'Nunian S, Gibson SM, et al. The results of CRAFT-1: a multi-center, double-blind, placebo-controlled crossover study of digoxin in symptomatic paroxysmal atrial fibrillation. *J Am Coll Cardiol.* 1993;21:478A. Abstract.

20. Lang R, Klein HD, Weiss E, et al. Superiority of oral verapamil therapy to digoxin in treatment of chronic atrial fibrillation. *Chest.* 1983;83:491.

21. Beasley R, Smith DA, McHaffie DJ. Exercise heart rates at different serum digoxin concentrations in patients with atrial fibrillation. *Br Med J.* 1985;290:9.

22. Ahuja RC, Sinha N, Saran RK, et al. Digoxin or verapamil or metoprolol for heart rate control in patients with mitral stenosis: a randomised cross-over study. *Int J Cardiol.* 1989;25:325.

23. Ellenbogen KA, German LD, O'Callaghan WG, et al. Frequency-dependent effects of verapamil on atrioventricular nodal conduction in man. *Circulation.* 1985;72:344.

24. Talajic M, Lemery R, Roy D, et al. Rate-dependent effects of diltiazem on human atrioventricular nodal properties. *Circulation.* 1992;86:870.

25. Salerno DM, Dias VC, Kleiger RE, et al. Efficacy and safety of intravenous diltiazem for treatment of atrial fibrillation and atrial flutter. *Am J Cardiol.* 1989;63:1046.

26. Heywood JT, Graham B, Margis GE, et al. The effects of intravenous diltiazem on rapid atrial fibrillation or flutter accompanied by congestive heart failure. *Am J Cardiol.* 1991;67:1150.

27. Ellenbogen KA, Roark SF, Smith MS, et al. Effects of sustained intravenous diltiazem infusion in healthy persons. *Am J Cardiol.* 1986; 58:1055.

28. Atwood JE, Myers JN, Sullivan MJ, et al. Diltiazem and exercise performance in patients with chronic atrial fibrillation. *Chest.* 1988;92:20.

29. Maragno I, Santostasi G, Gaion RM, et al. Low- and medium-dose diltiazem in chronic atrial fibrillation: comparison with digoxin and correlation with drug plasma levels. *Am Heart J.* 1988;116:385.

30. Lundström T, Rydén L. Ventricular rate control and exercise performance in chronic atrial fibrillation: effects of diltiazem and verapamil. *J Am Coll Cardiol.* 1990;16:86.

31. The Multicenter Diltiazem Post-Infarction Trial Research Group. The effect of diltiazem on morbidity and reinfarction after myocardial infarction. *N Engl J Med.* 1988;319:385.

32. Shenasa M, Kus T, Fromer M, et al. Effect of intravenous and oral calcium antagonists (diltiazem and verapamil) on sustenance of atrial fibrillation. *Am J Cardiol.* 1988;62:403.

33. Kumagai K, Matsuo K, Ono M, et al. Effects of verapamil on electrophysiological properties in paroxysmal atrial fibrillation. *PACE Pacing Clin Electrophysiol.* 1993;16:309.
34. James MA, Channer KS, Papouchado M, et al. Improved control of atrial fibrillation with combined pindolol and digoxin therapy. *Eur Heart J.* 1989;10:83.
35. Lundström T, Moor E, Rydén L. Differential effects of xamoterol and verapamil on ventricular rate regulation in patients with chronic atrial fibrillation. *Am Heart J.* 1992;124:917.
36. Ang EL, Chan WL, Cleland JGF, et al. Placebo controlled trial of xamoterol versus digoxin in chronic atrial fibrillation. *Br Heart J.* 1990; 64:256.
37. Lewis RV, McMurray J, McDevitt DG. Effects of atenolol, verapamil, and xamoterol on heart rate and exercise tolerance in digitalised patients with chronic atrial fibrillation. *J Cardiovasc Pharmacol.* 1989; 13:1.
38. Matsuda M, Matsuda Y, Yamagishi T, et al. Effects of digoxin, propranolol, and verapamil on exercise in patients with chronic isolated atrial fibrillation. *Cardiovasc Res.* 1991;25:453.
39. Kay GN, Bubien RS, Epstein AE, et al. Effect of catheter ablation of the atrioventricular junction on quality of life and exercise tolerance in paroxysmal atrial fibrillation. *Am J Cardiol.* 1988;62:741.
40. Heinz G, Siostrzonek P, Kreiner G, et al. Improvement in left ventricular systolic function after successful radiofrequency His bundle ablation for drug refractory, chronic atrial fibrillation and recurrent atrial flutter. *Am J Cardiol.* 1992;69:489.

Chapter 11

Editorial Comments

Kenneth A. Ellenbogen, MD

Sir William Harvey was one of the first physicians to describe the atrial contribution to cardiac output when he noted in the 1600s, "If you cut the tip of the (frog) heart with a scissors, you will see blood gush out at each beat of the auricles."[1] Subsequently, a large number of investigators have further delineated the contribution of the atria to ventricular filling. Studies in both animals and humans have shown that an appropriately timed atrial contraction can increase cardiac output by 18% to 60%. Many factors influence the effectiveness of atrial systole, including the vigor of atrial contraction, heart rate, left atrial volume and pressure, left ventricular end-diastolic pressure, left ventricular stiffness, state of the autonomic nervous system, and the site of ventricular activation.[2,3] Nevertheless, a substantial percentage of patients are unable to maintain sinus rhythm after multiple trials of antiarrhythmic agents, and further therapy is directed at heart rate control.

In fact, "atrial fibrillation may be the rhythm of choice" in certain groups of patients. Most clinicians agree that patients who have been in atrial fibrillation for long periods of time (>1 year), patients unable or unwilling to take chronic antiarrhythmic drug therapy, patients in whom antiarrhythmic drugs have been associated with life-threatening proarrhythmia or systemic toxicity, and patients in whom antiarrhythmic drugs prove to be ineffective are unlikely to benefit from efforts to restore and maintain sinus rhythm. Additionally, patients with very large atria (>6 to 7 cm) may be another group in whom sinus rhythm is unlikely to be restored.

From DiMarco JP, Prystowsky EN (eds): *Atrial Arrhythmias: State of the Art.* Armonk, NY, Futura Publishing Company, Inc., © 1995.

What Is Optimal Heart Rate Control?

Optimal heart rate control has never been adequately defined. A number of recent clinical trials of intravenous β-blockers and calcium channel blockers have defined "adequate heart rate control" as a ventricular response at rest of <100 beats per minute or a >20% decrease in baseline heart rate.[4,5] The definition of heart rate control should differ depending on whether one is analyzing acute (eg, short-term or immediate) heart rate control or chronic (eg, long-term or outpatient) heart rate control. In the acute situation, heart rate control can be greatly affected by the state of the autonomic nervous system. Digoxin exerts its atrioventricular (AV) nodal conduction slowing effects by enhancing vagal tone to the AV node. Increased sympathetic tone due to stress or exercise can significantly diminish or even completely abolish the AV nodal conduction slowing effects of digoxin. In one study, the AV nodal blocking effects of 0.5 mg of oral digoxin were completely abolished at peak exercise. Clinically, Goldman et al[6] described this phenomenon with digoxin when he noted that amounts of digoxin sufficient to achieve "therapeutic" drug levels and good heart rate control in outpatients were often inadequate to slow the ventricular response in patients with serious or complicating illnesses. In this group of patients, digoxin concentrations of 2.5 to 6 ng/mL are often required to obtain heart rate control if conditions such as infections, hypoxia, or recent surgery are present. Drugs that bind to sodium or calcium channels may show decreased electrophysiological effects with increased sympathetic tone. Nayebpour et al[7] showed that preservation of rate-dependent AV nodal slowing by diltiazem was greater in dogs that received combined muscarinic and adrenergic blockade. The relationship between diltiazem concentration and prolongation of AV nodal Wenckebach cycle length was three times greater in autonomically blocked dogs.

Few studies have attempted to rigorously describe what is meant by the phrase "optimal heart rate control." In a study of 60 patients with atrial fibrillation, Rawles[8] measured stroke volume by continuous-wave Doppler examination from the sternal notch. For each patient, he attempted to construct a linear relationship between ventricular rate (preceding two RR intervals) and cardiac output (stroke volume from Doppler examination). If the slope was positive, then he considered the heart rate to be "controlled," and if the slope was negative (eg, a reduction in ventricular rate would lead to increased cardiac output), then the ventricular rate was "uncontrolled." He studied 26 patients with "idiopathic" atrial fibrillation, 13 with mitral valve disease, 19 with ischemic heart disease or hypertension, 1 with thyrotoxicosis, and 1 with a pulmonary embolus. Ventricular rate was controlled in every patient whose rate was <90 beats per minute, uncontrolled in every patient whose rate was >140 beats per minute, and controlled in 73% when the ventricular rate was between 90 and 140 beats per minute. The calculated maximal cardiac output occurred over a wide range of heart rates. Rawles suggested that because of the loss of atrial contraction, the ventricular rate needs to be at least 20% higher than in sinus rhythm to maintain a normal cardiac output. This does not imply that patients benefit from higher rates, since other considerations, such as mean left atrial pressure, presence of coronary artery disease, and myocardial oxygen demand, must be considered.

Further insight into "optimal heart rate control" is suggested by work from the pacing literature. Narahara et al[9] measured left ventricular volumes and ejection fraction with radionuclide techniques during chronic ventricular pacing in a group of 22 patients. Seventeen of the 22 patients had complete heart block with no intrinsic cardiac rhythm at baseline or during exercise. They found that patients with cardiomegaly responded differently from patients with normal ventricular function. The mean cardiac index was highest during ventricular pacing at rates of 70 to 90 beats per minute for patients with cardiomegaly, whereas in patients with normal-sized left ventricles, there was no difference in cardiac index with ventricular pacing at rates of 50 to 100 beats per minute. Patients with cardiomegaly maximized their cardiac output within a narrow range of heart rates. From an extensive review of animal and clinical pacing studies, Geddes and Wessale[10] concluded that most patients have a range of heart rates during which stroke volume and cardiac output increase and then plateau as the pacing rate is increased. Following the plateau phase (which may be brief or absent in some individuals), cardiac output and stroke volume then decrease as the paced rate is further increased. They concluded that the best resting pacing rate is during this plateau phase, which in patients with left ventricular dysfunction or during exercise may be difficult to determine because it is relatively small. These reports emphasize the importance of individualizing heart rate control. The presence of underlying cardiac pathophysiology will further define the range of optimal heart rates for a given patient.

Why Heart Rate Control?

Most patients with a rapid ventricular response have symptoms: palpitations, shortness of breath, chest pain, dizziness, lack of energy, and poor exercise tolerance. One objective of heart rate control is to provide symptom relief. Salerno et al[11] examined the improvement of symptoms in 50 patients who were randomized to receive a bolus of placebo or one of several doses of intravenous diltiazem. Seventy-six percent of patients experienced symptoms at baseline that were thought to be related to their arrhythmia, and 64% of patients felt better after receiving an intravenous bolus of diltiazem. Increasing doses of diltiazem produced an increasing chance of a therapeutic response and were also correlated with an improvement in symptoms.

Another important reason for achieving heart rate control is to prevent the development of a tachycardia-induced caridomyopathy. The effect of acute tachycardia on left ventricular function in patients with a wide variety of supraventricular arrhythmias has been well described in the cardiology literature, primarily as isolated case reports.[12-16] Tachycardia-induced cardiomyopathy has been described in patients with ectopic atrial tachycardia, AV reciprocating tachycardia, and rapid atrial flutter and atrial fibrillation. Two recent reports have highlighted the existence of this entity in patients with atrial fibrillation. One series from the Mayo Clinic reported 10 patients with atrial fibrillation and severe left ventricular dysfunction who had ventricular rate control achieved pharmacologically (n=5) or conversion to sinus rhythm (n=5) and developed improvement in ventricular function and functional class.[17] This report emphasizes that improvement in ventricular function is gradual, occurring over a 1- to 12-month period. The initial heart rate in these patients varied from 120 to 180 beats per minute. The authors do not estimate how frequently tachycardia-induced cardiomyopathy occurred in their population. Heinz et al[18] describe a group of 10 patients with atrial fibrillation and flutter whose ventricular rate was >120 beats per minute despite therapy with digitalis, verapamil, sotalol, β-blockers, and combination therapy. The patients underwent successful radiofrequency ablation of the His bundle, and a decline in end-systolic dimension was noted, with an improvement in LV function that was most marked in patients with impaired LV function at baseline. Scheinman also reported an improvement in left ventricular function in 4 of 5 patients with an ejection fraction of <35% undergoing DC catheter ablation of the AV junction for rapid atrial fibrillation.

Another report from Van Gelder et al[19] reported on 16 patients of a consecutive series of 120 patients with atrial fibrillation. Eight patients developed recurrent atrial fibrillation and were not evaluated further, and the other 8 patients remained in sinus rhythm. A significant improvement in left ventricular function occurred about 1 month after restoration of sinus rhythm. The authors suggested that some patients with atrial fibrillation may have an intrinsic cardiomyopathy. Of the 8 patients reported on in this study, the mean resting heart rate varied from 90 to 160 beats per minute, with 3 patients having heart rates >150 beats per minute. The issue of whether atrial fibrillation alone, despite adequate heart rate control, leads to a cardiomyopathy has not been well studied. Improved exercise performance after cardioversion from atrial fibrillation to sinus rhythm has been reported by a number of groups. Improved exercise tolerance with increased oxygen uptake and cardiac output are generally observed with exercise after sinus rhythm has been restored, and the reasons are most likely multifactorial.[20-22] Potential reasons include a reduced heart rate during exercise in sinus rhythm providing greater diastolic filling time, coronary flow, and reduced myocardial oxygen demand; return of atrial contraction leading to improved tricuspid and mitral valve closure; and appropriately timed and organized atrial systole.

Damiano et al[23] developed a model of left ventricular dysfunction based on these clinical observations. They paced the atria of 12 adult dogs at 190 beats per minute and measured serial chamber sizes and left ventricular ejection fraction with radionuclide angiography. A decrease in ejection fraction was noted at 1 week, which became markedly depressed by 4 weeks. No further decline in ejection fraction was noted at 3 months. End-diastolic volume increased progressively after 2 weeks of pacing, and stroke volume was significantly depressed by the third week of pacing. These functional changes during rapid atrial pacing were not noted during acute (eg, short-lived) increases in the atrial pacing rate. The reversibility of these changes was studied by allowing 5 animals to recover for 12 weeks and repeating the serial radionuclide angiograms. Ejection fraction returned to control levels after a 2-week recovery; however, end-diastolic volume did not completely return to normal.

Multiple questions remain that are left unanswered by these studies. The mean heart rate at which one can develop a cardiomyopathy, the duration of time it takes to develop the cardiomyopathy, and the amount of time it takes for the cardiomyopathy to resolve are unknown. Finally, the frequency with which tachycardia-induced cardiomyopathy develops in patients with poorly controlled heart rates is unknown.

How To Achieve Heart Rate Control?

The previous chapter reviewed the efficacy of the three classes of agents for heart rate control: digoxin, β-blockers, and calcium channel blockers. The maximum acute efficacy reported with any single agent appears to be about 60% to 80% and is probably slightly higher in the chronic, long-term clinically stable outpatient. In a retrospective review of clinical outcomes and costs associated with heart rate control, loss of heart rate control was associated with a longer hospital stay in 50% of 115 patients from 18 academic medical centers.[24]

A sizable group of patients remains whose heart rate is poorly controlled with monotherapy. In those patients, combination therapy has been shown to have synergistic effects. Multiple combinations of AV nodal blocking drugs have been studied. The best-studied combinations digoxin and diltiazem or verapamil[25,26] and digoxin plus β-blockers.[26,27] Both of these combinations have the advantage of better heart rate control with exercise. Several studies of combination therapy of digoxin and calcium channel blockers have shown either no change or an improvement in exercise tolerance. A recent study has also documented the safety of combination β-blocker and calcium channel blocker therapy. Wiesfeld and colleagues[28] demonstrated the hemodynamic tolerability, safety, and efficacy of high-dose intravenous diltiazem in patients on oral metoprolol. Many questions remain, and Zarowitz and Gheorghiade[29] recently called for a prospective controlled trial comparing digoxin with combination therapy of digoxin and β-blockers or calcium channel blockers to determine the best "pharmacological" control of heart rate. Emphasizing the lack of consistency in therapy of atrial fibrillation, Roberts et al[24] noted that adenosine was administered to 11% of patients with atrial fibrillation, combination therapy was initiated in 41% of patients, and only one third of patients received an initial digoxin dose >0.25 mg. In addition, 40% of patients receiving combination therapy for heart rate control had a second drug given within 2 hours of the first digoxin dose. These observations emphasize the lack of consistent and pharmacodynamically sound therapy to slow the ventricular response, further underlining the need to develop a treatment algorithm for this situation.

Comparison of Treatment Strategies

The superiority of heart rate control and anticoagulation (when appropriate) compared with maintenance of sinus rhythm with antiarrhythmic drugs has never been prospectively studied. A recently proposed VA cooperative study (CSP 399) designed to study this question is currently under review by the executive committee on cooperative studies. The study design consists of two phases. The first phase is a prospective comparison of amiodarone, quinidine, and placebo for maintenance of sinus rhythm. The outcome measurements are recurrence of atrial fibrillation, death, cardiac arrest, stroke, congestive heart failure, and sustained ventricular tachycardia. The second phase of this study tests two different treatment strategies. It will compare heart rate control and continuous anticoagulation with the previously determined most effective antiarrhythmic drug for maintenance of sinus rhythm. The end point will be a composite encompassing sudden death, total mortality, thromboembolic phenomena, disabling stroke, and development or exacerbation of heart failure. This phase of the study is also designed to examine the quality of life as well as the physiological consequences of restoring and maintaining sinus rhythm by serial treadmill exercise testing and serial echocardiography to determine atrial size and function.

Conclusions

It should be appreciated that significant questions remain about what constitutes optimal heart rate control, how it is measured, and how it is best achieved. Future prospective studies that compare treatment strategies and closely follow defined patient populations should help define the scope of tachycardia-induced cardiomyopathy and instruct us as to how important it is to maintain sinus rhythm.

References

1. Harvey W; Franklin, trans. *Movement of Heart and Blood in Animals. An Anatomical Essay.* Oxford, England: Blackwell Scientific; 1957:34.
2. Reynolds DW. Hemodynamics of cardiac pacing. In: Ellenbogen KA, ed. *Cardiac Pacing.* Boston, Mass: Blackwell Scientific Publishing; 1992:120–161.
3. Buckingham TA, Janosik DL, Pearson AC. Pacemaker hemodynamics: clinical implications. *Prog Cardiovasc Dis.* 1992;34:347.
4. Ellenbogen KA, Dias VC, Plumb VJ, et al. A placebo controlled trial of continuous intravenous diltiazem infusion for 24-hour heart rate control during atrial fibrillation and atrial flutter: a multicenter study. *J Am Coll Cardiol.* 1991;18:891.
5. The Esmolol Multicenter Study Research Group. Efficacy and safety of esmolol vs propranolol in the treatment of supraventricular tachyarrhythmias: a multicenter double-blind clinical trial. *Am Heart J.* 1985; 110:913.
6. Goldman S, Probst P, Selzer A, et al. Inefficacy of "therapeutic" serum levels of digoxin in controlling the ventricular rate in atrial fibrillation. *Am J Cardiol.* 1975;35:651.
7. Nayebpour M, Talajic M, Jing W, et al. Autonomic modulation of the frequency-dependent actions of diltiazem on the atrioventricular node in anesthetized dogs. *J Pharmacol Exp Ther.* 1990;253:353.
8. Rawles JM. What is meant by a "controlled" ventricular rate in atrial fibrillation? *Br Heart J.* 1990;63:157.
9. Narahara KA, Blettel ML. Effect of rate on left ventricular volumes and ejection fraction during chronic ventricular pacing. *Circulation.* 1983; 67:323.
10. Geddes LA, Wessale JL. Cardiac output, stroke volume, and pacing rate: a review of the literature and a proposed technique for selection of the optimum pacing rate for an exercise responsive pacemaker. *J Cardiovasc Electrophysiol.* 1991;2:408.
11. Salerno DM, Goldenberg IF, Schroeder JS, et al. The dose-response relationship of intravenous diltiazem to rate control and symptom relief in patients with atrial fibrillation and atrial flutter: a double-blind, placebo-controlled, randomized multicenter study. *J Am Coll Cardiol.* 1991;17:56A.
12. Brill IC. Congestive heart failure arising from uncontrolled auricular fibrillation in the otherwise normal heart: follow-up notes on a previously reported case. *Am J Med.* 1947;2:544.
13. Phillips E, Levine SA. Auricular fibrillation without other evidence of heart disease: a cause of reversible heart failure. *Am J Med.* 1949;7:478.

14. McLaran CJ, Gersh BJ, Sugrue DD, et al. Tachycardia induced myocardial dysfuction: a reversible phenomenon? *Br Heart J.* 1985;53:323.
15. Packer DL, Bardy GH, Worley SJ, et al. Tachycardia-induced cardiomyopathy: a reversible form of left ventricular dysfunction. *Am J Cardiol.* 1986;57:563.
16. Lemery R, Brugada P, Cheriex E, et al. Reversibility of tachycardia-induced left ventricular dysfunction after closed-chest catheter ablation of the atrioventricular junction for intractable atrial fibrillation. *Am J Cardiol.* 1987;60:1406.
17. Grogan M, Smith HC, Gersh BJ, et al. Left ventricular dysfunction due to atrial fibrillation in patients initially believed to have idiopathic dilated cardiomyopathy. *Am J Cardiol.* 1992;69:1570.
18. Heinz G, Siostrzonek P, Kreiner G, et al. Improvement in left ventricular systolic function after successful radiofrequency His bundle ablation for drug refractory, chronic atrial fibrillation and recurrent atrial flutter. *Am J Cardiol.* 1992;69:489.
19. Van Gelder IC, Crijns HJGM, Blanksma PK, et al. Time course of hemodynamic changes and improvement of exercise tolerance after cardioversion of chronic atrial fibrillation unassociated with cardiac valve disease. *Am J Cardiol.* 1993;72:560.
20. Lipkin DP, Frenneaux M, Stewart R, et al. Delayed improvement in exercise capacity after cardioversion of atrial fibrillation to sinus rhythm. *Br Heart J.* 1988;59:572.
21. Atwood JE, Myers J, Sullivan M, et al. The effect of cardioversion on maximal exercise capacity in patients with chronic atrial fibrillation. *Am Heart J.* 1989;118:913.
22. Alam M, Thorstrand C. Left ventricular function in patients with atrial fibrillation before and after cardioversion. *Am J Cardiol.* 1992;69:694.
23. Damiano RJ Jr, Tripp HF Jr, Asano T, et al. Left ventricular dysfunction and dilatation resulting from chronic supraventricular tachycardia. *J Thorac Cardiovasc Surg.* 1987;94:135.
24. Roberts SA, Diaz C, Nolan PE, et al. Effectiveness and costs of digoxin treatment for atrial fibrillation and flutter. *Am J Cardiol.* 1993;72:567.
25. Roth A, Harrison E, Mitani G, et al. Efficacy and safety of medium- and high-dose diltiazem alone and in combination with digoxin for control of heart rate at rest and during exercise in patients with chronic atrial fibrillation. *Circulation.* 1986;73:316.
26. David D, Segni ED, Klein HO, et al. Inefficacy of digitalis in the control of heart rate in patients with chronic atrial fibrillation: beneficial effect of an added beta adrenergic blocking agent. *Am J Cardiol.* 1979;44:1378.
27. Sarter BH, Marchlinski FE. Redefining the role of digoxin in the treatment of atrial fibrillation. *Am J Cardiol.* 1992;69:71G.
28. Wiesfeld ACP, Remme WJ, Look MP, et al. Acute hemodynamic and electrophysiologic effects and safety of high-dose intravenous diltiazem in patients receiving metoprolol. *Am J Cardiol.* 1992;70:997.
29. Zarowitz BJ, Gheorghiade M. Optimal heart rate control for patients with chronic atrial fibrillation: are pharmacologic choices truly changing? *Am Heart J.* 1992;123:1401.

Chapter 12

Anticoagulation to Prevent Stroke in Atrial Fibrillation

Daniel E. Singer, MD

Introduction

Over the past decade we have come to appreciate that atrial fibrillation (AF) markedly increases the risk of stroke and that long-term anticoagulation largely reverses this increased risk. This chapter reviews in detail the initial set of five randomized clinical trials (RCTs) of antithrombotic therapy in AF, reports on preliminary analyses of additional relevant RCTs, indicates the implications of these studies for clinical practice, and provides an assessment of future research needs. This discussion applies to those patients for whom return to permanent sinus rhythm is no longer a therapeutic goal.

For consideration of anticoagulation, AF has historically been categorized as rheumatic or nonrheumatic (NRAF). AF in the setting of rheumatic heart disease, primarily mitral stenosis, has long been a widely accepted risk factor for stroke.[1] The assumption has been that AF coupled with mitral stenosis greatly increases stasis of blood in the atrium and promotes thrombus formation and subsequent emboli. Lifelong anticoagulation has been standard therapy for such patients, although the clinical studies supporting this management strategy are fairly weak.[1] Presumably, the clear consensus in favor of anticoagulants in rheumatic AF results from the dramatic presentation of stroke or visceral embolus in these predominantly younger patients.

The vast majority of patients with AF have NRAF associated with aging. These patients often have other conditions, such as hyperten-

From DiMarco JP, Prystowsky EN (eds): *Atrial Arrhythmias: State of the Art*. Armonk, NY, Futura Publishing Company, Inc., © 1995.

sion or coronary artery disease, that themselves predispose to stroke. When a stroke occurred in such patients, it was unclear whether NRAF itself led to the stroke, and, even if it did, whether the efficacy of anticoagulants would be worth their risk in such elderly patients.

The Framingham Heart Study,[2] in particular, highlighted the important link between NRAF and stroke. The Framingham Study estimated the prevalence of AF as approximately 2% for individuals in their sixties, rising to 10% for those > 80 years old. The risk of stroke was increased fourfold to fivefold throughout this age range, even as the risk of stroke among those without AF rose with age. From the prevalence of AF and its increased risk for stroke, one can estimate that AF accounts for 15% of all strokes, or about 70,000 strokes each year in the United States.[2, 3]

Randomized Trials of Warfarin to Prevent Stroke in Atrial Fibrillation

To test whether the increased risk of stroke due to AF was reversible, five randomized trials of warfarin were begun independently in the mid 1980s.[4-8] The trials include the Copenhagen Atrial Fibrillation, Aspirin, Anticoagulation Trial (AFASAK), the Boston Area Anticoagulation Trial for Atrial Fibrillation (BAATAF), the Stroke Prevention in Atrial Fibrillation trial (SPAF), the Canadian Atrial Fibrillation Anticoagulation trial (CAFA), and the Veterans' Administration Stroke Prevention in Nonrheumatic Atrial Fibrillation trial (SPINAF). All were primary prevention trials, with a very small fraction of patients having had a prior stroke. All were stopped early because of the demonstrated efficacy of warfarin.

AFASAK

AFASAK[4] was a three-armed trial comparing warfarin at a target international normalized ratio (INR) of 2.8 to 4.2 (roughly corresponding to a prothrombin time ratio [PTR] of 1.7 to 2.0), aspirin at 75 mg/d, and an aspirin placebo. AFASAK's target INR corresponded to a fairly high intensity of anticoagulation. As with BAATAF and SPAF, AFASAK did not blind warfarin therapy. AFASAK was probably the closest to a community trial of warfarin. Patients were identified at two outpatient electrocardiography laboratories used by general practitioners. Of 1842 eligible patients, 1007 entered the trial, a very high recruitment fraction. Slightly more than half of the patients were men (Table 1). The median age was in the mid 70s. A high proportion of patients had hypertension. More than 50% were reported as having heart failure, although the specificity of this diagnosis is not clear.

Three hundred thirty-six subjects were assigned to placebo (ie, aspirin placebo), 336 to aspirin, and 335 to warfarin. Thirty-eight percent of patients assigned to warfarin withdrew from the study after an average follow-up of < 1 year. This high percentage of withdrawals may have resulted from AFASAK's high recruitment fraction; more highly selected samples of patients might have been more compliant. AFASAK reported 4 outcome events (here, ischemic strokes plus systemic emboli) in the warfarin group, 20 in the aspirin group, and 21 on placebo (90% of these outcomes were is-

TABLE 1. Clinical Characteristics of Patients at Entry to Randomized Trials*

Feature	AFASAK	BAATAF	SPAF	CAFA	SPINAF
Male,%	54	70	70	73	100
Age	75†	68	66	67	67
AF >1 y,%	...	68	72	82	86‡
PAF, %	0	16	34	7	0
Hx stroke, %	4	3	8§	4§	0
HBP, %	31	51	55	34	62
Diabetes, %	10	16	19	10	20
Angina, %	16	25	10	20	23
Hx MI, %	8	16	6	12	21
CHF, %	51	28	19	20	30

*These are the features of the control or placebo groups from each trial. AF = atrial fibrillation; PAF = paroxysmal or intermittent AF; Hx = history of; HBP = hypertension; MI = myocardial infarction; CHF = congestive heart failure. Abbreviations of trials as in text.

† The mean age is provided except for AFASAK, which provided the median.

‡ Duration of AF was not provided by AFASAK. For SPINAF, 86% had AF > 6 months.

§ In SPAF and CAFA, percentages are for history of stroke and/or transient ischemic attack.

chemic strokes), corresponding to an annual rate of 1.6% in warfarin versus 5.6% in the placebo group (Table 2.). There were two major hemorrhages on warfarin, including one fatal intracerebral bleed. The marked benefit of warfarin coupled with the low rate of major hemorrhage led to the early stopping of the trial.

Two additional points about AFASAK are worth noting. First, there was subsequent disagreement about the event rates reported for an intention-to-treat analysis. If patients who withdrew from therapy are included in the analysis, the number of thromboembolic events becomes 10 vs 21 vs 25 for warfarin, aspirin, and placebo, respectively ($P \approx .05$). In contrast, only three patients in the warfarin arm who sustained a thromboembolic event were actually taking warfarin, and of these, two had briefly discontinued war-

TABLE 2. Results of the First Five Randomized Trials of Warfarin for Atrial Fibrillation*

	AFASAK	BAATAF	SPAF	CAFA	SPINAF
Warfarin					
Subjects, n	335	212	210	187	260
Events, n	4	2	6	5	4
Person-years	250	487	260	200	456
Annual rate, %	1.6	0.41	2.3	2.5	0.88
Control					
Subjects, n	336	208	211	191	265
Events, n	21	13	18	11	19
Person-years	373	435	244	212	440
Annual rate, %	5.6	3.0	7.4	5.2	4.3
Preventive efficacy, %	71	86	69	52	79
95% CI, %	23–90	51–96	27–85	(−36)–87	52–90
Intracranial hemor-rhage rate due to warfarin	0.40	0.21	0	0.50	0.22

*The definition of outcome events varied somewhat in the different trials, but ischemic strokes accounted for the vast majority of events. All trials other than SPINAF also counted peripheral "non–central nervous system" emboli. Intracranial hemorrhages are presented in the last row of this table. Person-years in the warfarin and control arms of AFASAK were inferred from data given in their report[4]; person-years were given explicitly in the other trials.[5–8] "Preventive efficacy" is the same as "risk reduction" and is calculated by (1-RR)X100, where RR is the relative risk, warfarin/control. The efficacy analysis is presented for CAFA, since that was their planned primary analysis; for all other trials, intention-to-treat results are provided.

farin, resulting in an INR well below target at the time of their event.

BAATAF

BAATAF[5] randomized 212 patients to "low-dose" warfarin (target PTR, 1.2 to 1.5) and 208 to control. Therapy was not blinded. Subjects in the control group could take aspirin, and approximately half did. Nearly three quarters of the patients were male (Table 1). The average age was 68 years. A small proportion of subjects had intermittent AF, most for several years. Half the subjects had no clinical heart disease other than AF, although many of these had hypertension or diabetes. Only 10% of BAATAF patients assigned to warfarin withdrew from therapy permanently.

BAATAF observed 13 strokes in the control arm vs two in the warfarin arm, for a preventive efficacy of 86% (Table 2). There were no other embolic events. There was one presumed subdural hematoma that was fatal in a patient on warfarin. Otherwise, the rate of serious bleeding was essentially the same in warfarin as in control. Eight of the 13 control patients who sustained a stroke were taking aspirin. Analyses to remove confounding in this nonrandomized assessment of aspirin estimated that the rate of stroke remained several-fold higher on aspirin than on warfarin.[9]

SPAF

SPAF[6] randomly assigned patients to warfarin (target PTR of 1.3 to 1.8), aspirin at 325 mg/d, or aspirin placebo (group 1). Warfarin therapy was not blinded. SPAF also studied patients who would not or could not take warfarin. These latter patients were separately randomized to aspirin at 325 mg/d or aspirin placebo (group 2). SPAF estimated that a relatively small fraction of eligible patients were actually recruited, a finding consistent with other American studies. Patients in the SPAF warfarin trial had a somewhat younger average age at entry, and a smaller proportion with congestive heart failure than in BAATAF. One third of the patients had intermittent AF, and the overwhelming majority had had AF for >1 year (Table 1).

SPAF observed that warfarin reduced the risk of ischemic stroke and systemic embolic events by 69%, from 7.4% to 2.3% per year (Table 2). Of the six patients in the warfarin arm who had strokes, four were not taking warfarin at the time of their stroke.

SPAF provided a mixed picture of the effectiveness of aspirin. It reported an overall reduction in risk of stroke and systemic emboli of 42%. However, this effect was markedly heterogeneous in the two separately randomized studies of aspirin. In the study that included warfarin as a possible therapy (group 1), only one outcome event was observed in the aspirin group, contrasted with 18 in placebo. In group 2, in which patients were assigned to either aspirin or aspirin placebo, there were 25 events on aspirin vs 28 in placebo (not statistically significant). The event rate on aspirin in group 2 (approximately 5% per year) was very similar to that reported in AFASAK, in which no effect of aspirin was seen. Subgroup analyses in SPAF suggested that aspirin did not confer benefit on patients > 75 years old and was not very effective at preventing serious strokes.

There was one fatal intracerebral hemorrhage on warfarin and one subdural hematoma with full recovery. Two patients in the placebo group had subdural hematomas (with full recovery). There was no increase in major bleeding from other anatomic sites with warfarin.

CAFA

CAFA[7] was a double-blind, placebo-controlled trial of low-dose warfarin (target INR, 2 to 3) in AF. After the AFASAK report and a preliminary report of the SPAF trial, the CAFA investigators decided to stop their trial to allow all patients access to warfarin. CAFA counted events (ie, nonlacunar strokes or non–central nervous system emboli) using an "efficacy" analysis, in which events occurring >28 days after therapy was stopped would not be counted. By this approach, there were 5 primary events in warfarin vs 11 in placebo, for a risk reduction of 52% (Table 2). Of these 5 events in the warfarin category, 2 occurred in patients who had discontinued the drug, and an additional 2 were in patients well below the anticoagulation target, with INRs of 1.1. Major bleeding occurred in 5 patients on warfarin, including 1 fatal intracranial hemorrhage, and in 1 patient on placebo (2.5% vs 0.5% per year).

SPINAF

SPINAF[8] was the only completed trial to provide a fully blinded assessment of warfarin. As a Department of Veterans Affairs study, it entered only men (Table 1). Patients with intermittent AF were not eligible. The entry characteristics of subjects in SPINAF suggested somewhat more cardiovascular disease but were generally similar to the other studies. SPINAF used a 12-hour cutoff to distinguish transient ischemic attacks from strokes, rather than the more usual 24-hour cutoff used by the other studies. In this study, warfarin at low dose (target PTR of 1.2 to 1.5) reduced the risk of stroke by 79% (Table 2). There was one nonfatal intracerebral hemorrhage in the warfarin-treated group vs none in the placebo group. There were six other major hemorrhages in warfarin vs four in placebo (all gastrointestinal hemorrhages).

Meta-analysis of the First Five RCTs

This group of studies, as a whole, provides a consistency of evidence that is truly distinctive among prevention trials. Warfarin removes most of the risk of stroke due to AF. It can do so at a low intensity of anticoagulation, and at least in the first set of trials, it can do so with little increase in major bleeding. Since all these trials stopped early, the number of events observed in each was small, resulting in imprecision in the estimates from the trials. The information value of these trials can be amplified by formally pooling their results. In particular, analyses of such pooled results can provide more precise estimates of the efficacy of warfarin (ie, tighter confidence intervals) and better identification of groups of patients at high and low risk of stroke. This sort of information is particularly important when such a potentially risky and demanding therapy is being considered.[10,11] A formal collaborative pooling of the primary data from the RCTs has now been accomplished and analyzed.[12] These analyses, which include some data not specifically included in the original trial reports, provide a pooled (meta-analytic) estimate of the efficacy (ie, risk reduction) of warfarin of 68% (95% confidence interval, 50% to 79%). This estimate was calculated on the basis of intention to treat (ie, by initial randomization status). Since a large fraction of all strokes counted in the warfarin group occurred among patients not actually taking warfarin at the time of the stroke, it is reasonable to assume that the true efficacy of warfarin is even higher. This assumption is bolstered by the fact that the trials providing the highest estimate of efficacy, BAATAF and SPINAF, observed no *non*anticoagulated strokes among patients assigned to warfarin. Since only 80% of the stroke risk faced by individuals with AF is attributable to AF itself (assuming a relative risk of 5), it is clear that nearly all this additional risk due to AF is prevented by anticoagulation.

The meta-analysis identified the following independent risk factors for stroke with AF: (1) prior stroke or transient ischemic attack (relative risk [RR] of 2.5); (2) age, RR=1.4 per decade; (3) hypertension, RR=1.6; and (4) diabetes, RR=1.7. Coronary heart disease and congestive heart failure were univariate risk factors but did not add significantly to the prediction of stroke once the other risk factors were included in the multivariate model. Analysis of echocardiographic features is currently incomplete. The annual risk of stroke ranged from 1.0% for those <65 years old with none of the other three clinical risk factors to 8.1% for those >75 years old with at least one other risk factor. The remarkable finding was that warfarin reduced the rates in all risk categories (assembled by age and at least one other clinical risk factor) to between 1.0% and 1.7% per year. Only for the youngest, lowest-risk group did warfarin not reduce the risk of stroke. In the other risk categories, warfarin reduced the absolute risk of stroke by 2.8% per year or more. In essence, the strongest risk factor for stroke was whether the patient was anticoagulated!

Second "Wave" of RCTs in AF

Since the completion of the meta-analysis, the results of two additional trials have been published, the SPAF II trial[13] and the

European Atrial Fibrillation trial (EAFT).[14] SPAF II was an extension of SPAF I group 1 with the aspirin placebo group removed, thereby limiting the comparison to warfarin at PTR of 1.3 to 1.8 (INR, 2 to 4.5) vs aspirin at 325 mg/d. With the beginning of SPAF II, patients were separately randomized according to age: ≤75 vs >75 years old. This was motivated by the finding in SPAF I that aspirin appeared to work only in the younger patients. The results of SPAF II stand in contrast with the earlier studies. In particular, there was a high rate of intracranial hemorrhage on warfarin: 0.5% per year in the younger group, and almost 2% per year in those >75 years old. Warfarin appeared to be modestly more effective than aspirin in preventing ischemic stroke in both age groups, but when the intracranial hemorrhages were added to the ischemic strokes, the aggregate rates of strokes with residual deficit were very similar in both the aspirin and warfarin groups: about 1.5% per year in the younger group and about 4.5% per year in the older group. This latter rate of "bad" events was more than double that seen in the warfarin arms of the earlier trials.

Problems in the design, execution, and analysis of SPAF II severely weaken its conclusions. Inclusion of the anomalous findings from SPAF I group 1 regarding aspirin likely results in an overestimate of the efficacy of aspirin in SPAF II, particularly in the patients ≤75 years old (the predominant age group for SPAF I group 1). Analyses removing the experience of SPAF I group 1 would show a substantial relative benefit of warfarin vs aspirin in the younger age group. Many of the events occurring in the warfarin groups occurred in patients who were not actually taking warfarin. Of 56 events occurring in patients on any antithrombotic therapy, 39 occurred in patients taking aspirin vs 17 in patients taking warfarin. This effect was seen in both age categories: 20 events vs 9 in the younger group and 19 vs 8 in the older group. These considerations make it likely that warfarin is substantially more effective than aspirin in preventing stroke. The fact that the relative risk of warfarin vs aspirin was the same in both age categories argues against the hypothesis that aspirin is more protective in younger age groups.

The increased rates of intracranial bleeding observed in SPAF II, particularly in the elderly, are clearly worrisome. However, the upper bound of the SPAF II INR target, INR 4.5, was the highest of any trial in AF, and there was a suggestion that increased anticoagulant intensity was associated with intracranial bleeding. All these concerns notwithstanding, SPAF II does raise important questions about the safety and net benefit of anticoagulation in older patients with AF. Unfortunately, it is these older patients who are at highest risk for stroke and for whom there is no evidence that aspirin is beneficial.

EAFT[14] was a trial of antithrombotic therapy for patients with AF who had already had a transient ischemic attack or minor stroke. The structure of the trial was similar to that of SPAF I. For patients who would or could accept anticoagulation, there was a three-armed design of oral anticoagulation at INR 2.5 to 4.0 vs aspirin at 300 mg/d vs aspirin placebo. For those who were not candidates for anticoagulation, the comparison groups were aspirin at 300 mg/d vs placebo. The rates of stroke in the placebo groups were much higher (12% per year) than those in the primary prevention trials. A large number of events were observed, producing relatively precise estimates of effect. Anticoagulation again reduced the risk of stroke by about two thirds. Aspirin had no significant effect (88 events in aspirin vs 90 in control), although the rate of stroke in those randomized to aspirin was slightly lower than in placebo (Table 3).

TABLE 3. Antithrombotic Therapy to Prevent Stroke in NRAF: Summary of Preventive Efficacy*

I. Anticoagulation			
	Trial	INR	Preventive Efficacy, %
	Pooled first 5 trials	≈1.4–4.5	68 (50–79)
	EAFT	2.5–4.0	66 (43–80)
II. Aspirin			
	Trial	mg/day	Preventive Efficacy, %
	AFASAK	75	18 [(-60)–58]
	SPAF 1, group 1	325	95 (65–99)
	SPAF 1, group 2	325	8 [(-67)–49]
	EAFT	300	14 [(-15)–36]

*Preventive efficacy refers to the estimate of the proportion of strokes prevented in each trial. The preventive efficacy for aspirin estimated in AFASAK uses nonpublished data provided to the meta-analysis[12]; the preventive efficacy for aspirin from the two SPAF 1 RCTs was calculated by reworking data presented in two publications.[6,26] The trials included as the "first five trials" are those summarized in Table 2; trial abbreviated titles are explained in the text.

Discussion

The clear message that comes through all these trials is that oral anticoagulation, in particular warfarin, dramatically reduces the risk of stroke in AF. In contrast, there is little evidence that aspirin has much efficacy in AF (Table 3). Only the SPAF study supports a beneficial effect of aspirin, and even in SPAF there is strong evidence to the contrary (ie, SPAF I group 2). Aspirin may provide a true small benefit (eg, risk reduction of 10% to 20%), but this awaits better definition from future studies.

Despite the dramatic efficacy of warfarin, it remains an often unattractive therapy for physicians and patients.[15] Patients who are feeling well are reluctant to undertake a lifelong regimen of a risky therapy that demands frequent blood tests for monitoring and ongoing concern about diet and other medications. Patients who do begin warfarin frequently quit. Quitting may result from patients' fatigue with the rigors of monitoring blood tests and medical visits or from a "minor" bleeding event that undermines patient enthusiasm.[16] More widespread use of warfarin and better sustained compliance would result from easier and safer, yet effective, antithrombotic regimens and from better targeting of warfarin therapy to those likely to benefit most.

Future research should define the lowest effective level of anticoagulation. Such low doses of warfarin should add safety and may allow less frequent monitoring. Newer ways of monitoring anticoagulation should be tested. These would include more mathematically sophisticated monitoring schedules to allow less frequent testing[17] as well as home-based (via fingerstick capillary blood samples) measurement of INRs to add convenience.[18] More widespread use of dedicated clinics to manage warfarin would add effectiveness and safety. Implementation of prothrombin time monitoring using INRs rather than PTRs would immediately improve the precision and safety of anticoagulation.[19] The prothrombin time test itself should be compared with better measures of in vivo effectiveness of anticoagulants.[20,21]

One hundred patients with AF need to be anticoagulated each year to prevent an average of three strokes, not all of which leave a permanent neurological deficit. We need to better identify those who will benefit most from anticoagulation. Further definition of risk factors for stroke in AF, particularly echocardiographic features, would naturally result from cumulative meta-analyses of results of new RCTs added to the old. In addition, better and more current definition of risk factors for bleeding on anticoagulation, particularly among patients anticoagulated outside of RCTS, would complete the data needed for rational decisions about individual patients with AF. These studies on risk factors for bleeding are emerging.[22-25]

For the time being, it appears that the only patients with AF who are at low enough risk to defer warfarin therapy are those who are relatively young (eg, <65 years old) and have no other risk factors for stroke as specified above. For all other patients with AF, life-long anticoagulation at low intensity, eg, INR of 2.0 to 3.0, is indicated. The past decade of RCTs has placed the burden of proof on the physician or patient who decides *not* to undertake long-term anticoagulant therapy.

Acknowledgment:

Some of the material presented in this paper appeared in earlier versions in previous publications by the author. These include Singer et al. "Preventing stroke in atrial fibrillation." *Coron Artery Dis.* 1992;3:753–760 (in particular Table 3), and Singer. "Overview of the randomized trials to prevent stroke in atrial fibrillation." *Ann Epidemiol.* 1993;3:563–567. Permission to represent relevant material is granted by Current Science Publication and Elsevier Science Inc, respectively, who hold the copyrights.

References

1. Dunn M, Alexander J, De Silva R, Hildner F. Antithrombotic therapy in atrial fibrillation. *Chest.* 1989;95(suppl):118S–127S.
2. Wolf PA, Abbott RD, Kannel WB. Atrial fibrillation: a major contributor to stroke in the elderly. *Arch Intern Med.* 1987;147:1561–1564.
3. United States Bureau of the Census. *Statistical Abstract of the United States: 1992.* 112th ed. Washington, DC:15.
4. Petersen P, Godtfredsen J, Boysen G, Andersen ED, Andersen B. Placebo-controlled, randomised trial of warfarin and aspirin for prevention of thromboembolic complications in chronic atrial fibrillation: the Copenhagen AFASAK study. *Lancet.* 1989;1:175–179.
5. The Boston Area Anticoagulation Trial for Atrial Fibrillation Investiga-

tors. The effect of low-dose warfarin on the risk of stroke patients with nonrheumatic atrial fibrillation. *N Engl J Med.* 1190;323:1505–1511.

6. Stroke Prevention in Atrial Fibrillation Investigators. Stroke prevention in atrial fibrillation study: final results. *Circulation.* 1991;84:527–539.

7. Connolly SJ, Laupacis A, Gent M, Roberts RS, Cairns JA, Joyner C. Canadian Atrial Fibrillation Anticoagulation (CAFA) study. *J Am Coll Cardiol.* 1991;18:349–355.

8. Ezekowitz MD, Bridgers SL, James KE, et al. Warfarin in the prevention of stroke associated with nonrheumatic atrial fibrillation. *N Engl J Med.* 1992;327:1406–1412.

9. Singer DE, Hughes RA, Gress DR, et al. The effect of aspirin on the risk of stroke in patients with atrial fibrillation: the BAATAF study. *Am Heart J.* 1992;124:1567–1573.

10. Singer DE. The randomized trials of warfarin for atrial fibrillation. *N Engl J Med.* 1992;327:1451–1453. Editorial.

11. Singer DE. Problems with stopping rules in trials of risky therapies: the case of warfarin to prevent stroke in atrial fibrillation. *Clin Res.* 1993;41:482–486.

12. Atrial Fibrillation Investigators: Laupacis A, Boysen G, Connolly S, Ezekowitz M, Hart R, James K, Kistler J, Kronmal R, Petersen P, Singer D. Atrial fibrillation: risk factors for embolization and efficacy of antithrombotic therapy. *Arch Intern Med.* 1994;154:1449-1457.

13. Stroke Prevention in Atrial Fibrillation Investigators. Warfarin versus aspirin for prevention of thromboembolism in atrial fibrillation: Stroke Prevention in Atrial Fibrillation II Study. *Lancet.* 1994;343:687–691.

14. European Atrial Fibrillation Trial Study Group. Secondary prevention in nonrheumatic atrial fibrillation after transient ischaemic attack or minor stroke. *Lancet.* 1993;342:1255–1262.

15. Kutner M, Nixon G, Silverstone F. Physicians' attitudes toward oral anticoagulants and antiplatelet agents for stroke prevention in elderly patients with atrial fibrillation. *Arch Intern Med.* 1991;151:1950–1953.

16. Lancaster TR, Singer DE, Sheehan MA, Oertel LB, Maraventano SW, Hughes RA, Kistler JP. The impact of long-term warfarin therapy on quality of life: evidence from a randomized trial. *Arch Intern Med.* 1991;151:1944–1949.

17. Kent DL, Vermes D, McDonell M, et al. A model for planning optimal follow-up for outpatients on warfarin anticoagulation. *Med Decis Making.* 1992;12:132–141.

18. White RH, McCurdy SA, von Marensdorff H, Woodruff DE Jr, Leftgoff L. Home prothrombin time monitoring following the initiation of warfarin therapy: a randomized, prospective study. *Ann Intern Med.* 1989; 111:730–737.

19. Hirsh J. Is the dose of warfarin prescribed by American physicians unnecessarily high? *Arch Intern Med.* 1987;147:769–771.

20. Furie B, Furie BC. Molecular and cellular biology of blood coagulation. *N Engl J Med.* 1992;326:800–806.

21. Bauer KA, Rosenberg RD. The pathophysiology of the prethrombotic state in humans: insights gained from studies using markers of hemostatic system activation. *Blood.* 1987;70:343–350.

22. Landefeld CS, Rosenblatt MW, Goldman L. Bleeding in outpatients treated with warfarin: relation to the prothrombin time and important remediable lesions. *Am J Med.* 1989;87:153–159.
23. Fihn SD, McDonell M, Martin D, et al. Risk factors for complications of chronic anticoagulation. *Ann Intern Med.* 1993;118:511–520.
24. van der Meer FJM, Rosendaal FR, Vandenbroucke JP, Briet E. Bleeding complications in oral anticoagulant therapy: an analysis of risk factors. *Arch Intern Med.* 1993;153:1557–1562.
25. Hylek EM, Singer DE. Risk factors for intracranial hemorrhage in outpatients taking warfarin. *Ann Intern Med.* 1994;120:897–902.
26. Stroke Prevention in Atrial Fibrillation Investigators. Preliminary report of the Stroke Prevention in Atrial Fibrillation Study. *N Engl J Med.* 1990;322:863–868.

Chapter 12

Editorial Comments

Valentin Fuster, MD, PhD; Robert G. Hart, MD;
and Jonathan Halperin, MD

Defining the Problems and Risk Stratification

To reemphasize Dr Singer's presentation, the high risks of thromboembolism in atrial fibrillation (AF) associated with mitral stenosis and prosthetic mitral valves have long been appreciated, but AF, even in the absence of these valvular disorders, carries a substantially increased risk of ischemic stroke.[1] However, the absolute rate of stroke varies importantly with patient age and coexistent cardiovascular disease.[2,3] Stratification of AF patients into those at high and low risk for thromboembolism is a crucial determinant of optimal antithrombotic prophylaxis.

Two studies included sufficient numbers of patients and strokes, analyzed by multivariable techniques, and provide the most reliable stratification schemes available (see Table 1): the SPAF I placebo patient[4] and the AF pooled analysis[2] that Singer alluded to. The differences in the two schemes (age >65 years vs heart failure) are not contradictory or even substantially conflicting, since clinical variables overlap (age is related to heart failure, hypertension, and diabetes). Interestingly, intermittent (ie, paroxysmal) AF was not an independent predictor of thromboembolic risk in either study. In sum, the five clinical variables listed in Table 1 are independently predictive of thromboembolic risk and are clinically useful to characterize AF patients at high and low risk for stroke.

Echocardiographic predictors of increased thromboembolic risk in AF are enlarged left atrial size (mitigated by mitral regurgitation) and, independently, impaired left ventricular function.[4-6]

From DiMarco JP, Prystowsky EN (eds): *Atrial Arrhythmias: State of the Art.* Armonk, NY, Futura Publishing Company, Inc., © 1995.

327

TABLE 1.   Risk Stratification in Atrial Fibrillation:* Independent
Predictors of Thromboembolic Risk

	SPAF I placebo patients[2]	AFI pooled analysis[2]
Number of Patients	568	1236
Number of Events	46	81
High-Risk Variables	Hx of hypertension	Hx of hypertension
	Prior stroke/TIA	Prior stroke/TIA
	Diabetes	Diabetes
	Recent heart failure	Age > 65 years
Thromboembolic Rate (95% CI)		
Low-risk	1.4%/yr (0.05–3.7)	1.0%/yr (0.3–3.1)
High-risk	>7%/yr	>5%/yr
Percentage of cohort "low-risk"	38%	15%

SPAF = Stroke Prevention in Atrial Fibrillation study
AFI = Atrial Fibrillation Investigators
*Large, prospectively acquired data sets analyzed by multivariable techniques. The SPAF I placebo data set[1] was included in the pooled analysis of clinical trials by the Atrial Fibrillation Investigators.[2]

Impaired left ventricular function may further contribute to stasis within the left atrium in AF patients.[7,8] Precordial echocardiographic findings can be combined with clinical risk stratifiers to identify AF patients with very low inherent rates of thromboembolism.[4] The predictive value of transesophageal echocardiographic findings (such as left atrial appendage thrombi and/or "smoke" type of diversities) for subsequent stroke has yet to be validated by adequate clinical studies; at present, data are insufficient to recommend routine transesophageal echocardiography to stratify thromboembolic potential in AF patients.

Antithrombotic Trials: Lessons Learned and Questions to be Answered

Singer reviewed each of the randomized trials in the prevention of stroke in AF. From these trials, three main concepts have evolved that deserve a brief comment.

Significant Efficacy of Oral Anticoagulation

Anticoagulation with oral vitamin K antagonists such as warfarin is highly effective for reducing ischemic stroke in AF patients. Five recent randomized clinical trials using INR ranges of approximately 1.0 to 4.2 showed a mean reduction in ischemic stroke of nearly 70% in patients assigned anticoagulation; on-therapy analysis indicated an even greater benefit.[2] The incremental risk of serious bleeding was <1%/y among anticoagulated patients selected for participation in these clinical trials and followed carefully on protocols. Low-intensity anticoagulation (INR, 2.0 to 3.0) clearly confers benefit.[2,9] Warfarin is very effective in subgroups of AF patients with a high inherent risk of thromboembolism (see Table 1).[2,10]

The Questionable Safety of Oral Anticoagulation

The safety and tolerability of chronic anticoagulation to conventional levels has not been well defined in the very elderly (>75 years old), the subgroup encompassing perhaps half of AF-associated stroke. All but one of the placebo-controlled clinical trials testing anticoagulation enrolled AF patients with a mean age in the late 60s.[2] The single placebo-controlled trial involving AF patients with a mean age of 75 years reported a 38% withdrawal rate from anticoagulation after 1 year.[11] The recently reported SPAF II trial comparing anticoagulation in AF patients ≤75 and >75 years old found that the risk of major hemorrhage during anticoagulation (INR range, 2.0 to 4.5; mean INR, 2.7) was substantially increased in AF patients >75 years old compared with younger AF patients anticoagulated to similar intensities.[10] While the very elderly have a greater risk of AF-associated stroke, the benefit of anticoagulation in SPAF II was offset somewhat by its greater toxicity in this age group. Indeed, in agreement with Singer's comments, lower-intensity anticoagulation may be as effective and is certainly safer,[9] and pending results of ongoing clinical trials, it seem sensible to seek a target INR of ≤2.0 in AF patients >75 years old.

The Questionable Efficacy of Aspirin

The efficacy of aspirin, an antiplatelet agent, for stroke prevention in AF patients is less clear and remains controversial.[2] The effect of aspirin in doses between 75 and 325 mg/d has been assessed in three randomized, placebo-controlled clinical trials with a statistically significant risk reduction of about 25% (range, 14% to 44%) in aspirin-treated patients, considering pooled data,[12,13] also including the recently reported European Atrial Fibrillation Trial (EAFT).[14] However, aspirin was significantly less effective than anticoagulation in two of these clinical trials[13,14] and also by secondary on-therapy analysis of SPAF II.[10] There is no compelling evidence that the specific dose of aspirin between 75 and 325 mg/d confers more or less benefit. In short, aspirin has some degree of efficacy for preventing AF-associated stroke, but it is clearly less than that of anticoagulation.

Conclusion: Who Should Receive Antithrombotics? Which one?

Primary Prevention of Stroke in AF Patients

Pending the completion of ongoing clinical studies, "low-risk" AF patients ≤75 years old can be given aspirin (325 mg/d) to prevent stroke; aspirin is particularly justified if risk factors for atherosclerotic disease or for noncardioembolic stroke are present. Patients at "high risk" for cardioembolic stroke (prior stroke/transient ischemic attack, heart failure, systolic hypertension, or increase in left atrial or left ventricular size by echocardiography) who can safely receive anticoagulation should be treated with warfarin. For "high-risk" AF patients ≤75 years old, an INR range of 2.0 to 3.0 is safe and effective; for those >75 years old, a lower target INR of ≤2.0 is recommended. AF patients who cannot safely receive anticoagulation should be given aspirin.

Secondary Prevention of Stroke in AF Patients

In AF patients with acute stroke, the risk of recurrent stroke (within 2 weeks) is relatively low. Initiating oral anticoagulation within a few days in submassive infarcts seems reasonable; a delay in starting warfarin of 1 week or more in AF patients with large infarcts may be prudent to avoid accentuating secondary brain hemorrhage. According to the EAFT, in AF patients with previous stroke or transient ischemic attack with or without carotid artery stenosis, long-term anticoagulation is an optimal treatment for secondary prevention for all who can safely receive it. The long-term rate of recurrent stroke is high, exceeding 10% per year. Although the EAFT documented an INR of 2.5 to 4.0 to be relatively safe, pending results of ongoing trials, lower INR as suggested in primary prevention may be optimal.

To quote Andrew Laupacis in a recent editorial[15]: "The past 5 years have seen enormous progress in the antithrombotic management of patients with atrial fibrillation. We now know that most patients benefit from anticoagulation therapy if the drug is monitored closely. Over the next 5 years the aims are to clarify the role of aspirin, the optimum intensity of anticoagulation, and whether a combination of low-dose warfarin and aspirin is better than conventional-dose warfarin alone."

References

1. Wolf PA, Abbott RD, Kannel WB. Atrial fibrillation as an independent risk factor for stroke: the Framingham Study. *Stroke.* 1991;22:983–988.
2. Atrial Fibrillation Investigators. Risk factors for stroke and efficacy of antithrombotic therapy in atrial fibrillation: analysis of pooled data from five randomized controlled trials. *Ann Intern. Med.* 1994;154:1449–1457.
3. Stroke Prevention in Atrial Fibrillation Investigators. Predictors of thromboembolism in atrial fibrillation, I: clinical features of patients at risk. *Ann Intern Med.* 1992;116:1–5.
4. Stroke Prevention in Atrial Fibrillation Investigators. Predictors of thromboembolism in atrial fibrillation, II: echocardiographic features of patients at risk. *Ann Intern Med.* 1992;116:6–12.
5. Kopekcy SL, Gersh BJ, McGoon MD, Whisnant JP, Holmes DR, Ilstrup DM, Frye RL. The natural history of lone atrial fibrillation: a population-based study over three decades. *N Engl J Med.* 1987;317:669–674.
6. Blackshear JL, Pearce LA, Asinger RW, Dittrich HC, Goldman ME, Zabalgoitia M, Rothbart RM, Halperin JL. Mitral regurgitation associated with reduced thromboembolic events in high risk patients with atrial fibrillation. *J Am Coll Cardiol.* In press.
7. Rosenthal MS, Halperin JL. Thromboembolism in nonvalvular atrial fibrillation: the answer may be in the ventricle. *Int J Cardiol.* 1992;37: 277–282.
8. Zabalgoitia M, Dipeshkumar KG, McPherson D, et al. Spontaneous echo contrast in severe left ventricular dysfunction: a risk factor for thromboembolism. *Circulation.* 1990;84 (suppl III):III–109. Abstract.

9. Veterans Affairs Stroke Prevention in Non-rheumatic Atrial Fibrillation Investigators. Warfarin in the prevention of stroke associated with non-rheumatic atrial fibrillation. *N Engl J Med.* 1992;327:1406–1412.
10. Stroke Prevention in Atrial Fibrillation Investigators. Warfarin versus aspirin for prevention of thromboembolism in atrial fibrillation: stroke prevention in atrial fibrillation II study. *Lancet.* 1994;343:687–691.
11. Petersen P, Boysen G, Godtfredsen J, Andersen ED, Andersen B. Placebo-controlled randomized trial of warfarin and aspirin prevention of thromboembolic complications in chronic atrial fibrillation. *Lancet.* 1989;1:175–179.
12. Stroke Prevention in Atrial Fibrillation Investigators. The Stroke Prevention in Atrial Fibrillation Study: final results. *Circulation.* 1991;84: 527–539.
13. Petersen P, Boysen G. Prevention of stroke in atrial fibrillation. *N Engl J Med.* 1990;323:482.
14. EAFT Study Group. European Atrial Fibrillation Trial: Secondary prevention of vascular events in patients with non-rheumatic atrial fibrillation and recent transient ischemic attack or minor stroke. *Lancet.* 1993;342:1255.
15. Laupacis A. Anticoagulatants for atrial fibrillation. *Lancet.* 1993;342: 1251.

Chapter 13

Electrical Therapy of Atrial Arrhythmias

Carlos A. Morillo, MD;
George J. Klein, MD, FRCPC, FACC;
and Raymond Yee, MD, FRCPC, FACC

Introduction

Atrial arrhythmias occur in all age groups and are associated with a multitude of causes. Antiarrhythmic drugs constitute the usual therapy when therapy is necessary, with electrical therapy generally considered in symptomatic patients refractory to medical therapy. Electrical therapy may be used to prevent tachycardia (ie, bradycardia pacing), terminate tachycardia (ie, antitachycardia pacing),[1-9] or eliminate the arrhythmogenic substrate (ie, catheter ablation[10-14] of diverse atrial arrhythmias). Atrial tachycardias are defined as supraventricular tachycardias in which the tachycardia mechanism resides entirely in the atria. The clinical diagnosis is made when the tachycardia persists even in the presence of atrioventricular (AV) nodal block such as produced by adenosine. Underlying cardiac or pulmonary disease is frequently observed in the adult with atrial tachycardia.[15,16] The onset of the tachycardia may be paroxysmal or nonparoxysmal, and termination of the tachycardia is generally not achieved by vagotonic maneuvers.

Focal ("Ectopic") Atrial Tachycardias

Focal ("ectopic") atrial tachycardia is an uncommon cause of superventricular tachycardia, accounting for <10% of supraventric-

From DiMarco JP, Prystowsky EN (eds): *Atrial Arrhythmias: State of the Art.* Armonk, NY, Futura Publishing Company, Inc., © 1995.

ular tachycardias studied in most electrophysiology laboratories.[16] Patients usually have a history of cardiac or pulmonary disease, although young adults and children may have the tachycardia in the absence of cardiopulmonary disease.[17–21] Tachycardia is regular and characterized by an ectopic P-wave morphology and rate between 100 and 240 beats per minute. Variable degrees of AV block or 1:1 AV conduction may be observed.[16,22,23]

The clinical presentation varies widely, symptomatic patients usually presenting with paroxysmal tachycardia. Exercise intolerance or congestive heart failure may be the predominant manifestation in patients with incessant tachycardia.[17–19]

The mechanism of the tachycardia is variable and may often be determined by programmed electrical stimulation. Failure to induce or terminate the tachycardia by programmed stimulation suggests that "abnormal automaticity" may be the underlying mecha-

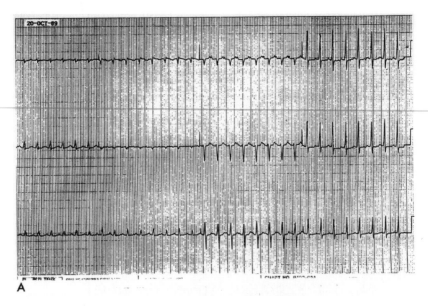

A

FIGURE 1A.   *Ectopic atrial tachycardia. The 12-lead ECG in a patient presenting with incessant atrial tachycardia and heart failure shows a narrow QRS complex tachycardia at a cycle length of 320 msec. P waves are visible as a sharp deflection superimposed on the T wave in lead V_1.*

nism.[15] Intra-atrial reentry is readily induced by programmed stimulation, and the diagnostic criteria include (1) consistent induction and termination of tachycardia by atrial extrastimuli at critical coupling intervals, (2) demonstration of intra-atrial conduction delay, (3) observation of abnormalities of conduction and refractoriness during baseline study, and (4) the demonstration of entrainment and reset during tachycardia.[16] Triggered activity may be an alternative mechanism, particularly when verapamil or adenosine terminates the tachycardia.

Experience with antitachycardia pacing therapy in patients with ectopic atrial tachycardia is confined to a handful of case reports.[3,4,7,24] Antitachycardia pacing is limited to those cases in which tachycardia is reproducibly terminated by programmed stimulation (usually, intra-atrial reentry). Catheter ablation using DC energy and, more recently, radiofrequency ablation of atrial foci have been demonstrated to be feasible and associated with acceptable success rates and satisfactory short-term outcome (Fig 1).[17,25,26] It is probable that catheter ablation will become the preferred nonpharmacological therapy for these arrhythmias.

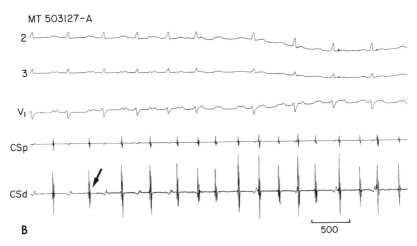

FIGURE 1B. *Ectopic atrial tachycardia. Surface ECG leads 2, 3, and V₁ and intracardiac electrograms from the proximal (CSp) and distal (CSd) coronary sinus electrodes are shown. Earliest atrial activation during tachycardia occurred at the CSd (arrow), demonstrating a left atrial focus.*

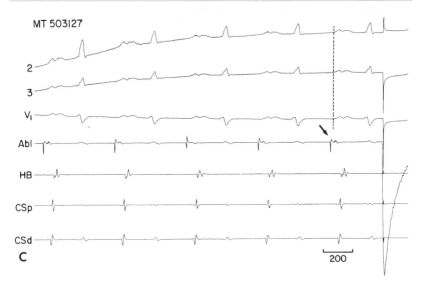

FIGURE 1C. *Atrial tachycardia ablation. Electrogram at the ideal site for radiofrequency catheter ablation is shown. The broken line indicates the onset of the P wave on the surface ECG. Atrial electrogram recorded by the distal pole of the ablation catheter (arrow) preceded the earliest atrial activation (CSd). Radiofrequency energy delivered at this site successfully terminated atrial tachycardia. Abl=ablation catheter; HB=His bundle electrogram; other abbreviations same as in B, D.*

Sinus Node Reentrant Tachycardia

Sinus node reentrant tachycardia is a supraventricular tachycardia with electrocardiographic and electrophysiological characteristics suggesting sinus node origin. Sinus node reentry is infrequently associated with clinical symptoms, and therapy is rarely indicated. In some refractory cases, radiofrequency ablation in the sinus node area has been reported to be successful.[25]

Atrial Flutter

Atrial flutter occurs more often in patients with structural heart disease and may be paroxysmal or, less frequently, chronic. Atrial flutter is characterized by an atrial rate between 240 and 300 beats per minute. The ventricular response rate is usually half the atrial rate. Atrial flutter has been classified according to electrocardiographic characteristics and response to programmed stimulation.

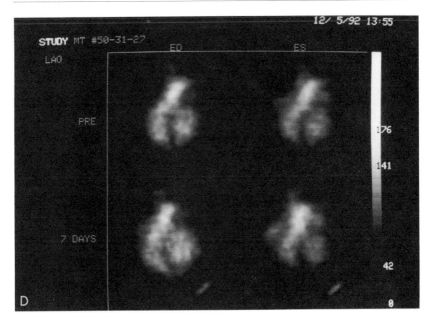

FIGURE 1D.   *Radionuclide angiograms of the same patient before ablation (Pre) and 7 days after the procedure. Ejection fraction was calculated at 23% before the ablation. A marked improvement was noted 7 days after the ablation with an ejection fraction of 52%. ED=end diastole; ES=end systole; LAO=left anterior oblique; Pre=preablation.*

Typical ("common") atrial flutter (type I) is characterized by negative flutter or F waves in the inferior limb leads (II, III, and aVF). The rate is usually around 300 beats per minute, and it can be entrained and terminated with atrial pacing.[27] In atypical atrial flutter (type II), F waves are positive in the inferior limbs, rate varies between 240 and 340 beats per minute, and rapid atrial pacing does not terminate the arrhythmia.

Recent studies in humans have established that the mechanism leading to typical atrial flutter is a large reentrant circuit in the right atrium.[28–31] The circuit proceeds from the coronary sinus os region ("counterclockwise") up the atrial septum and returns via the crista terminalis to the coronary sinus orifice region (Fig 2). The area of slow conduction has been identified in the low posteroseptal right atrium by the presence of prolonged low-amplitude fragmented electrical activity and long stimulus–to–P wave intervals during pacing entrainment.[32–34] The mechanism of atypical flutter has been suggested to be similar, with the circuit proceeding in the "clockwise" direction.[35]

H.P. 318737

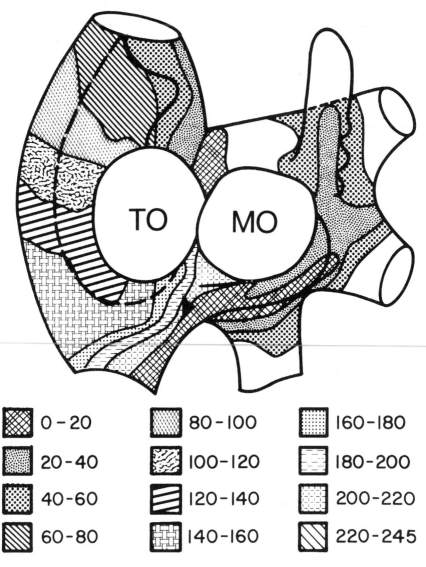

▨	0-20	▨	80-100	▦	160-180
▧	20-40	▨	100-120	▦	180-200
▦	40-60	▨	120-140	▦	200-220
▨	60-80	▦	140-160	▨	220-245

FIGURE 2.   *Atrial flutter isochronal map. Diagrammatic representation of the atrial epicardial surface is shown. Earliest activation site is shown at the coronary sinus ostium (arrowhead). The circuit proceeds from the coronary sinus ostium region ("counterclockwise") up the atrial septum and returns via the crista terminalis to the coronary sinus orifice region. TO=tricuspid orifice; MO=mitral orifice.*

Experience with antitachycardia pacing for the management of refractory atrial flutter is limited.[5,36] Such therapy is feasible only in patients with type I atrial flutter, proven to be reproducibly terminated by pacing at electrophysiological study. DC ablation and radiofrequency catheter ablation guided to the posterior and/or inferior coronary sinus ostium have been reported recently, with promising results (Fig 3).[37–39] Although longer follow-up periods are necessary to estab-

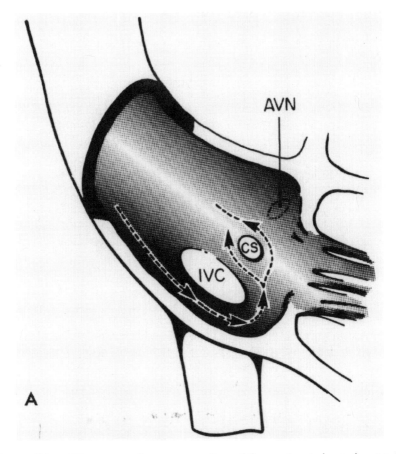

FIGURE 3A.   *Diagrammatic representation of the anatomic basis for atrial flutter ablation with a longitudinal view of the right atrium as if the right atrial free wall had been removed. Radiofrequency energy is delivered between the tricupsid annulus and the inferior limit of the coronary sinus (CS) as well as the posterior coronary sinus orifice and the inferior vena caval (IVC) regions. AVN=atrioventricular node.*

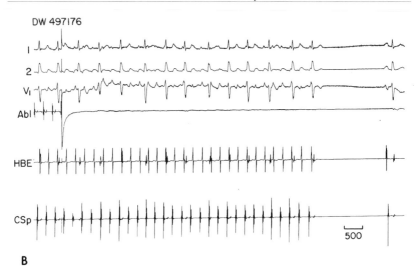

B

FIGURE 3B. *Atrial flutter radiofrequency ablation. ECG surface leads 1, 2, and V₁ and three intracardiac electrograms are shown. Radiofrequency energy delivered immediately posterior and inferior to the coronary sinus ostium terminates atrial flutter (last beat). Abl=ablation catheter; CSp= proximal coronary sinus; HBE=His bundle electrogram.*

lish long-term benefits, it is probable that catheter ablation will become the preferred electrical therapy for this arrhythmia.

Atrial Fibrillation

Although atrial fibrillation (AF) is by far the most prevalent sustained arrhythmia, therapeutic interventions directed at controlling and preventing the recurrence of AF have not been entirely satisfactory.[40-44] AF may be paroxysmal or chronic and is commonly associated with hypertension, congestive heart failure, rheumatic valvular disease, or no underlying heart disease (lone AF).[45] AF may also be classified as "primary" or "secondary." Primary AF occurs directly in the absence of other preceding arrhythmia. In secondary AF, another tachycardia, such as AV nodal reentrant or AV reentrant tachycardia, consistently precedes and precipitates AF (Fig 4). In the latter instance, therapy is generally directed at the inciting arrhythmia.

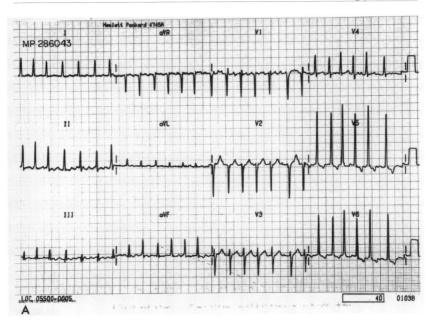

Figure 4A. *Idiopathic atrial fibrillation. Twelve-lead ECG in a 35-year-old patient with paroxysmal atrial fibrillation with rapid ventricular response (mean, 159 beats per minute) is shown.*

Electrocardiographically, AF is identified by absence of discrete organized atrial activity, the presence of a variable RR interval, and an irregular baseline between QRS complexes. The atrial "rate" varies between 350 and 550 beats per minute, with a widely variable ventricular response.

The basic electrophysiological mechanisms underlying the genesis and maintenance of AF remain incompletely understood. Historically, two main hypotheses have been proposed, namely, a rapidly firing atrial focus (or foci) or multiple reentrant circuits.[46–50] It is possible that the two mechanisms may coexist. Recent studies from Allessie et al[50] support the multiple-wavelet hypothesis. These studies suggest that multiple wavelets resulting from random intra-atrial reentry of the leading-circle type form the basis of AF.[50] We recently developed a reproducible model of sustained AF in the dog.[51] In this model, chronic rapid atrial pacing was maintained for 6 weeks, after which sustained AF was readily inducible in 80% of the dogs.[51] AF was associated with biatrial myopathy and marked

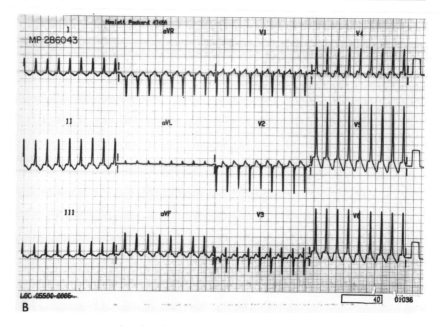

FIGURE 4B.   Twelve-lead ECG during electrophysiology study. Narrow complex tachycardia at a rate of 320 msec induced by programmed electrical stimulation is shown. The tachycardia always precipitated atrial fibrillation in this patient.

changes in atrial vulnerability. An area confined to the left posterior atrium was uniformly documented to have a shorter AF cycle length (Fig 5). Multiple cryoablation applications at this site significantly prolonged the atrial cycle length, terminating the arrhythmia or converting it into atrial flutter in most animals. In the same model, left atrial multipoint rapid pacing using a mesh electrode with an area of 6 cm^2 was performed during AF (unpublished). Rapid pacing at short intervals resulted in local capture of AF (Fig 6), although AF could not be terminated by this technique. Similar results limited to smaller captured areas in the left atrium have recently been reported.[52]

These findings suggest that the mechanism leading to AF in this model may be related to an area localized to the posterior left atrium. The ability of this area to sustain rapid atrial rates may be related to the maintenance of chronic AF. Further support for this hypothesis may be derived from analysis of the epicardial electrograms obtained

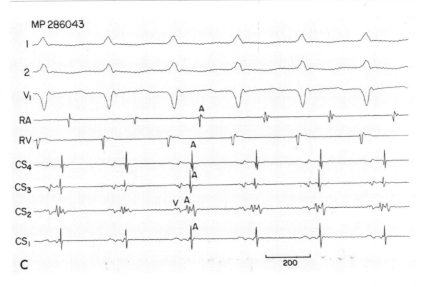

FIGURE 4C. *Electrophysiology study. Surface ECG leads 1, 2, and V_1 and six intracardiac electrograms during tachycardia are shown. Earliest retrograde activation occurred in the distal coronary sinus (CS_2), followed by the proximal coronary sinus (CS_3), indicating the presence of a concealed left lateral accessory pathway. Radiofrequency ablation of the pathway achieved control of the patient's atrial fibrillation. A=atrial electrogram; CS_1, CS_2=distal coronary sinus; CS_3, CS_4=proximal coronary sinus; RA=right atrial electrogram; RV=right ventricular apex electrogram.*

before discharge from patients undergoing "corridor" surgery for AF at our institution. This operation effectively divides the atria into three electrically isolated regions, two in the right atrium and one in the left atrium. Thirteen patients have undergone this operation between 1985 and 1993. Persistence of AF in the excluded left atrium was observed in 9 (70%) of the 13 patients. In contrast, AF in the right excluded atrium was documented in only 1 patient.[53] Early reports using surgical left atrial isolation in patients with AF also documented fibrillation in the excluded left atrium.[54] The explanation for this finding is unclear. However, a shorter refractory period in the left atrium has been experimentally documented.[55] The cycle length of local activation during AF correlates with local refractoriness,[56,57] and we recently reported a significantly shorter mean left AF cycle length (LA, 81 ± 8 msec vs RA, 94 ± 9 msec) in our experimental model,[51] consistent with

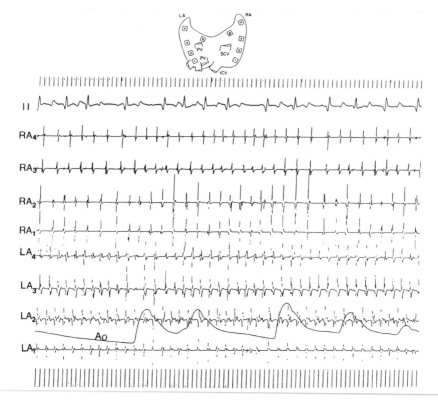

FIGURE 5.   *Experimental atrial fibrillation. Sustained atrial fibrillation induced by programmed stimulation in a dog. Surface ECG lead II and eight bipolar epicardial electrograms are shown. Upper part of the figure shows a diagram that depicts the distribution of the epicardial electrodes on the right and left atria. Shortest mean atrial fibrillation cycle length was localized to the posterior left atria (80 msec; LA_1, LA_2) compared with 99 msec in the right atria. Ao=aortic pressure; IVC=inferior vena cava; LA_1, LA_2=left posterior atria; LA_3, LA_4=left atrial appendage; PV=pulmonary veins; RA_1, RA_2=right posterior atria; RA_3, RA_4=right atrial appendage; SVC=superior vena cava.*

that reported by Allessie et al.[52] Therefore, it is possible to speculate that shorter refractory periods in the left atrium capable of sustaining faster atrial rates, associated with an anatomic obstacle (ie, pulmonary veins), may provide the "generator" necessary to maintain AF in some patients.

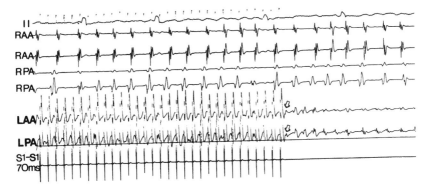

FIGURE 6. *Multiple-site pacing. ECG lead II and six bipolar epicardial electrograms in a dog with sustained atrial fibrillation are shown. Multipoint pacing of the left atrial wall and left posterior region using a 6-cm² mesh electrode at a cycle length of 70 msec is shown. Regional capture of the left atria is achieved, but no effect on the right atrial fibrillation interval was observed. Cessation of pacing (arrows) did not terminate atrial fibrillation. LAA=left atrial appendage; LPA=left posterior atria; RAA= right atrial appendage; RPA=right posterior atria; S1-S1=atrial pacing interval.*

Therapy for AF

A major goal of therapy is directed toward the control of ventricular response and reduction of the hemodynamic consequences of AF. Restoration and maintenance of sinus rhythm are the primary goal when possible.

Pacing Therapy

Pacing therapy may be useful for the prevention of AF, especially when onset of AF is consistently related to preceding bradycardia. The importance of pacing mode in patients with a pacemaker implanted for sinus node dysfunction or AV node disease has recently been emphasized.[1,58–62] In nonrandomized studies, the incidence of AF as well as morbidity and mortality appear to be decreased with physiological pacing (DDD or AAI) compared with ventricular pacing (VVI or DVI) modes.[58-61] Hesselson et al[61] recently reported the effects of single-chamber pacing in over 900 patients, followed for a period of 7 years. Overall, AF developed in 14% of patients, 4% with DDD pacing mode, 8% DVI, and 19% VVI. Mortality was significantly higher in patients with VVI and DVI pacemakers: 50% and 38%, respectively, compared with 22% in those with a DDD pacemaker. In a recent retrospective study,[62] the occurrence of AF in a series of patients with a DDD pacemaker was 10%. The risk of developing AF was higher in those patients with a prior history of AF and sick sinus syndrome. Other nonrandomized comparative studies have reported a lower incidence of thromboembolic stroke when AAI or DDD pacing modes were used, compared with VVI.[58-60] It has been suggested that the higher occurrence of AF may be related to an increased release of atrial natriuretic peptide triggered by atrial stretching due to retrograde flow through intermittently incompetent atrioventricular valves.[63,64]

It is possible that physiological pacing in patients requiring pacing may be an important measure to prevent the occurrence of AF. This remains to be confirmed by prospective randomized trials comparing physiological to ventricular pacing therapy.

Control of Ventricular Response

Control of the ventricular rate is the primary objective in patients with established AF. Ventricular pacing may have a role in this regard. Witttkampf and de Jongste[65] recently observed that right ventricular pacing in patients with AF eliminated spontaneous RR intervals shorter than the pacing cycles. Pacing at a fixed rate slightly faster than the mean ventricular response during AF abolished >95% of spontaneous ventricular activity. Heart rate was consequently regularized to the actual pacing rate. These investigators have developed an automatic pacing algorithm capable of regularizing the ventricular response in patients with AF.[66] The role of this pacing method remains theoretical, and long-term efficacy is unknown.

Radiofrequency catheter modification of the posterior AV node input has also been described as a potential method of achieving ventricular rate control.[67,68] This is based on the observation that "slow-pathway" conduction in patients with AV node reentry can be ablated in this region. The theoretical basis is that the posterior input region has a shorter refractory period even in patients without overt dual-pathway physiology. The role and long-term efficacy of this approach require further investigation.

The preferred nonpharmacological method for rate control in most patients with established drug-refractory AF is currently radiofrequency catheter ablation of the AV node. Reported success rates range between 62% and 94%, with a recurrence rate of 5%.[69–73] This technique has a low incidence of complications and may be safely performed without general anesthesia. The major limitations of this procedure are that ablation of the AV node has no effect on the incidence of thromboembolic complications, the atrial contribution to hemodynamics is lost, and permanent pacing is required.

Electrical Cardioversion

Transthoracic electrical cardioversion remains the standard method of terminating AF in drug-refractory patients. This is usually most effective in patients with AF or recent onset (<3 months' duration) and in patients presenting with acute AF associated with poor hemodynamic tolerance.[74] Successful conversion to normal sinus rhythm is achieved in up to 90% of patients and may be related to the duration of AF and underlying cardiac disease. Maintenance of sinus rhythm depends on atrial size, progression of heart disease, co-morbid conditions, and appropriate selection of antiarrhythmic therapy.

Recently, results of transvenous catheter atrial defibrillation in animals and humans have been reported.[75–80] Levy et al[78] reported limited success rates unless high energies were delivered between a transvenous catheter positioned in the right atrium and a chest wall electrode. In contrast, Cooper et al[77] used an animal model and reported high success rates with a biphasic waveform (1.3 ± 0.4 J) delivered between two transvenous electrodes placed in the right atrium and coronary sinus. The major obstacles to the use of such therapy include the concern of inadvertent induction of ventricular fibrillation and the pain associated with cardioversion even with energies as low as 0.5 J. The potential role of an implantable atrial defibrillator remains to be elucidated.

Summary and Conclusions

Electrical therapy of atrial arrhythmias has rapidly expanded, and newer indications are foreseen in the future. Many atrial arrhythmias may be treated by radiofrequency catheter ablation, and the role of catheter ablation will undoubtedly increase. AF remains the ultimate challenge.

References

1. Gross JN, Sackstein RD, Furman S. Cardiac pacing and atrial arrhythmias. *Cardiol Clin.* 1992;10:609–617.
2. Attuel P, Pellerin D, Mugica J, et al. DDD pacing: an effective treatment modality for recurrent atrial arrhythmias. *PACE Pacing Clin Electrophysiol.* 1988;11:1647–1654.
3. Fisher JD, Kim SG, Mercando AD. Electrical devices for treatment of arrhythmias. *Am J Cardiol.* 1988;61:45A–57A.
4. Goyal SL, Lichstein E, Gupta PK, et al. Refractory reentrant atrial tachycardia: successful treatment with a permanent radio frequency triggered atrial pacemaker. *Am J Med.* 1975;58:586–590.
5. Wyndham CR, Wu D, Denes P, et al. Self-initiated conversion of paroxysmal atrial flutter utilizing a radio-frequency pacemaker. *Am J Cardiol.* 1978;1119–1122.
6. Peters RW, Scheinman MM, Morady F, et al. Long-term management of recurrent paroxysmal tachycardia by burst pacing. *PACE Pacing Clin Electrophysiol.* 1985;8:35–44.
7. den Dulk K, Bertholet M, Brugada P, et al. Clinical experience with implantable devices for control of tachyarrhythmias. *PACE Pacing Clin Electrophysiol.* 1984;7:548–556.
8. Abinader EG. Recurrent supraventricular tachycardia: success and subsequent failure of termination by implanted endocardial pacemaker. *JAMA.* 1976;236:2203–2205.
9. Luderitz B, d'Alnoncourt CN, Steibeck G, et al. Therapeutic pacing in tachyarrhythmias by implanted pacemakers. *PACE Pacing Clin Electrophysiol.* 1982;5:366–371.
10. Gürsoy S, Schlüter M, Kuck KH. Radiofrequency current catheter ablation for control of supraventricular arrhythmias. *J Cardiovasc Electrophysiol.* 1993;4:194–205.
11. Gallagher JJ, Svenson RH, Kasell JH, et al. Catheter technique for closed chest ablation of the atrioventricular conduction system. *N Engl J Med.* 1982;306:194–200.
12. Warin JF, Haissaguerre M, Lemetayer P, et al. Catheter ablation of accessory pathways with a direct approach: results in 35 patients. *Circulation.* 1988;78:800–815.

13. Hassaguerre M, Warin JF, Lemateyer P, et al. Closed-chest ablation of retrograde conduction in patients with atrioventricular nodal reentrant tachycardia. *N Engl J Med*. 1989;320:426–433.
14. Huang SK, Bharati S, Graham AR, et al. Closed chest catheter desiccation of the atrioventricular junction using radiofrequency energy: a new method of catheter ablation. *J Am Coll Cardiol*. 1987;9:349–358.
15. Wu D, Denes P, Amat-y-Leon F. Clinical, electrocardiographic and electrophysiologic observations in patients with paroxysmal supraventricular tachycardia. *Am J Cardiol*. 1978;41:1045–1051.
16. Wathen MS, Klein GJ, Yee R, et al. Classification and terminology of supraventricular tachycardia. *Cardiol Clin*. 1993;11:109–120.
17. Gillette P, Wampler D, Garson A, et al. Treatment of atrial automatic tachycardia by ablation procedures. *J Am Coll Cardiol*. 1985;6:405–409.
18. Goldreyer B, Gallagher JJ, Damato A. The electrophysiologic demonstration of ectopic atrial tachycardia in man. *Am Heart J*. 1973;85:205–215.
19. Keane J, Plauth W, Nadas A. Chronic ectopic tachycardia of infancy and childhood. *Am Heart J*. 1972;84:748–757.
20. Levine H, Smith C. Repetitive paroxysmal tachycardia in adults. *Cardiology*. 1970;55:2–21.
21. Parkinson J, Papp C. Repetitive paroxysmal tachycardia. *Br Heart J*. 1947;9:241–262.
22. Klein G, Sharma A, Yee R, et al. Classification of supraventricular tachycardias. *Am J Cardiol*. 1987;60:27D–31D.
23. Lown B, Wyatt N, Levine H. Paroxysmal atrial tachycardia with block. *Circulation*. 1960;21:129–143.
24. Arbel ER, Cohen CH, Langendorf R, et al. Successful treatment of drug-resistant atrial tachycardia and intractable congestive heart failure with permanent coupled atrial pacing. *Am J Cardiol*. 1978;41:336–340.
25. Kay GN, Chong F, Epstein A, et al. Radiofrequency ablation for treatment of primary atrial tachycardias. *J Am Coll Cardiol*. 1993; 21:901–909.
26. Tracy CM, Swartz JF, Fletcher RD, et al. Radiofrequency catheter ablation of ectopic atrial tachycardia using paced activation sequence mapping. *J Am Coll Cardiol*. 1993;21:910–917.
27. Waldo AL, McLean WAH, Karp RB, et al. Entrainment and interruption of atrial flutter with atrial pacing: studies in man following open heart surgery. *Circulation*. 1977;56:737–745.
28. Klein GJ, Guiraudon GM, Sharma AD, et al. Demonstration of macroreentry and feasibility of operative therapy in the common type of atrial flutter. *Am J Cardiol*. 1986;57:587–591.
29. Disertori M, Inama G, Vergara G, et al. Evidence of a reentry circuit in the common type of atrial flutter in man. *Circulation*. 1983;67:434–440.
30. Olshansky B, Okumura K, Henthorn R, et al. Atrial mapping of human atrial flutter demonstrates reentry in the right atrium. *J Am Coll Cardiol*. 1988;7:194A.
31. Chauvin M, Brechenmacher C, Voegtlin JR. Application de la cartographie endocavitaire a l'étude du flutter auriculaire. *Arch Mal Coeur*. 1983;76:1020–1030.

32. Cosio FG, Arribas F, Palacios J, et al. Fragmented electrograms and continuous electrical activity in atrial flutter. *Am J Cardiol.* 1986;57: 1309–1314.

33. Cosio FG, Arribas F, Barbero JM, et al. Validation of double spike electrograms as markers of conduction delay or block in atrial flutter. *Am J Cardiol.* 1988;61:775–780.

34. Olshansky B, Okumura K, Hess PG, et al. Demonstration of an area of slow conduction in human atrial flutter. *J Am Coll Cardiol.* 1990;16: 1639–1648.

35. Cosio FG, Goicolea A, Lòpez-Gil M, et al. Atrial endocardial mapping in the rare form of atrial flutter. *Am J Cardiol.* 1990;66:715–720.

36. Barold SS, Wyndham CRC, Kappenberger LL, et al. Implanted atrial pacemakers for paroxysmal atrial flutter: long-term efficacy. *Ann Intern Med.* 1987;107:144–151.

37. Saoudi N, Atallah G, Kirkorian G, et al. Catheter ablation of atrial myocardium in human type I atrial flutter. *Circulation.* 1990;81:762–771.

38. Feld GK, Fleck RP, Chen PS, et al. Radiofrequency catheter ablation for the treatment of human type 1 atrial flutter. *Circulation.* 1992;86: 1233–1240.

39. Cosio FG, López-Gil M, Goicolea A, et al. Radiofrequency ablation of the inferior vena cava–tricuspid valve isthmus in common atrial flutter. *Am J Cardiol.* 1993;71:705–709.

40. Cox JL, Schuessler RB, D'Agostino HJ, et al. The surgical treatment of atrial fibrillation. *J Thorac Cardiovasc Surg.* 1991;101:569–583.

41. Kannel WB, Wolf PA. Epidemiology of atrial fibrillation. In: Falk RH, Podrid PJ, eds. *Atrial Fibrillation: Mechanisms and Management.* New York, NY: Raven Press; 1992:81–92.

42. Kannel WB, Abbott RD, Savage DD, et al. Epidemiologic features of atrial fibrillation: the Framingham Study. *N Engl J Med.* 1982;306: 1018–1022.

43. Podrid PJ, Falk RH. Management of atrial fibrillation: an overview. In: Falk RH, Podrid PJ, eds. *Atrial Fibrillation: Mechanisms and Management.* New York, NY: Raven Press; 1992:389–411.

44. Feld GK. Atrial fibrillation: is there a safe and highly effective pharmacological treatment? *Circulation.* 1990;82:2248–2250.

45. Leather RA, Kerr CR. Atrial fibrillation in the absence of overt cardiac disease. In: Falk RH, Podrid PJ, eds. *Atrial Fibrillation: Mechanisms and Management.* New York, NY: Raven Press; 1992:93–108.

46. Scher D. Studies on auricular tachycardia caused by aconitine administration. *Proc Soc Exp Biol Med N Y.* 1947;64:233–239.

47. Moe GK, Abildskov JA. Atrial fibrillation as a self-sustaining arrhythmia independent of focal discharge. *Am Heart J.* 1959;58:59–70.

48. Moe GK. On the multiple wavelet hypothesis of atrial fibrillation. *Arch Int Pharmacodyn Ther.* 1962;140:183–188.

49. Allessie MA, Rensma PL, Brugada J, et al. Pathophysiology of atrial fibrillation. In: Zipes DP, Jalife J, eds. *Cardiac Electrophysiology: From Cell to Bedside.* Philadelphia, Pa: WB Saunders Co; 1990:548–559.

50. Allessie MA, Lammers WJEP, Bonke FIM, et al. Experimental evaluation of Moe's multiple wavelet hypothesis of atrial fibrillation. In: Zipes

DP, Jalife J, eds. *Cardiac Electrophysiology and Arrhythmias.* New York, NY: Grune & Stratton; 1985:265–276.

51. Morillo CA, Klein GJ, Jones DL. Experimental atrial fibrillation: evidence for a focal mechanism. *J Am Coll Cardiol.* 1993;21:111A.

52. Allessie M, Kirchof C, Scheffer GJ, et al. Regional control of atrial fibrillation by rapid pacing in conscious dogs. *Circulation.* 1991;84:1689–1697.

53. Leitch JW, Klein GJ, Yee R, et al. Sinus node-atrio-ventricular node isolation: long term results with the corridor operation for atrial fibrillation. *J Am Coll Cardiol.* 1990;17:970–975.

54. Williams JM, Ungerleider RM, Lofland GK, et al. Left atrial isolation: a new technique for the treatment of supraventricular arrhythmias. *J Thorac Cardiovasc Surg.* 1980;80:373–380.

55. Rensma PL, Allessie MA, Lammers WJEP, et al. Length of excitation wave and susceptibility to reentrant atrial arrhythmias in normal conscious dogs. *Circ Res.* 1988;62:395–410.

56. Lammers WJEP, Allessie MA, Rensma PL, et al. The use of fibrillation cycle length to determine spatial dispersion in electrophysiological properties and to characterize the underlying mechanism of fibrillation. *New Trends Arrhythmias.* 1986;2:109–112.

57. Opthof T, Ramdat-Misier AR, Coronel R, et al. Dispersion of refractoriness in canine ventricular myocardium: effects of sympathetic stimulation. *Circ Res.* 1991;68:1204–1215.

58. Rosenqvist M, Brandt J, Schuller H. Long-term pacing in sinus node disease: the effects of stimulation mode on cardiovascular morbidity and mortality. *Am Heart J.* 1988;116:16–22.

59. Zanini R, Facchinetti A, Gallo G, et al. Morbidity and mortality in patients with sinus node disease: comparative effects of atrial and ventricular pacing. *PACE Pacing Clin Electrophysiol.* 1990;13:2076–2079.

60. Stangl K, Seitz K, Wirtzfeld A, et al. Differences between atrial single chamber pacing (AAI) and ventricular single chamber pacing (VVI) with respect to prognosis and antiarrhythmic effect in patients with sick sinus node syndrome. *PACE Pacing Clin Electrophysiol.* 1990;13:2080–2085.

61. Hesselson AB, Parsonnet V, Bernstein AD, et al. Deleterious effects of long-term single-chamber ventricular pacing in patients with sick sinus syndrome: the hidden benefits of dual-chamber pacing. *J Am Coll Cardiol.* 1992;19:1542–1549.

62. Gross JN, Moser S, Benedek ZM, et al. DDD pacing mode survival in patients with a dual-chamber pacemaker. *J Am Coll Cardiol.* 1992;19:1536–1541.

63. Stangl K, Weil J, Laule M, et al. Influence of AV synchrony on the plasma levels of atrial natriuretic peptide (ANP) in patients with total AV block. *PACE Pacing Clin Electrophysiol.* 1988;11:1176–1181.

64. Travill C, Meurig Williams TD, Vardas P, et al. Hypotension in pacemaker syndrome is associated with marked atrial natriuretic peptide (ANP) release. *PACE Pacing Clin Electrophysiol.* 1989;12:1182.

65. Wittkampf FHM, de Jongste MJL. Rate stabilization by right ventricu-

lar on-demand pacing in patients with atrial fibrillation. *PACE Pacing Clin Electrophysiol.* 1986;9:1147–1153.

66. Wittkampf FHM, de Jongste MJL, Lie HI, et al. Effect of right ventricular pacing on ventricular rhythm during atrial fibrillation. *J Am Coll Cardiol.* 1988;11:539–545.

67. Kuck KH, Kunze KP, Schlüter M, et al. Transcatheter modulation by radiofrequency current of atrioventricular nodal conduction in patients with atrial fibrillation. In: Lüderitz B, Saksena S, eds. *Interventional Electrophysiology.* Mt Kisco, NY: Futura Publishing Co, Inc: 1991:271–277.

68. Fleck RP, Chen PS, Boyce K, et al. Radiofrequency modification of atrioventricular conduction by selective ablation of the low posterior septal right atrium in a patient with atrial fibrillation and a rapid ventricular response. *PACE Pacing Clin Electrophysiol.* 1993;16:377–381.

69. Yeung-Lai-Wah J, Alison JF, Lonergan L, et al. High success rate of atrioventricular node ablation with radiofrequency energy. *J Am Coll Cardiol.* 1991;18:1753–1758.

70. Langberg JJ, Chin M, Schamp DJ, et al. Ablation of the atrioventricular junction with radiofrequency energy using a new electrode catheter. *Am J Cardiol.* 1991;67:142–147.

71. Huang SK, Bharati S, Graham AR, et al. Closed chest catheter desiccation of the atrioventricular junction using radiofrequency energy: a new method of catheter ablation. *J Am Coll Cardiol.* 1987;9:349–358.

72. Jackman WM, Wang XZ, Friday KJ, et al. Catheter ablation of atrioventricular junction using radiofrequency current in 17 patients: comparison of standard and large-tip catheter electrodes. *Circulation.* 1991; 83:1562–1576.

73. Olgin JE, Scheinman MM. Comparison of high energy direct current and radiofrequency catheter ablation of the atrioventricular junction. *J Am Coll Cardiol.* 1993;21:557–564.

74. Falk RH, Podrid PJ. Electrical cardioversion of atrial fibrillation. In: Falk RH, Podrid PJ, eds. *Atrial Fibrillation: Mechanisms and Management.* New York, NY: Raven Press; 1992:181–195.

75. Dunbar DN, Tobler HG, Fetter J, et al. Intracavitary electrode catheter cardioversion of atrial tachyarrhythmias in the dog. *J Am Coll Cardiol.* 1986;7:1015–1027.

76. Kumagai K, Yamanouchi Y, Tashiro N, et al. Transesophageal long energy synchronous transcatheter cardioversion of atrial flutter/fibrillation in the dog. *Am Heart J.* 1992;123:417-420.

77. Cooper RAS, Alferness CA, Smith WM, et al. Internal cardioversion of atrial fibrillation in sheep. *Circulation.* 1993;87:1673–1686.

78. Levy S, Lacombe P, Cointe R, et al. High energy transcatheter cardioversion of chronic atrial fibrillation. *J Am Coll Cardiol.* 1988;12:514–518.

79. Levy S, Camm J. An implantable atrial defibrillator: an impossible dream? *Circulation.* 1993;87:1769–1772.

80. Powell AC, Garan H, McGovern BA, et al. Low energy cardioversion of atrial fibrillation in the sheep. *J Am Coll Cardiol.* 1992;20:707–711.

Chapter 13

Editorial Comments

Jerry C. Griffin, MD

In the past decade, the implanted ventricular defibrillator has moved from the status of a case report[1] to a commonly used modality in the treatment of ventricular arrhythmias.[2] Drs Morillo, Klein, and Yee included a number of reports suggesting that prevention of atrial bradycardia and the maintenance of AV synchrony by use of currently available pacemakers lessen the risk of atrial fibrillation. In addition, they cited two new and novel techniques around which an implanted device might be developed for the management of recurring or paroxysmal atrial fibrillation. The work of Allessie et al [3-5] suggests that highly specialized methods of pacing might be able to entrain the atrium and "extinguish" an episode of atrial fibrillation, while Mirowski and Mower[6] first demonstrated the ability to selectively defibrillate the atria by use of catheter electrodes. The purpose of this comment is to review the strengths and weaknesses of these innovative approaches.

Regional Entrainment

In a series of experiments, Allessie and colleagues[3,4] have demonstrated that atrial fibrillation is a result of multiple circulating wavelets and that an excitable gap exists in atrial tissue during atrial fibrillation. In a recent study,[5] they were able to capture a portion of a fibrillating left atrium by delivering high-energy pacing pulses at or near the median activation cycle length of the atrium. The window of entrainment was small, with a mean of 16 msec, and the rate of pacing rapid, with a median cycle length of 98 msec. To achieve capture early in the relative refractory period, the pacing

From DiMarco JP, Prystowsky EN (eds): *Atrial Arrhythmias: State of the Art*. Armonk, NY, Futura Publishing Company, Inc., © 1995.

stimulus was delivered at a voltage six times the atrial threshold measured at a coupling interval of 300 msec. The zone of influence of a single capturing stimulus appeared to be small, roughly 5 cm in diameter. Pacing from a single stimulation site did not achieve capture of all or a critical amount of atrial tissue, nor did it result in termination of the arrhythmia.

At present, the translation of these concepts into an implantable device would encounter several obstacles. Although the number of pacing sites that would be required for termination of atrial fibrillation is unknown, it could be as many as 6 to 10 for atria as large as those of humans. To reach a sixfold margin with chronic atrial electrodes, each pacing site would have to be supplied with considerable voltage. The electrodes would probably have to be distributed over both the right and left atria so as not to leave a critical mass of fibrillating myocardium. Such an electrode system would probably have to be placed by thoracotomy. A transvenous lead system is unlikely, since both atria will probably have to be stimulated. Currently, the only transvenous access to the left atrium is via the coronary sinus. A lead placed there would service only the base of the left atrium and at the same time place the ventricle at risk from rapid high-energy pacing.

Transvenous Atrial Defibrillation

Mirowski and Mower first reported transvenous atrial defibrillation in 1974. Their work in both animals and humans is summarized in a recent article.[6] Other early attempts using internal, transvenous, low-energy shocks[7,8] enjoyed little success, probably because of the suboptimal placement of the electrodes. In these series, both electrodes were placed on the right side of the heart. Neither incorporated any part of the left atrium in the current path.

Most recent studies of atrial defibrillation in humans have used high-energy shocks delivered between an electrode in the right atrium and a skin electrode.[9,10] Typically, a single shock was delivered to convert fibrillation, usually at 200 to 300 J, and thresholds were not measured. Short-term success rates exceeded those for transthoracic defibrillation. Other than occasional transient atrioventricular block, no other traumatic complications or ventricular fibrillation were reported.

Keane et al[11] returned to the idea of low-energy atrial defibrillation using a right atrium–to–coronary sinus shock vector. In that study, patients having a recent onset of atrial fibrillation were cardioverted with a mean energy of 3.4 J.

There is also a growing body of work in animals related to low-energy transvenous atrial defibrillation. Powell et al[12] and Kumagai et al[13] evaluated internal atrial defibrillation in animal models of atrial fibrillation. Although they used different models and different lead fields, they were able to successfully defibrillate the atria with energies <5 J. In all three studies, the left atrium was incorporated in the lead field.

The most extensive study of atrial defibrillation using intravascular electrodes was performed by Cooper et al.[14] They tested a variety of electrode positions, all incorporating the left atrium into the current path. Leads were placed in the coronary sinus, in the left pulmonary artery, and on the left chest wall. The best vector was between the right atrium and the great cardiac vein, just beneath the left atrial appendage. Biphasic shock waveforms performed better than monophasic. The best biphasic waveform had equal durations of 3 msec for each phase. With the optimal lead location and waveform, atrial defibrillation thresholds were 1.3 ±0.4 J. Shock delivery was synchronous with the R wave, and no episodes of ventricular arrhythmia were initiated when that was the case.

We investigated the issue of ventricular proarrhythmia resulting from shocks delivered to the atrium (G. Ayers et al, unpublished data.) A right atrium–to–coronary sinus shock vector was used. Sixteen adult sheep were studied; half (group A) were shocked just below atrial defibrillation threshold and half (group B) at twice threshold. Shocks were delivered according to four protocols: (1) a shock synchronous with the last paced beat of an eight-stimulus sequence (S1); (2) a shock synchronous with a programmed premature stimulus (S2) following an eight-beat drive (S1); (3) a shock synchronous with an S3 following an S2 delivered at the longest interval not allowing sinus escape after an eight-beat drive (S1), a short-long-short sequence; and (4) a shock synchronous with a native beat conducted in atrial fibrillation (Fig 1). Each beat had to occur during a 50-msec window beginning at some programmed in-

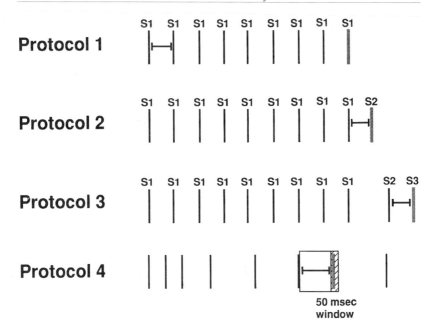

FIGURE 1. *Pacing and shock timing in a study by G. Ayers et al (unpublished data) are illustrated. Single verticle lines represent paced beats (protocols 1 to 3) or native beats (protocol 4). Shock delivery was synchronous with beats represented by shaded lines. In protocol 4, shocks were delivered in atrial fibrillation. A delay was programmed following each beat (open box). If the next beat fell within 50 msec (hatched box) after the delay point was reached, a shock was delivered (shaded line). The horizontal I beam indicates the cycle length, which was decremental in successive runs.*

terval following the previous beat. In each case, after delivery of a shock, either the programmed paced beat or the window was moved closer toward refractoriness, and the shock was repeated. Intravenous epinephrine was used to achieve minimum refractory periods in the ventricle. When the cycle length preceding shock delivery was ≤300 msec, a ventricular arrhythmia was induced after 11 of 964 shocks (Table 1). When the preceding cycle length was >300 msec, no ventricular arrhythmias were seen (895 shocks). There was no difference in the likelihood of proarrhythmia between subthreshold and twice-threshold shocks.

TABLE 1.   Shocks Resulting in Ventricular Fibrillation, Preceding
CL in msec

Group/Protocol	I	II	III	IV
A		230	280	240
		240		
B	250	230	260	198
	300	230		
		250		

The obstacles confronting selective transvenous atrial defibrillation have recently been summarized by Levy and Camm.[15] They cite
pain, detection, and ventricular proarrhythmia as the three major issues. Although certain factors may modulate the degree of perception
of a defibrillating shock, threshold energy requirements will most
likely determine whether pain is a limiting factor. Current animal
threshold levels may be nearing the region at which the level of discomfort is tolerable. Atrial fibrillation will undoubtedly pose a greater
challenge to automated detection than its ventricular counterpart. Bal-
ancing that is the lack of urgency. An acceptable time for detection and
conversion can probably be measured in minutes rather than seconds.
Multiple tests can be applied if necessary, and in sequential order of
sensitivity, specificity, or complexity. The most serious concern is that
for ventricular proarrhythmia. The association between capacitor discharge stimulation of the ventricles during the relative refractory period and ventricular fibrillation has been shown, even for pacing stimuli.[16] Ventricular arrhythmias, including fibrillation, will sometimes
occur if unsynchronized shocks are delivered in the relative refractory
period of the ventricles[12,14] (also G. Ayers, unpublished data). However,
even accurately synchronized shocks may fall during the relative refractory period (of the preceding beat) if the preceding RR interval is
sufficiently short. Thus, it is important that R-wave synchronization be
accurate and shocks be inhibited during periods of tachycardia.

References

1. Mirowski M, Reid PR, Mower MM, et al. Termination of malignant ventricular arrhythmias with an implanted automatic defibrillator in
   human beings. *N Engl J Med*. 1980;303:322–324.

2. Dreifus LS, Fisch C, Griffin JC, et al. Guidelines for implantation of cardiac pacemakers and antiarrhythmia devices. *J Am Coll Cardiol.* 1991; 18:1–13.
3. Allessie MA, Rensma PL, Brugada J, Smeets JL, Penn OC, Kirchhof CJ. Pathophysiology of atrial fibrillation. In: Zipes DP, Jalife J, eds. *Cardiac Electrophysiology: From Cell to Bedside.* Philadelphia, Pa: WB Saunders Co; 1990:548–558.
4. Allessie MA, Kirchhof CJHJ, Scheffer GJ, Chorro FJ, Brugada J. Regional control of atrial fibrillation by rapid pacing in conscious dogs. *Circulation.* 1991;84:1689–1697.
5. Kirchhof C, Chorro F, Scheffer GJ, Brugada J, Konings K, Zetelaki Z, Allessie M. Regional entrainment of atrial fibrillation studied by high-resolution mapping in open-chest dogs. *Circulation.* 1993;88:736–749.
6. Mirowski M, Mower MM. An automatic implantable defibrillator for recurrent atrial tachyarrhythmias. In: Touboul P, Waldo AL, eds. *Atrial Arrhythmias: Current Concepts and Management.* St Louis, Mo: Mosby Yearbook; 1990:419–421.
7. Nathan AW, Bexton RS, et al. Internal transvenous low energy cardioversion for the treatment of cardiac arrhythmias. *Br Heart J.* 1984;52:377–384.
8. Hartlzer GO, Kallok MJ. Low energy transvenous intracavitary cardioversion of tachycardias. In: Steinbach K, ed. *Cardiac Pacing: Proceedings of the VIIth World Symposium on Cardiac Pacing.* Darmstadt, Germany: Steinkopff; 1983:853–858.
9. Levy S, Lacombe P, Cointe R, Bru P. High energy transcatheter cardioversion of chronic atrial fibrillation. *J Am Coll Cardiol.* 1988;12: 514–518.
10. Levy S, Lauribe P, Dolla E, Kou W, Kadish A, Calkins H, Pagannelli F, Moyal C, Bremondy M, Schork A, Shyr Y, Das S, Shea M, Gupta N, Morady F. A randomized comparison of external and internal cardioversion of chronic atrial fibrillation. *Circulation.* 1992;86:1415–1420.
11. Keane D, Sulke N, Cooke R, Jackson G, Sowton E. Endocardial cardioversion of atrial flutter and fibrillation. *PACE Pacing Clin Electrophysiol.* 1993;16:928.
12. Powell A, McGovern B, Garan H, Holden H, Ruskin J. Low energy atrial defibrillation in a sheep model of atrial fibrillation. *J Am Coll Cardiol.* 1991;17:248(A).
13. Kumagai K, Yamanouchi Y, et al. Low energy synchronous transcatheter cardioversion of atrial flutter/fibrillation in the dog. *J Am Coll Cardiol.* 1990;16:497–500.
14. Cooper RAS, Alferness CA, Smith WM, Ideker RE. Internal cardioversion of atrial fibrillation in sheep. *Circulation.* 1993;87:1673–1686.
15. Levy S, Camm J. An implantable atrial defibrillator: an impossible dream? *Circulation.* 1993;87:1769–1772.
16. Mehra R, Furman S. Vulnerability of the mildly ischemic ventricle to cathodal, anodal, and bipolar stimulation. *Circ Res.* 1977;41:159–166.

Chapter 14

Current Indications: Surgical Intervention for Atrial Arrhythmias

James E. Lowe, MD

The indications for surgical intervention for atrial arrhythmias have changed dramatically over the past 5 years with the widespread use and proven success of radiofrequency catheter ablation techniques. Disabling reentrant arrhythmias resulting from the Wolff-Parkinson-White syndrome, concealed accessory atrioventricular (AV) connections, and AV node reentry can usually be eliminated without surgery. However, patients with automatic atrial tachycardia who have failed either medical therapy or radiofrequency catheter ablation attempts and select patients with atrial flutter / fibrillation should be considered for operative intervention to prevent specific long-term complications resulting from each of these arrhythmias.

The purpose of this chapter is to review operative techniques and surgical results for control of these two specific atrial arrhythmias.

Automatic Atrial Tachycardia

Automatic atrial tachycardia (AAT) is an uncommon arrhythmia recognized since the early days of electrocardiography; it was first reported by Lewis in 1909.[1] AAT results from either a single extranodal automatic focus (also referred to as chronic ectopic atrial tachycardia) or increased automaticity or possibly reentry of the sinoatrial node (inappropriate sinus tachycardia).[2]

AAT must be distinguished from multifocal atrial tachycardia, which is usually secondary to an acute or chronic illness.[3] The treatment of multifocal atrial tachycardia is medical and directed toward

From DiMarco JP, Prystowsky EN (eds): *Atrial Arrhythmias: State of the Art.* Armonk, NY, Futura Publishing Company, Inc., © 1995.

controlling the underlying acute or chronic illness causing the arrhythmia. In contrast, patients with AAT have a primary atrial myocardial abnormality that can be cured by either radiofrequency catheter ablation or by an appropriate electrophysiologically guided operation. Numerous patients with AAT have been reported, and the majority cannot be controlled with medical therapy alone.[2] Recently, it has been shown experimentally in our laboratory, as well as clinically, that many patients with AAT developed a tachycardia-induced dilated cardiomyopathy and congestive heart failure.[4,5] Elimination of the tachycardia by either medical, catheter, or surgical intervention usually leads to marked improvement in ventricular function and elimination of congestive heart failure.[2]

Clinical Review

Recently, the clinical courses of all patients with AAT presenting to the Electrophysiology Service at Duke University Medical Center were reviewed.[2] Patients with multifocal atrial tachycardia were excluded. From 1979 to the present, 18 patients, 8 male and 10 female, ranging in age from 13 to 63 years (mean age, 28.1 ± 2.9 years) were diagnosed as having AAT. There were 14 right atrial and 4 left atrial ectopic sites. In addition to our experience, a total of 118 additional patients previously reported in the literature were also available for analysis, and the results of medical and surgical therapy were compared.[2] Although a number of recent reports suggest that radiofrequency catheter ablation for AAT may be highly effective, insufficient numbers of patients have been reported for statistical comparison of surgical therapy with radiofrequency catheter ablation for AAT. However, it is becoming increasingly obvious that the majority of patients referred for surgery in the future will have undergone attempted radiofrequency catheter ablation.

Diagnosis

AAT can usually be diagnosed by the standard ECG followed by an electrophysiological study to confirm the site of the automatic focus.[3] Typically, the surface ECG shows an incessant, narrow, complex SVT (Fig 1). In patients with inappropriate sinus tachycardia, P waves remain unchanged, and in patients with chronic ectopic atrial tachycardia, the P-wave morphology differs from that observed during si-

I, II, III   aVR, aVL, aVF   V₁, V₂, V₃   V₄, V₅, V₆

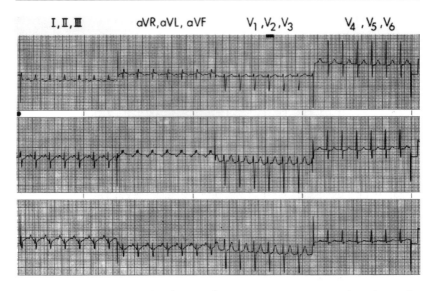

FIGURE 1.   *Surface 12-lead ECG showing an ectopic atrial tachycardia with a cycle length of 500 msec in a patient with a left atrial focus. Although the P waves in leads II, III, and aVF are upright, those in I and aVL are inverted, consistent with an atrial origin. Reproduced with permission from Lowe JE, et al. Ectopic atrial tachycardia.* Semin Thorac Cardiovasc Surg. *1989;1:58.*

nus rhythm. The "ectopic" P wave spontaneously initiates the tachycardia. Often, a "warm-up" phase is also identified, which is characterized by a shortening of the tachycardia cycle length over the first 3 to 5 beats to a final steady cycle length. Attempts to slow the rate with vagal maneuvers are usually unsuccessful.

During EP study, premature extrastimuli and rapid atrial pacing do not initiate the tachycardia, which serves to distinguish chronic ectopic atrial tachycardia and inappropriate sinus tachycardia from reentrant arrhythmias. The tachycardia can be reset with either premature atrial extrastimuli or DC countershock. Rapid atrial pacing often results in overdrive suppression, with a gradual return of the original ectopic accelerated rate once pacing has been discontinued. Mapping is necessary to exclude the presence of reentry phenomena, such as AV node reentrant tachycardia or concealed extranodal bypass tracts. In addition, the goal of mapping is to identify the site of ectopic activity to allow for possible catheter or surgical ablation.[6,7] (Fig 2).

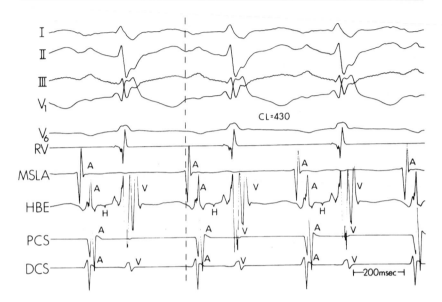

FIGURE 2.   *Endocardial recordings from the same patient as in Fig 1 with an ectopic atrial tachycardia originating in the left atrium. The recordings represent the surface ECG leads I, II, III, V_1, and V_6. Also shown are bipolar electrograms from the RV, MSLA approached from a patent foramen, HBE, and the PCS and DCS positions. The earliest site of local atrial activity, recorded from the left atrial catheter, precedes the onset of the surface P waves as represented by the dashed line. RV=right ventricle; MSLA=midlateral left atrium; HBE=His bundle electrogram; PCS=proximal coronary sinus; DCS=distal coronary sinus. Reproduced with permission from Lowe JE, et al. Ectopic atrial tachycardia. Semin Thorac Cardiovasc Surg. 1989;1:58.*

Operative Technique and Results

Because our study extended more than 10 years, drug regimens changed according to available medications and preferences of referring cardiologists.[2] Surgical intervention was undertaken if the tachycardia was not adequately controlled with medication, especially in patients who had tachycardia-induced cardiomyopathy and congestive heart failure. At follow-up, all patients were questioned regarding symptoms, current medications, and other treatment received in the interim since operation.

Of the 18 patients, one was not given a medical trial because it was thought that his arrhythmia could best be treated surgically. Otherwise, all patients initially received medical treatment, which was unsuccessful in 12 of 17. Three of these 12 did not undergo an operation (one was asymptomatic, one had psychological problems making her a poor surgical candidate, and one declined surgical intervention and subsequently was lost to follow-up). Two patients were referred for surgery after failed radiofrequency catheter ablation attempts. A total of 9 patients underwent operative treatment with isolation procedures, cryoablation, or excision of the ectopic foci, or some combination of these.[2]

Fig 3 shows excision of a portion of the right atrium containing a diverticulum that was the site of origin of AAT. This particular patient was a 34-year-old man who presented with chronic congestive

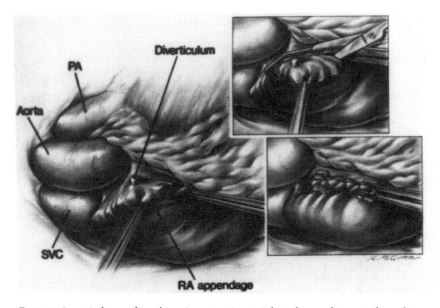

FIGURE 3. *A focus for chronic ectopic atrial tachycardia was found to originate in a small right atrial (RA) diverticulum. The diverticulum and surrounding right atrium were easily excised and repaired primarily without the need of cardipulmonary bypass. PA=pulmonary artery; SVC=superior vena cava. Reproduced with permission from Hendry PJ, et al. Surgical treatment of automatic atrial tachycardias. Ann Thorac Surg. 1990; 49:253.*

heart failure and an ejection fraction of 14%. Following operative cure, the patient was functional class I, with a ejection fraction of 40%. Excision of the sinus node was used for patients with inappropriate sinus tachycardia (Fig 4). Cryoablation or isolation procedures were used for foci in areas not amenable to easy and safe excision—for example, around the coronary sinus or pulmonary veins (Figs 5 and 6).

A 20-year-old man with AAT presented with a massively dilated heart with a left ventricular ejection fraction of 15%. A portion of the right atrium containing the focus was excised, and the defect was repaired with a rotation flap (Fig 7).

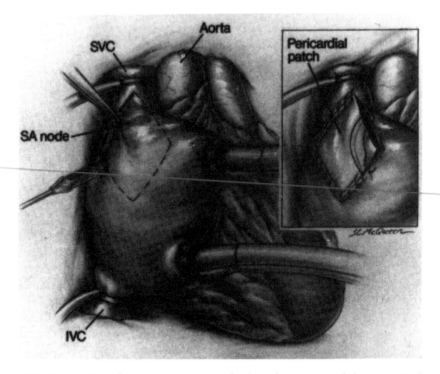

FIGURE 4.   *A wide excision was applied to the region of the sinoatrial (SA) node for surgical treatment of inappropriate sinus tachycardia. IVC=inferior vena cava; SVC=superior vena cava. The large defect created in the right atrial wall was repaired with a large pericardial patch. Reproduced with permission from Hendry PJ, et al. Surgical treatment of automatic atrial tachycardias. Ann Thorac Surg. 1990;49:253.*

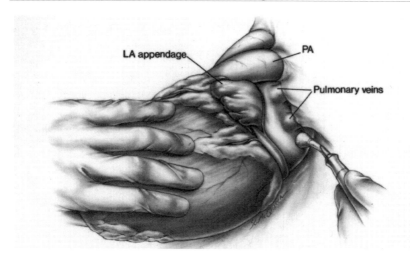

FIGURE 5. *Cryoablation was used to ablate a small focus of ectopic atrial tachycardia near the left inferior pulmonary vein. LA=left atrial; PA=pulmonary artery. Reproduced with permission from Hendry PJ, et al. Surgical treatment of automatic atrial tachycardias.* Ann Thorac Surg. *1990;49:253.*

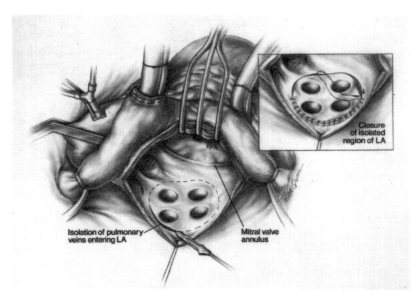

FIGURE 6. *Intraoperative mapping confirmed a focus of ectopic atrial tachycardia that appeared to be originating between the insertion of the pulmonary veins into the posterior left atrium (LA). Because the exact site was uncertain, a partial left atrial isolation procedure was used. Reproduced with permission from Lowe JE, et al. Ectopic Atrial Tachycardia.* Semin Thorac Cardiovasc Surg. *1989;1:58.*

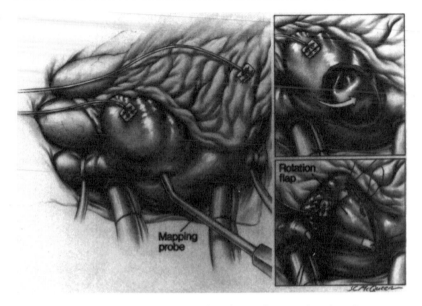

FIGURE 7.   A focus of ectopic atrial tachycardia was localized to an area over the right atrial free wall by use of a bipolar mapping probe. The area was widely excised and the defect repaired with a rotation flap of the remaining right atrium, including the right atrial appendage. Reproduced with permission from Hendry PJ, et al. Surgical treatment of automatic atrial tachycardias. Ann Throac Surg. 1990;49:253.

Eight patients had successful postoperative outcomes, as defined by the presence of sinus rhythm. The treatment success rate was significantly better for our surgical group (88.9%, 8/9) than for our medical group (33.3%, 6/18, P<.01).

Histological study was performed on excised portions of atrium containing the ectopic foci in 6 of the 9 surgically treated patients.[2] In 3 patients with chronic ectopic atrial tachycardia, only one had any identifiable abnormality, which consisted of focal thinning and bleb formation (Fig 3). Tissue excised from the 3 patients with inappropriate sinus tachycardia showed an increased number of lipofuscin-laden vacuoles by electron microscopy, with otherwise normal sinoatrial node tissue.[8]

Long-term follow-up was obtained in 7 of 8 surgically treated patients, all of whom were in sinus rhythm at the time of discharge. One patient with chronic ectopic atrial tachycardia was in sinus rhythm 6 months after surgery but has since been lost to follow-up.

Of the remaining 4 patients with chronic ectopic atrial tachycardia before surgery, all continue to be asymptomatic when recently contacted 3 to 7 years after operation.[2]

Interestingly, of the 3 patients with inappropriate sinus tachycardia, only one was completely free from arrhythmias.[2] Two new foci of supraventricular tachycardia developed in 1 patient, and a junctional tachycardia necessitating AV node catheter ablation and pacemaker insertion had developed in another. Of the 6 patients with chronic ectopic atrial tachycardia who had cardiomyopathy, 4 underwent follow-up radionuclid scans to assess left ventricular function. The mean preoperative ejection fraction was 19% compared with 46% at 4 to 6 weeks after surgery ($P<.05$).[2]

The only death in the entire series occurred in a young woman in whom supraventricular tachycardia developed during pregnancy. One year later, at age 16 years, she was evaluated for severe congestive heart failure and ectopic atrial tachycardia, which was refractory to medical therapy. She suffered cardiac arrest during the induction of anesthesia and was resuscitated on cardiopulmonary bypass. Her focus was thought to arise from the left atrial appendage, but despite excision of the left atrial appendage, ablation of the AV node, and pacemaker insertion, she continued to have supraventricular tachycardia and chronic congestive heart failure. Her clinical course suggested that she had multifocal atrial tachycardia and not AAT. She died 3 days after surgery of complications of her chronic congestive heart failure.

Including our experience with 18 patients, a total of 136 patients with AAT have been reported.[2] Seventy-six patients underwent surgical treatment with either isolation or excisional procedures, with an overall success rate of 87%. Assuming that all patients were treated initially with drug therapy, then the actual success rate for medical treatment is only 34% (46/136). Comparing cure rates between the surgical group and the medically treated group, there was a significant difference favoring surgery ($P<.001$).

Comment

In our experience, in 100% (6/6) of the patients undergoing operation for chronic ectopic atrial tachycardia, left ventricular dysfunction was documented before operation (mean ejection fraction, 19%). Interestingly, none of the 3 patients with inappropriate sinus tachycardia had a cardiomyopathy. The patients who underwent surgical treatment for chronic ectopic atrial tachycardia were therefore at higher risk for complications than those who underwent operation for other supraventricular tachycardia syndromes during the same time period, such as ablation of accessory pathways in the Wolff-Parkinson-White syndrome. Overall, 53.3% (8/15) of our patients with chronic ectopic atrial tachycardia had documented left ventricular dysfunction, which is comparable to the incidence of 54% to 63% previously reported.[9,10] It is now clear that elimination of the tachycardia leads to marked improvement in ventricular function, as seen in our patients who underwent postoperative radionuclide ventriculograms.[2]

Despite the introduction of new antiarrhythmic medications, the overall cure rate with medical therapy does not appear to have improved over the past 10 years. The overall success rate for medical therapy in our experience was only 33.3%.

Although surgical therapy is highly effective for patients with chronic ectopic atrial tachycardia, the outcome is less predictable for those who have inappropriate sinus tachycardia.[2] One of our patients with inappropriate sinus tachycardia remains totally asymptomatic 5 years after operation. A second patient returned 3 years after operation with supraventricular tachycardia related to two new ectopic atrial foci. She was found to have an electrolyte imbalance caused by diuretic abuse, which was thought to be a contributing factor. In the third patient, a junctional tachycardia developed a few days after operation. It persisted intermittently for 6 years, at which time she underwent catheter ablation of the AV node and permanent pacemaker insertion. Our experience in the subgroup of patients with AAT who have inappropriate sinus tachycardia supports the findings of Guiraudon and colleagues[11] who also noted disappointing long-term results in this group. It is thought that these patients may have diffuse atrial electrical abnormalities and that operation alone might not be curative.

It is important to stress that there is no single best surgical procedure that can be applied to all patients with AAT.[2] Each operation must be individualized according to the site of origin of the focus causing tachycardia confirmed by preoperative and intraoperative mapping. Surgical cure can be accomplished with low morbidity and mortality and should be offered to those patients whose tachycardia is not easily controlled with drugs as well as those who have failed radiofrequency catheter ablation. It should be emphasized that a dilated cardiomyopathy and congestive heart failure will eventually develop in substantial numbers of patients with AAT that is not controlled.[2] Interestingly, in our experience, severe impairment of preoperative left ventricular ejection fraction did not result in an increased operative mortality. Therefore, few patients should ever be denied surgical intervention.

Recently, high rates of success have been reported with radiofrequency catheter ablation techniques.[12-16] Preliminary evidence suggests that some patients with AAT have discrete areas of atrial abnormality that can be successfully ablated with radiofrequency energy. However, it is clear that other patients with AAT have large and rather diffuse areas of patient abnormality that may require operative isolation or excision to effect a lasting cure.[17]

Atrial Fibrillation

Atrial fibrillation (AF) is the most common of all sustained cardiac arrhythmias, occurring in 0.4% of the general population in the United States.[18-23] The reported prevalence increases with age and may occur in 2% to 10% of individuals >60 years old.[24,25] AF is a perplexing clinical problem in that morbidity and mortality are determined by the presence or absence of valvular heart disease, age, left ventricular function, and concomitant illnesses. The most dreaded complication is embolic stroke which, even in the absence of valvular heart disease, occurs in 5% of patients with AF each year.[26] A number of important recent clinical studies have shown that the incidence of stroke can be significantly reduced but not eliminated by anticoagulation with warfarin or aspirin.

Current pharmacological treatment of AF is inadequate in that it commonly fails to restore sinus rhythm and usually can only attempt to achieve control of the ventricular response rate. Patients continue to experience annoying subjective symptoms secondary to an irregular heart rate or impaired hemodynamic function due to loss of AV synchrony and remain at significant risk for embolic stroke.[25]

A major impediment to the development of more effective therapies for patients with AF was a lack of understanding of the basic electrophysiological mechanisms resulting in the arrhythmia. On the basis of the experimental studies of Boineau and Allessie and confirmed in clinical studies by Cox,[27-30] it is now accepted that AF results from multiple macroreentrant circuits that depolarize atrial myocardium in changing patterns (Figs 8 and 9).

NORMAL ATRIAL ACTIVATION

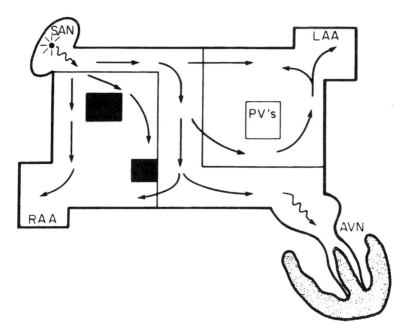

FIGURE 8.   *During normal sinus rhythm, the electrical impulse is generated within the sinoatrial node (SAN) and propagates across the right and left atria and the atrial septum to the atrioventricular node (AVN) and thence to the ventricles. Note that under normal circumstances, there is a collision of two portions of the sinus impulse beneath the pulmonary veins (PV's) posteriorly (upper portion of the left atrium). RAA and LAA=right and left atrial appendages. Reproduced with permission from Reference 30.*

Until recently, operative His bundle ablation introduced by Sealy et al[31] in 1991 and catheter ablation introduced by Scheinman et al[32] in 1982 were the only nonpharmacological means to control the ventricular response rate in patients with AF refractory to medical therapy. His bundle ablation requires insertion of a permanent pacemaker and does nothing to restore AV synchrony or reduce the risk of thromboembolic stroke (Fig 10). These disadvantages of His bundle ablation combined with a better understanding of the electrophysiological mechanisms resulting in AF provided the impetus

ATRIAL FIBRILLATION
(Multiple Macro-Reentrant Circuits)

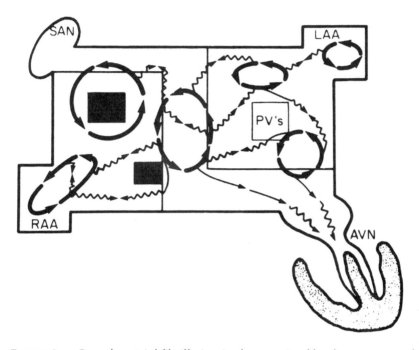

FIGURE 9.   *Complex atrial fibrillation is characterized by the presence of multiple macroreentrant circuits (heavy arrows) and variable passive atrial conduction (thin arrows). Abbreviations as in Fig 8. Reproduced with permission from Reference 30.*

for the development of operative approaches for attempted cure of AF in select patients.

Operative Techniques and Results

In 1985, Guiraudon et al[33] introduced the first operation designed to restore regular rhythm in patients with AF. The "corridor" procedure creates an isolated band of muscle that includes both the sinoatrial and AV nodes (Fig 11). This "corridor" allows the sinus

CATHETER ABLATION OF HIS BUNDLE

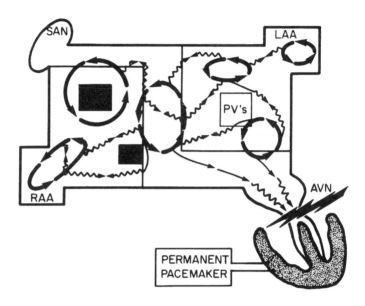

FIGURE 10.   *Schematic representation of the results of catheter ablation of the His bundle for atrial fibrillation. Since the atria continue to fibrillate, the atrial kick is not restored and the vulnerability to thromboembolism remains unchanged. Abbreviations as in Fig 8. Reproduced with permission from Reference 30.*

node to result in ventricular activation through the AV node–His bundle complex, resulting in a regular ventricular rhythm without permanent pacemaker implantation. However, the corridor procedure also isolates both atria from the ventricles. Therefore, the atrial component to diastolic ventricular filling is lost and cardiac hemodynamic function is not restored to normal. In addition, both isolated atria can continue to fibrillate, and the patient remains susceptible to the development of left atrial thrombus and subsequent embolic stroke. In effect, therefore, the corridor procedure offers no advantages over catheter ablation of the His bundle and has the disadvantage of increased surgical morbidity.

In 1987, Cox and Boineau, on the basis of a series of elegant experimental studies as well as intraoperative atrial mapping studies

CORRIDOR PROCEDURE

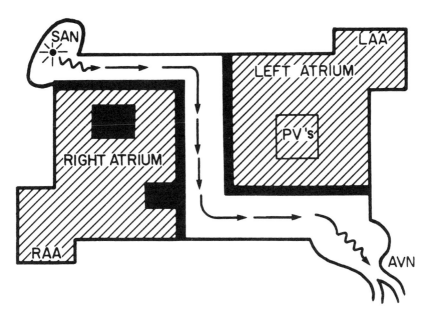

FIGURE 11. *Schematic representation of the results of the corridor procedure for the surgical treatment of atrial fibrillation. Technically speaking, a sinus rhythm may follow this procedure in that the sinus node impulse drives the ventricles. However, because of loss of both right atrial and left atrial synchrony with the respective ventricles, the hemodynamic abnormalities associated with atrial fibrillation are not improved. In addition, the vulnerability to the development of left atrial thrombi is not alleviated. Abbreviations as in Fig 8. Reproduced with permission from Reference 30.*

in patients with AF, introduced the "maze" procedure; they recently reviewed their 5-year experience.[34] Since experimental studies have shown that AF is due to interatrial reentry, multiple reentrant wavelets within the atria are maintained by the inhomogeneity of tissue refractoriness within atrial myocardium.[27] The maze procedure creates a "maze" of electrical propagation routes involving the entire atrial myocardium. However, there is only one site of entrance, the sinoatrial node, and only one site of exit, the AV node. The maze procedure allows the normal impulse from the sinoatrial node to propagate and activate the entire atrial myocardium except for the excised atrial appendages and atrial myocardium surrounding the isolated pulmonary veins[34] (Figs 12 and 13).

The maze procedure divides two of the three major pathways of conduction between the sinoatrial and AV nodes: the crista terminalis and the anterior limbus of the fossa ovalis. Therefore, the electrical impulse leaving the sinoatrial node can propagate only along

MAZE PROCEDURE
FOR ATRIAL FIBRILLATION

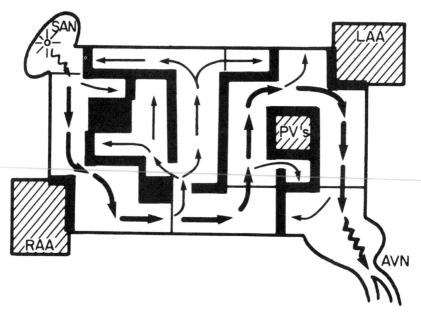

FIGURE 12.   *Because atrial fibrillation is characterized by the presence of multiple macroreentrant circuits that are fleeting in nature and can occur anywhere in the atria, a surgical procedure based on the principle of a maze was developed. Both atrial appendages are excised, and the pulmonary veins are electrically activated by providing for multiple blind alleys off the main conduction route between the sinoatrial node and the AV node, thereby preserving atrial transport function postoperatively. Abbreviations as in Fig 8. Reproduced with permission from Reference 30.*

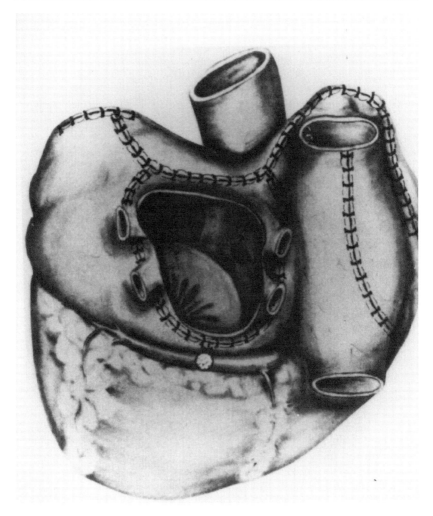

FIGURE 13. *The maze procedure shown on a three-dimensional representation of the heart. Note the presence of the transmural cryolesion of the coronary sinus at the site of the posterior inferior left atriotomy. Also note the bridge of tissue in the region of the atrioventricular node that allows conduction of the atrial impulse to the ventricles. Both atrial appendages have been excised. The only completely isolated portions of the atrium are the orifices of the pulmonary veins. Reproduced with permission from Reference 30.*

a posterior and inferior direction to the AV node. The impulse also travels anteriorly around the lateral base of the atrium onto the anterior surface of the right atrium. It then continues propagation in a right-to-left direction to the left atrium and enters the anterior aspect of the atrial septum. Depolarization continues around the base of the lateral left atrium onto the posterior surface of the left atrium, where again it is blocked superiorly and inferiorly. The atrial septum activates in an anterior-to-posterior direction beneath the septal incision to break through on the epicardial surface posteriorly. Depolarization then spreads to the posterior inferior right atrium, posterior inferior left atrium, and posterior superior left atrium between the right superior pulmonary vein and the superior vena cava. After activation of the posterior surface of the atria, the electrical impulse cannot propagate further in any direction.

The maze procedure prevents the development of macroreentrant AF because the multiple atrial incisions are placed such that it is not possible for an electrical wave front to originate in any one area of the atrium and then return to, or reenter, the original site of origin without crossing one of the atriotomies. In addition, the atrial incisions are placed close enough to one another that there is not enough atrial myocardium between incisions to allow development of a macroreentrant circuit.[34]

However, during the postoperative period, nearly 50% of patients develop transient atrial flutter/fibrillation. For a temporary period following surgery, the effective refractory period of the atria shortens secondary to a variety of factors, including elevated levels of serum catecholamines, pericarditis, and surgical trauma. This temporary milieu allows smaller than normal reentrant circuits to form within the "mazes," and transient atrial flutter/fibrillation can occur[34] (Fig 14).

From September of 1987 through July of 1993, 92 patients have undergone the maze procedure for AF at Barnes Hospital in St Louis. Approximately half of the patients suffered from paroxysmal or intermittent AF, and the remaining patients had chronic AF. Surgical indications included arrhythmia intolerance in 63%, drug intolerance in 17%, and previous stroke or transient ischemic attack in 20%. There were three operative deaths (3%). Major postoperative complications included postoperative bleeding requiring reexploration (7%) and postoperative fluid retention. Although not yet proven, it is believed that the pathogenesis of postoperative fluid retention is secondary to a decrease in atrial natriuretic peptide

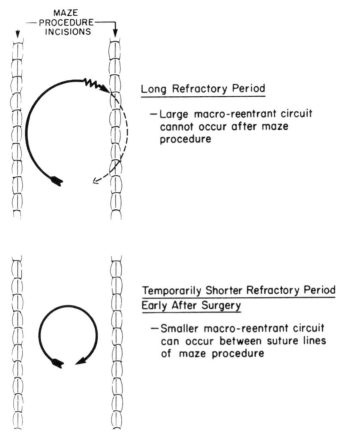

MAZE
— PROCEDURE —
INCISIONS

Long Refractory Period

— Large macro-reentrant circuit
cannot occur after maze
procedure

Temporarily Shorter Refractory Period
Early After Surgery

— Smaller macro-reentrant circuit
can occur between suture lines
of maze procedure

FIGURE 14. *Electrophysiological basis of recurrence of atrial fibrillation in the early postoperative period and of the disappearance of atrial fibrillation after the atria have healed following the maze procedure. In both normal and diseased atria, the refractory period is relatively long, thus limiting the minimum size that a macroreentrant circuit can be. The maze procedure abolishes atrial fibrillation by positioning atriotomies close enough together to prevent the development of such large macroreentrant circuits (upper panel). However, in the early postoperative period, the refractory period of the atrium is decreased, allowing the formation of macroreentrant circuits that are small enough to occur between the suture lines of the maze procedure (lower panel), resulting in perioperative atrial flutter or fibrillation. Once the atria have healed after operation (>3 months), the refractory period returns to preoperative ranges and the atria can no longer fibrillate. Reproduced with permission from Reference 34.*

caused by the multiple atriotomies.[34] At the present time, all patients receive spironolactone after surgery, which has prevented the development of postoperative pulmonary edema.

As described earlier, approximately 50% of patients treated with the maze procedure developed perioperative atrial arrhythmias at some time during the first 3 months following operation. Fortunately, like other types of perioperative AF, these arrhythmias disappeared after the atriotomies healed, and they did not require long-term antiarrhythmic therapy. Importantly, after surgery, return of atrial transport function has been documented by transesophageal echocardiography.[34]

Initial results after the maze operation are promising. Thus far, there has been only a 2 %recurrence of AF (mean follow-up, 22 ± 13 months). Therefore, AF has been abolished in 98% of patients who have undergone the procedure.[34] Arrhythmias have been controlled by the maze procedure alone in 89% of patients and by surgery plus one medication in 9% of patients. AV synchrony has also been restored in 98% of patients by restoration of sinus rhythm in 60% and by pacemaker implantation in 38% of patients with abnormal sinoatrial nodes (uncovering of sick sinus syndrome after surgery; this also includes patients with preoperative pacemakers).

Recently, similar results have been reported by McCarthy and associates[35] from the Cleveland Clinic in 14 patients treated between January 1, 1991, and the end of May 1992. There was one operative death (7%), and 2 patients required pacemaker implantation for sick sinus syndrome (14%). Five patients (36%) developed postoperative fluid retention requiring aggressive treatment with diuretics.

Comment

It is estimated that more than 200 maze procedures have been performed worldwide. Compelling evidence shows that the procedure does indeed abolish macroreentrant AF and that near normal atrial transport can be restored.[34] We can hope that sufficient follow-up will establish that thromboembolic strokes can be nearly eliminated in long-term survivors without the risks of chronic anticoagulation.

Presently, only select patients are candidates for the maze procedure. Based on the reported experiences of Cox at Barnes Hospital[34] and McCarthy at the Cleveland Clinic,[35] current indications for the MAZE Procedure include (1) documented prior thromboembolic stroke of cardiac origin in patients with paroxysmal or chronic atrial fibrillation; (2) patient intolerance of paroxysmal or chronic atrial fibrillation with debilitating symptoms; (3) drug intolerance; and (4) select patients with AF undergoing mitral valve repair or other cardiac procedures.

Absolute and relative contraindications for the maze procedure include (1) well-tolerated paroxysmal or lone atrial fibrillation in patients <60 years old (low risk for thromboembolism with normal overall life expectancy); (2) age >70 years (relative contraindication); (3) impaired left ventricular function (relative contraindication); and (4) comorbid disease such as severe chronic obstructive pulmonary disease or renal insufficiency.

Patients considered as candidates for the maze procedure should understand that (1) the operation is extensive and the surgical mortality is approximately 3%; (2) transient but significant postoperative morbidity can occur, including bleeding requiring reexploration, postoperative fluid retention requiring diuretics, and transient atrial flutter/fibrillation requiring short-term use of antiarrhythmic medications; (3) permanent dual-chamber pacemaker implantation may be required after unmasking of coexistent sick sinus syndrome; and (4) the long-term results regarding maintenance of atrial transport function and risk of atrial thrombus formation and subsequent embolic stroke remain unknown.

A final observation regarding the maze procedure should be made. The development of this operation by Cox and Boineau is a splendid example of how basic, well-designed investigative work can result in innovative and effective new clinical therapy even for the most challenging of clinical problems, such as the treatment of atrial fibrillation.

References

1. Lewis T. Paroxysmal tachycardia, the result of ectopic impulse formation formation. *Heart.* 1909–1910;1:262.
2. Lowe JE. Surgery for automatic atrial tachycardias. *Cardiac Surgery: State of the Art Reviews.* 1990;4:197–205.
3. Lowe JE, Hendry PJ, Packer DL, et al. Surgical management of chronic ectopic atrial tachycardia. *Semin Thorac Cardiovasc Surg.* 1989;1:58–66.

4. Damiano RJ, Tripp HF, Asano T, et al. Left ventricular dysfunction and dilatation resulting from chronic supraventricular tachycardia. *J Thorac Cardiovasc Surg.* 1987;94:135–143.
5. Packer DL, Bardy GH, Worley SJ, et al. Tachycardia-induced cardiomyopathy: a reversible form of left ventricular dysfunction. *Am J Cardiol.* 1986;57:563–570.
6. Garson G, Gillette PC. Electrophysiologic studies of supraventricular tachycardia in children, I: clinical-electrophysiologic correlations. *Am Heart J.* 1981;102:223–250.
7. Wu D, Denes P, Amat-y-Leon F, et al. Clinical, electrocardiographic and electrophysiologic observations in patients with paroxysmal supraventricular tachycardia. *Am J Cardiol.* 1978;41:1045–1051.
8. Lowe JE, Hartwich T, Takla M, et al. Ultrastructure of electrophysiologically identified human sinoatrial nodes. *Basic Res Cardiol.* 1988; 83:401–409.
9. Morgan CL, Nadas AS. Chronic ectopic tachycardia in infancy and childhood. *Am Heart J.* 1964;67:617–627.
10. Gillette PC, Wampler DG, Garson A Jr, et al. Treatment of atrial automatic tachycardia by ablation procedures. *J Am Coll Cardiol.* 1985;6: 405–409.
11. Guiraudon GM, Klein GJ, Sharma AD, et al. Surgical treatment of supraventricular tachycardia: a five-year experience. *PACE Pacing Clin Electrophysiol.* 1986;9:1376–1380.
12. Walsh EP, Saul JP, Hulse JE, et al. Transcatheter ablation of ectopic atrial tachycardia in young patients using radiofrequency current. *Circulation.* 1992;86:1138–1146.
13. Case CL, Gillette PC, Oslizlok PC, et al. Radiofrequency catheter ablation of incessant, medically resistant supraventricular tachycardia in infants and small children. *J Am Coll Cardiol.* 1992;20:1405–1410.
14. Lau YR, Gillette PC, Wienecke MM, et al. Successful radiofrequency catheter ablation of an atrial ectopic tachycardia in an adolescent. *Am Heart J.* 1992;123:1384–1386.
15. Kall JG, Wilber DJ: Radiofrequency catheter ablation of an automatic atrial tachycardia in an adult. *PACE Pacing Clin Electrophysiol.* 1992;15: 281–287.
16. Kay GN, Chong F, Epstein AE, et al. Radiofrequency ablation for treatment of primary atrial tachycardias. *J Am Coll Cardiol.* 1993;21: 901–909.
17. Anderson KP. Management of ectopic atrial tachycardia. *J Am Coll Cardiol.* 1993;22:93–94.
18. Cameron A, Schwartz MJ, Kronmal RA, et al. Prevalence and significance of atrial fibrillation in coronary artery disease (CASS registry). *Am J Cardiol.* 1988;61:714–717.
19. Diamantopoulos EJ, Anthopoulos L, Nanas S, et al. Detection of arrhythmias in a representative sample of the Athens population. *Eur Heart J.* 1987;8(suppl D):17–19.
20. Onundarson PT, Thorgeirsson G, Jonmundsson E, et al. Chronic atrial fibrillation: epidemiologic features and 14 year follow-up: a case control study. *Eur Heart J.* 1987;8:521–527.

21. Hirosawa K, Sekiguchi M, Kasanuki H, et al. Natural history of atrial fibrillation. *Heart Vessels Suppl.* 1987;2:14–23.
22. Savage DD, Garrison RJ, Castelli WP, et al. Prevalence of submitral (annular) calcium and its correlates in a general population-based sample (the Framingham Study). *Am J Cardiol.* 1983;51:1375–1378.
23. Cox JL, Schuessler RB, D'Agostino JH Jr, et al. The surgical treatment of atrial fibrillation, III: development of a definitive surgical procedure. *J Thorac Cardiovasc Surg.* 1991;101:569–583.
24. Alpert JS, Petersen P, Godtfredwen J. Atrial fibrillation: natural history, complications, and management. *Annu Rev Med.* 1988;39:41–52.
25. Cox JL, Boineau JP, Schuessler RB, et al. A review of surgery for atrial fibrillation. *J Cardiovasc Electrophysiol.* 1991;2:541–561.
26. Halperin JL, Hart RG. Atrial fibrillation and stroke: new ideas, persisting dilemmas. *Stroke.* 1988;19:937–941.
27. Boineau JP, Schuessler RB, Mooney CR, et al. Natural and evoked atrial flutter due to circus movement in dogs: role of abnormal atrial pathways, slow conduction, nonuniform refractory period distribution and premature beats. *Am J Cardiol.* 1980;45:1167–1181.
28. Allessie MA, Bonke FIM, Schopman FJG. Circus movement in rabbit atrial muscle as a mechanism of tachycardia, III: the "leading circle" concept: a new mode of circus movement in cardiac tissue without the involvement of an anatomical obstacle. *Circ Res.* 1977;41:9–18.
29. Allessie MA, Lammers WJEP, Bonke FIM, et al. Experimental evaluation of Moe's multiple wavelet hypothesis of atrial fibrillation. In: Zipes DP, Jalife J, eds. *Cardiac Electrophysiology and Arrhythmias.* Orlando, Fl.: Grune & Stratton; 1985:265–275.
30. Cox JL, Canavan TE, Schuessler RB, et al. The surgical treatment of atrial fibrillation, II: intraoperative electrophysiologic mapping and description of the electrophysiologic basis of atrial flutter and atrial fibrillation. *J Thorac Cardiovasc Surg.* 1991;101:406–426.
31. Sealy WC, Gallagher JJ, Kasell JH. His bundle interruption for control of inappropriate ventricular responses to atrial arrhythmias. *Ann Thorac Surg.* 1981;32:429.
32. Scheinman MM, Morady F, Hess DS, et al. Catheter-induced ablation of the atrioventricular junction to control refractory supraventricular arrhythmias. *JAMA.* 1982;248:851–855.
33. Guiraudon GM, Campbell CS, Jones DL, et al. Combined sinoatrial node atrioventricular node isolation: a surgical alternative to His bundle ablation in patients with atrial fibrillation. *Circulation.* 1985;72 (suppl III):III–220.
34. Cox JL, Boineau JP, Schuessler RB, et al. Five-year experience with the maze procedure for atrial fibrillation. *J Thorac Cardiovasc Surg.* 1993;56:814–823.
35. McCarthy PM, Castle LW, Maloney JD, et al. Initial experience with the maze procedure for atrial fibrillation. *J Thorac Cardiovasc Surg.* 1993; 105:1077–1087.

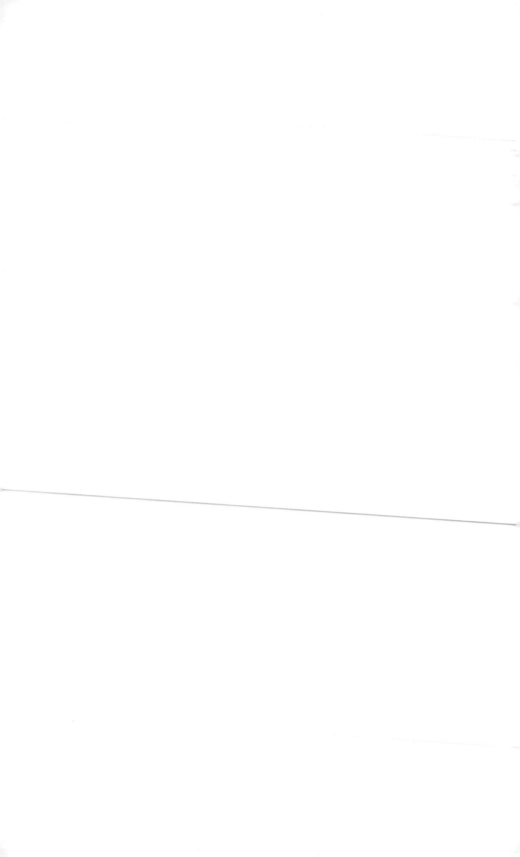

Chapter 14

Editorial Comments

Richard N.W. Hauer, MD

Introduction

The chapter by Lowe covers primarily the surgical treatment of automatic atrial tachycardia (AAT) and atrial fibrillation (AF). As indicated by the author, results of surgical therapy are poor in some other atrial arrhythmias. One of these is inappropriate sinus tachycardia. This means a more rapid rate than expected during given physiological circumstances. Patients with this disorder may be highly symptomatic. Of the three patients with inappropriate sinus tachycardia operated on at Duke University Medical Center, only one remained totally asymptomatic 5 years after operation.[1] Guiraudon and coworkers[2] also noted disappointing long-term results in these patients. In our own series, we attempted surgical treatment in a single patient with inappropriate sinus tachycardia. About 15 cm^2 of the atrial wall in the sinus node area was excised. The excised tissue was replaced by an epicardial patch. After the procedure, the patient had a normal rate and remained asymptomatic for several weeks only. The tachycardia recurred and showed a P-wave vector similar to that observed before surgery. We agree with the presumption that these patients may have diffuse atrial electrical abnormalities, which make successful surgical intervention less likely. For the same reason, patients with multifocal atrial tachycardia are not ideal candidates for surgery.

Automatic Atrial Tachycardia

In contrast to the poor surgical results in patients with inappropriate sinus tachycardia, surgical therapy for AAT is quite suc-

From DiMarco JP, Prystowsky EN (eds): *Atrial Arrhythmias: State of the Art*. Armonk, NY, Futura Publishing Company, Inc., © 1995.

cessful. Lowe describes a success rate of 87% in 76 patients from various centers. Successful surgical treatment is completely dependent on careful activation mapping to localize the site of origin of the arrhythmia. It is expected that some histological abnormality may be present at the arrhythmogenic site. However, few data are available on the histological substrate. In the report by Lowe, histological examination was carried out in only 3 of the 9 patients undergoing surgery for AAT. Only 1 of these patients showed an identifiable abnormality, which consisted of focal thinning and bleb formation. The mechanism of the tachycardia is another point of interest. AAT suggests a correct understanding of the mechanism. However, most information is obtained from indirect criteria inferred from behavior of the arrhythmia during programmed electrical stimulation. For the ultimate proof of the mechanism of arrhythmogenesis, microelectrode recording is needed in many cases. To the best of my knowledge, only two reports are available in which intracellular recordings were included in the measurements. The described mechanisms were triggered activity in diseased atrial myocardium and automaticity occurring in normal myocardium, respectively.[3,4] Since enough relevant information is still lacking on this subject, the name chronic ectopic atrial tachycardia is a better choice for this arrhythmia.

In the series of the Cardiac Arrhythmia Unit of the Heart-Lung Institute in Utrecht, three patients underwent surgical treatment for AAT. The sites of origin of the arrhythmias were localized in the right and left atrial appendages and in the left free wall, respectively. Treatment consisted of excision of the atrial appendages and cryosurgery in the patients with a free wall location. Treatment was successful in all cases.

Our last patient, with the site of origin close to the apex of the left atrial appendage, is of special interest, since information is available on the mechanism of her arrhythmia as well as the histology at the arrhythmogenic site. After intraoperative mapping, the left atrial appendage was excised and studied in the tissue bath in the experimental laboratory. Microelectrode studies revealed phase 4 depolarization during tachycardia at the site at which the origin of the arrhythmia was localized intraoperatively. Since phase 4 depolarization started from a depressed transmembrane potential, arrhythmogenesis was due to abnormal automaticity. Histological examination showed that spontaneous activity arose in an area with abnormal cells, characterized by an amorphous pale-staining eo-

sinophilic cytosol without nuclei. This area was surrounded by normal myocardium. Fibrosis was absent. The electrophysiologically
and histologically abnormal area was remarkably small, and only a
part of the atrial appendage was affected. If this case represents the
typical situation in patients with AAT, successful treatment with
map-guided surgery or even catheter ablation is understandable.

Atrial Fibrillation

AF may be associated with many clinically important sequelae,
including (1) palpitation arising from the irregular heartbeat and/or
rapid heart rate, (2) depressed exercise tolerance, (3) signs of congestive heart failure, and (4) thromboembolic sequelae. Antiarrhythmic drugs are the first step in the therapeutic management,
which should be directed toward restoration of normal sinus
rhythm. If drug therapy is successful, proarrhythmic effects are absent, and the drug is well tolerated, then this first therapeutic step
is also the best. In addition, it is widely available and has an acceptable chance of success in experienced hands. If drugs fail, however, nonpharmacological therapy should be considered.

Catheter ablation can offer ablation of the His bundle. In experienced hands, interruption of the His bundle is successful in close
to 100% of the cases. In our series, interruption failed in only 2 of
80 patients. Both patients underwent cardiac surgical procedures
years before ablation. His bundle ablation can, of course, offer no
cure. However, successful His bundle ablation is usually associated
with disappearance of palpitations, decrease or disappearance of
signs of heart failure, and marked improvement of exercise capa-
bilities. The use of radiofrequency current obviates the need for
anesthesia, and usually the patient can be discharged within several
days. The negative points are requirement of pacemaker insertion
and continuation of anticoagulant therapy to prevent thromboembolic sequelae.

The role of surgical treatment of AF is controversial. With the
corridor procedure, pacemaker implantation can be avoided in case
of absence of concomitant sinus node dysfunction. The ventricular
rate is still under control of the sinus node and is modulated by the
autonomic nervous system for adaptation to physiological demands. However, in four of nine patients with the corridor opera-

tion described by Leitch et al,[5] implantation of a permanent pacemaker was needed. In addition, in two of these nine patients, AF in the corridor recurred. Finally, since AF is still present, the procedure does not protect against thromboembolic complications. Compared with the less invasive radiofrequency His bundle ablation combined with implantation of a rate-responsive pacemaker, the corridor operation offers no obvious advantage.

The maze procedure is extensively discussed in the paper by Lowe. Compared with the corridor operation, the maze procedure has the advantage of restoration of sinus rhythm and termination of fibrillation in both atria. Theoretically, the major advantage of this technique is maintenance of atrial transport function and particularly a decrease of the incidence of thromboembolic complications. However, these potentially favorable aspects are not yet proven.

References

1. Lowe JE. Surgery for automatic atrial tachycardias. *Cardiac Surgery: State of the Art Reviews.* 1990;4:197–205.
2. Guiraudon GM, Klein GJ, Sharma AD, et al. Surgical treatment of supraventricular tachycardia: a five-year experience. *PACE Pacing Clin Electrophysiol.* 1986;9:1376–1380.
3. Wyndham CRC, Arnsdorf MF, Levitsky S, et al. Successful surgical excision of focal paroxysmal atrial tachycardia: observations in vivo and in vitro. *Circulation.* 1980;62:1365–1372.
4. Rossi L. Histopathologic correlates of atrial arrhythmias. In: Touboul P, Waldo AL, eds. *Atrial Arrhythmias: Current Concepts and Management.* St Louis, Mo: Mosby Year Book Inc; 1990:27.
5. Leitch JW, Klein G, Yee R, et al. Sinus node-atrioventricular node isolation: long-term results with the "corridor" operation for atrial fibrillation. *J Am Coll Cardiol.* 1991;17:970.

Chapter 15

Current Concerns and Future Directions in the Pharmacological Treatment of Atrial Fibrillation

*Andrea Natale, MD; Zalmen Blanck, MD;
Sanjay Deshpande, MD; Anwer Dhala, MD;
Mohammed Jazayeri, MD; Jasbir Sra, MD;
and Masood Akhtar, MD*

Introduction

Although the appreciation of atrial fibrillation dates back more than 300 years, this common rhythm disorder remains a troublesome and often difficult management problem. Despite recent advances in the therapy of patients with atrial fibrillation and a great expansion in the therapeutic armamentarium, treatment of atrial fibrillation with antiarrhythmic drugs is far from satisfactory. A substantial number of patients still have considerable disability and even a shortened life span. Since atrial fibrillation represents the most common arrhythmia seen by clinicians and it is the most common arrhythmia to cause admission to the hospital,[1] it is clear that effective and additional remedies are needed. Atrial fibrillation in the 1990s is fundamentally a different disorder from what it was during most of this century. Thirty to 50 years ago, the most frequent cause of atrial fibrillation was valvular heart disease, particularly mitral insufficiency and stenosis. At the present time, since treatment and prevention of this condition have advanced dramatically, its importance as a cause of atrial fibrillation has waned, and hypertensive heart disease and cardiac failure appear to be the most common associated disorders.[2] In addition, a condition

From DiMarco JP, Prystowsky EN (eds): *Atrial Arrhythmias: State of the Art.* Armonk, NY, Futura Publishing Company, Inc., © 1995.

characterized by the absence of any structural heart disease and named "lone or idiopathic" atrial fibrillation is increasingly recognized and constitutes at least 10% of all causes of this dysrhythmia. In the 1990s, however, despite the advent of potent new antiarrhythmic drugs, the major therapeutic challenge for the physician still remains the maintenance of sinus rhythm. It is not uncommon that we have to reconsider our initial therapeutic goal and redirect our efforts to the less ideal amelioration of symptoms and reduction of mortality and morbidity.

From Pathophysiology to Drug Therapy

As the clinical features of atrial fibrillation have evolved during recent decades, so has our understanding of the pathophysiology and the mechanism of this disorder. Currently, the perpetuation of atrial fibrillation is attributed, as proposed in 1962 by Moe,[3] to the presence of multiple meandering reentrant wavelets. The maintenance of fibrillation depends on the number of wavelets, which, in turn, depends on the atrial tissue mass and the average wavelength of the wavelets. Since the wavelength reflects the product of conduction velocity and refractory period, the effects of various antiarrhythmic medications can be anticipated by their ability to modulate the electrical property of myocardial cells and the propagation of the electrical impulse. Therefore, drugs that shorten the wavelength must be regarded as proarrhythmic, whereas agents that prolong the wavelength possess antifibrillatory properties. Investigations in animals and human patients[4] suggest that action potential prolongation in the absence of conduction slowing might be more effective in terminating atrial fibrillation and atrial flutter. On the other hand, compounds that produce decreased conduction velocity in addition to prolonging refractoriness must cause a larger prolongation of the refractory period to increase the wavelength sufficiently to stop atrial fibrillation. Awareness of the electrical model that accounts for the maintenance of atrial fibrillation does not always facilitate the choice of the most effective pharmacological agent. The lack of correspondence between experimental and clinical effects of drugs stems from the multiple facets of the arrhythmogenic substrates and their relationships with a myriad of other factors. In addition, it is difficult to correlate in vitro findings with the net in vivo effect in humans. The ideal situation would be the ability to select an antiarrhythmic agent that has specific activity against arrhythmia mechanisms involving particular cardiac tissues. In other words, the pharmacological therapy for an arrhythmia would depend on both the mechanism and the site of the arrhythmia. Unfortunately, this is not the case, and the selection of antiarrhythmic agents is usually empirical. Such a shortcoming originates from a limited understanding of drug / substrate interaction in vivo, the lack of a proper model to study modulation of the antiarrhythmic properties by a multitude of variables in vivo, and reliance on the current classification of antiarrhythmic drugs based on the electrophysiological effects of these compounds on action potential duration and conduction velocity in healthy tissue at normal stimulation rates. Is the present understanding of this dysrhythmia sufficient to embark on the development of new drugs? How can we achieve this goal if we do not have an appropriate pathophysiological model to study new drugs? Before we carry out clinical studies, we must know what we are treating and what the target is. At the cellular level, complex biochemical and structural transformations intervene, triggered by both mechanical and neurohumoral stimuli. However, the atrium is more than a collection of cells; it is a highly organized structure integrated in the cardiovascular loop. Even though the electrophysiological substrate forms the basis of the arrhythmia, the autonomic nervous system, the heart itself by its mechanical status, and a variety of other processes condition the expression, clinical pattern, and manifestations of the arrhythmia. Recognition of these provocative and modulating factors is particularly important and has therapeutic consequences that have been ignored and now need to be acknowledged to identify more specific therapeutic interventions. It is essential to distinguish between antiarrhythmic action and electrophysiological effects of drugs. Whether specific properties are antiarrhythmic depends on the mechanism of the arrhythmia, the type of antiarrhythmic action, and the interaction with a specific arrhythmic substrate.

It is difficult to organize the antiarrhythmic agents into a classification that may help to predict the electrophysiological effects of drugs on a specific arrhythmogenic tissue. This reflects a complex interplay of different variables, including, among others, alteration in circulating catecholamines or in autonomic tone,[5] the influence of drugs on passive membrane properties, and propagation across anisotropic tissue[6] (Table 1). To better comprehend the intricate in-

TABLE 1.   Factors Regulating the Effects of Antiarrhythmic Drugs

Heart rate (tachycardia-dependent effects)
Resting membrane potential
Type of myocardial tissue (conduction system vs working myocardium)
Associated conditions (ischemia, hypoxia, fibrosis, electrolytic imbalance, acidosis, inflammatory process)
Intrinsic tissue properties
Alteration of autonomic tone
Orientation of myocardial fibers
Arrhythmogenic substrate
Regional differences of drug tissue concentrations

teraction between substrate, triggering factors, and pharmacological agents and to provide informed inputs into the genesis of new chemical entities, we need to develop adequate models that closely reflect the clinical syndrome. In this respect, the growing conviction that the autonomic nervous system frequently modulates normal and abnormal electrophysiological mechanisms of rhythmicity[5] may delineate one profile of the next generation of antiarrhythmic agents, which ideally should provide a broader spectrum of properties to comply with the complexity of this rhythm disorder. In the meantime, the possibility of adjunctive therapies or the selection of agents with sympathovagal modulating effects should generally be entertained. The refinement of our understanding of the pathophysiology of atrial fibrillation may also indicate the way to innovative therapeutic strategies. In this domain, evidence of inflammatory infiltration of the atrial tissue similar to that observed in acute myocarditis has recently been reported.[7,8] It is conceivable that in a subgroup of patients, atrial fibrillation is the expression of an atrial myopathy preceded by some form of inflammatory process, possibly linked to a viral infection. It is not excluded that the development of more sensitive and simpler techniques to identify this cohort might promote treatment algorithms based on anti-inflammatory and immunosuppressant agents. In summary, although we currently have little knowledge of the mechanisms accounting for the electrical derangement of atria in atrial fibrillation, our understanding continues to grow and in the future will certainly provide information for a more efficient identification of new therapeutic measures.

Drug Therapy: What We Have and What We Should Have

Antiarrhythmic drugs have been used to convert atrial fibrillation and to maintain sinus rhythm since the work of Frey in 1918 and Lewis in 1922 using quinidine. While in other tachyarrhythmias, we have witnessed a substantial metamorphosis of the therapeutic approach, pharmacological agents still remain the first-line therapy for atrial fibrillation. When should therapy be undertaken? What are the indications? The following seems to represent the current status of our knowledge. The objective of treatment for atrial fibrillation, as for almost any disease, is threefold: prevention, relief of symptoms, and improvement of prognosis. Two possible treatment strategies can be considered. The simplest, although less than ideal, strategy is to slow atrioventricular nodal conduction and thus slow the ventricular response. The more difficult, but closer to ideal, treatment is to restore and to maintain normal sinus rhythm so as to preserve the atrial contribution to cardiac output and allow physiological and appropriate heart rate acceleration. In addition to the treatment of atrial fibrillation per se, attention must also be directed toward (1) accurate identification and correction of causes or associated conditions, (2) treatment of congestive heart failure when present, and (3) prevention of possible thromboembolism. The current availability of multiple pharmacological therapies gives the clinician great latitude in treating atrial fibrillation but also imposes the burden of choosing the most appropriate drug for a specific patient to ensure the optimum risk-benefit relation. The question of long-term antiarrhythmic pharmacological therapy often arises. The benefits of therapy must therefore be balanced by the known adverse effects of antiarrhythmic medications and the growing concern regarding the impact of those drugs in long-term treatment. We have to make a decision based on what level of symptoms and the frequency of recurrence we are treating. In particular, in patients who have frequent and disabling paroxysmal atrial fibrillation or those with left ventricular dysfunction or diastolic dysfunction, the maintenance of sinus rhythm can be quite important, and prophylactic therapy is clearly indicated. On the other hand, in those patients with less frequent or asymptomatic bouts, the only major concern remains the risk of thromboembolic events.

Maintenance of Sinus Rhythm

There is some evidence (see Allessie's chapter in this book) that prolonged episodes of atrial fibrillation increase the likelihood of persistent arrhythmia, suggesting the need to prevent even brief paroxysms. The decision to initiate a specific antiarrhythmic therapy implies that all potentially reversible factors have been managed optimally. An extensive list of studies has appeared that examined the role of different types of pharmacological agents for control of atrial fibrillation. Although we have learned that generally all class IA, IC, and III agents are more or less effective in terms of delaying or preventing recurrence of atrial fibrillation, several problems remain unsolved that need to be addressed for a more rational and appropriate approach to this rhythm disorder. A variety of study designs have been used that may have affected trial outcomes and influenced our perception of individual agent effectiveness.[9,10] We have learned that interpretable information concerning the efficacy and safety of therapeutic interventions can be most readily obtained from large-scale controlled clinical trials. Although major benefits have apparently accrued to patients with atrial fibrillation from the availability of new drugs, so far no clear data exist concerning the comparative efficacy of these agents. In general, there is no evidence that one of these compounds is superior to another or whether there are any important differences among them to justify any specific choice. Indeed, a rationale for a therapeutic hierarchy is not available, and for the moment, pharmacological agent selection remains crude and is still based on trial and error. Recently, emphasis has been placed on the antifibrillatory value of class III drugs such as sotalol and amiodarone.[11-17] The efficacy profile of these medications, along with clinical and experimental evidence that lengthening of the action potential duration and refractioriness, even in the absence of any change in conduction velocity, constitutes an important mechanism for termination and prevention of atrial fibrillation,[18] prompted the development of a newer generation of pure class III antiarrhythmic agents currently under clinical investigation. However, the characteristics of the so-called pure class III agents such as semetilide, dofetilide, and ibutilide should be differentiated from the more complex effects exerted by compounds such as amiodarone and sotalol. In addition, those agents that exhibit the sole effect of lengthening the action potential duration and the refractory period without any addition properties may produce, given the appropriate clinical circumstances, an appreciable incidence of torsade de pointes. It is possible that a more complex antiarrhythmic profile, such as shown by amiodarone, may be more desirable in the next antifibrillatory compounds. Relative to the use of amiodarone and sotalol, it must also be emphasized that when class III agents were used in comparative randomized studies,[11–16] their alleged superiority was not convincingly demonstrated (Table 2). Furthermore, despite a better adverse effect profile with the use of low-dose amiodarone,[17] the lack of prospectively collected long-term safety data with routine screening for side effects and cumulative toxicity should temper enthusiasm for the use of amiodarone in atrial fibrillation.

TABLE 2. Results of Randomized Comparative Study With Class III Agents for Atrial Fibrillation

Series	No. of Patients	Effectiveness, %	Follow-up, months
Vitolo[11]			
Amiodarone	28	79	6
Quinidine	26	46	6
Martin[12]			
Amiodarone	43	79	16
Disopyramide	27	55	16
Szyszka[13]			
Amiodarone	56	40	12
Quinidine	78	43	12
Propafenone	43	38	12
Verapamil	68	43	12
Digoxin	70	22	12
Placebo	56	20	12
Zehender[14]			
Amiodarone	12	92	3
Quinidine and			
verapamil	11	91	3
Reimold[15]			
Sotalol	50	30	12
Propafenone	50	37	12
Juul–Möller[16]			
Sotalol	97	49	6
Quinidine	86	42	6

In any case, although results with this medication may give reason for guarded optimism, larger comparative efficacy trials with random allocation to different therapeutic strategies are clearly required to identify the compound that will assume a major role as antifibrillatory agent.

Control of Ventricular Rate

Despite the use of powerful drugs, some patients return in atrial fibrillation or proceed from an initial partial or complete response to a more refractory and persistent dysrhythmia. In this subgroup, control of ventricular response represents a reasonable strategy. In this regard, we have become aware or have rediscovered that digitalis, the former mainstay of therapy, may now play a subsidiary role. At present, we have the choice of a number of β-blockers and two calcium channel blockers that probably have equal potency in acute and chronic control of ventricular response during atrial fibrillation. However, β-blockers may overcorrect the heart rate, resulting in excessive slowing and consequent decrease in cardiac output and exercise tolerance. Calcium channel blockers, on the other hand, do not blunt the heart rate to the same extent, and they are very effective at smoothing out the swings of heart rate that we usually observe in patients with atrial fibrillation. This notwithstanding, the use of both classes of medications is limited by the presence of a variety of side effects and, more importantly, the known negative inotropic action. In an attempt to improve the safety of calcium channel blocking drugs, newer compounds with a more favorable profile, such as diltiazem, have been developed. The ideal agent for control of patients with atrial fibrillation should be effective both at rest and during exercise, should possess no contraindications, should produce minimal side effects, and should be available in an affordable, once-daily formulation.

Adverse Reaction With Drug Therapy

One specific aspect of pharmacology, ie, toxicity profile, merits a special mention. Ever since therapy with quinidine, the archetype of antiarrhythmic compounds, was introduced, it has been argued whether the possible advantages of conversion to sinus rhythm in cases of atrial fibrillation compensate for the disadvantages and the risks. Frequently, the physician is faced with the dichotomy that seemingly reasonable and effective therapeutic maneuvers evoke, under certain circumstances, unexpected and even potentially deleterious effects. The main areas of concern with respect to drugs used to treat atrial fibrillation are adverse reaction in left ventricular function and a number of proarrhythmic effects, including (1) a worsening or change of a preexisting rhythm disorder, such as an increase in the frequency and duration of atrial fibrillation paroxysm, enhanced AV nodal conduction or increase of ventricular response related to slowing of atrial rate, or a change from atrial fibrillation to atrial flutter with a more rapid ventricular response; (2) development of new ventricular arrhythmias such as torsade de pointes and monomorphic ventricular tachycardia; and (3) occurrence of bradyarrhythmia resulting from depression of sinus node function or atrioventricular conduction. Although this complication of drug therapy has been well established and is of particular concern in patients with extensive heart disease and markedly impaired left ventricular function,[9,10,19] little is actually known about it and, despite much speculation, the mechanism by which drugs facilitate arrhythmias remains unresolved. It is essential that we understand the mechanism of this process so that we may potentially obviate the untoward effects while retaining the positive therapeutic value of these agents. Regarding this issue, attempts were made to establish a correlation between ion-channel activity and proarrhythmic action.[20] No clear pattern of correlation emerged, emphasizing that it may be exceedingly difficult to relate ion-channel data with clinical in vivo observations. The same is true in dealing with the antiarrhythmic actions of various agents. Clearly, more experimental data are required to determine whether any specific effect at the molecular level might account for their varying spectrum of antiarrhythmic and proarrhythmic actions in animal models and in humans. Until more information is available, it now seems prudent to be more circumspect when considering the initiation of drug therapy for atrial fibrillation.

Compatibility of Implantable Devices With Drug Therapy

In the era of technology, another aspect deserving of consideration is the possibility of interaction between antiarrhythmic drugs and implantable devices. A considerable proportion of patients subjected to defibrillator implant for ventricular tachycardia/ventricular fibrillation experience atrial fibrillation. In addition, treatment of atrial fibrillation by initiation of antiarrhythmic therapy may aggravate or precipitate conduction system impairment that necessitates pacing therapy. Clinical observations have shown that antiarrhythmic drugs, for the most part, are able to produce an increase of defibrillation energy requirements[21–25] and pacing threshold.[26–28] Furthermore, medications can interact with the arrhythmogenic substrate in the ventricle and make ventricular tachycardia episodes refractory to previously successful termination algorithms. It is also true that antiarrhythmic drugs can lengthen the tachycardia cycle beyond the detection rate of the device. In this setting, there is a demand for novel therapeutic entities that produce either no effects or a decrease of defibrillation energy requirements. Preliminary experimental results seem to indicate that class III agents might provide such benefits.[29,30] A newer upcoming generation of devices, implantable atrial defibrillators, will raise additional questions to be addressed and create further ground for potential interactions with pharmacological agents. Some data[31] seem to suggest that internal synchronized cardioversion of atrial fibrillation is more likely to precipitate ventricular fibrillation if the RR interval before the shock is short. Shorter intervals do not allow sufficient time for repolarization from prior QRS complex to complete; therefore, at the time of the shock, a portion of the myocardial tissue will still be vulnerable. In this context, medications that prolong the refractory period such as class III agents are most undesirable, whereas compounds with selective blocking effect on the atrioventricular node will minimize the probability of this event and make atrial defibrillation somewhat safer. It is clear that several issues remain unsettled (Table 3) and need to be resolved to provide a basis for developing adjunctive therapies and to achieve the maximal benefit from pharmacological treatment. However, major advances in therapeutics in all probability will come not from present drug development strategies but rather from the understanding of the molecular basis of arrhythmogenesis.

Future Directions

Although it is clear that several of the old and newer antiarrhythmic agents are efficacious in preventing recurrence of atrial

TABLE 3.   Unsettled and Critical Issues for More Efficient
Pharmacological Treatment

Large randomized comparative trials
  Efficacy
  Safety
  Cost
  Quality of life
Innovative compounds
  Convenient dosing
  No negative inotropism
  Minimal systemic toxicity
  Effective after substrate changes
  Minimal potential for proarrhythmia
  Compatibility with implantable devices
Better characterization of patient subgroups
More specific definition of different physiopathologies
Understanding of drug/substrate/trigger interaction
Comprehension of proarrhythmic mechanisms
Role of sympathovagal balance
Molecular/genetic basis

fibrillation, the best mode of initial therapy is not known with any certainty. When we ultimately understand arrhythmogensis, the nature of the channels that govern the movement of various ions, and the interaction of drugs with different "phases" of the channels, perhaps we will be able to select the mode of therapy that is most appropriate for each patient. Understanding and identification of specific entities of atrial fibrillation are desirable as well and might have important implications in tailoring therapy to this very heterogeneous rhythm disturbance. Better methods are needed for selecting high-risk patients, for categorizing them according to the therapeutic modality most ideal for them, and for assessing the antiarrhythmic effects of drugs. Further studies are required to better identify those patients who should be spared prolonged and frustrating serial trials of multiple antiarrhythmic agents. In this population, rate control with medications certainly represents an acceptable choice and needs to be compared with nonpharmacological approaches designed to achieve the same goal. In addition, these observations also highlight the demand for safer and more effective pharmacological agents. Ideally, selective prolongation of refractoriness in the atrial myocardium may have potential for a better safety and efficacy profile in limiting ventricular proarrhythmias and increasing compatibility with implantable devices. Initial estimates of the efficacy of newer investigational medications are encouraging, but additional safety data need to be accumulated. In the future, the interaction of modern molecular biology and the practice of medicine will probably revolutionize our approach to drug control of atrial fibrillation. Although cardiology has been slow to embrace the technique of recombinant DNA in the past few years, molecular cardiology techniques have suddenly blossomed and may offer a refreshing approach and an advantage over existing methodologies. Molecular biology provides an unexplored opportunity to investigate various biological processes in a manner hitherto not possible with the indirect techniques of biochemistry, biophysics, and physiology. The ability to perform in vivo structure-function analysis of a selected molecule will pave the way for the ongoing development of new therapeutic agents. The power of recombinant techniques to modify and specifically determine in vivo function of a single protein provides the means to develop specific drugs more rapidly and to minimize or alter their side effects. At present, most of the antiarrhythmic drugs are directed against the sodium channel. In the future, the awareness of a multitude of different regulatory channels and the ability to clone and sequence cardiac tissue–specific proteins responsible for the function of these ionic channels will promote the beginning of the era of recombinant DNA engineered therapy. Analysis of the structure-activity relationships of the electrophysiological effects of traditional and experimental antiarrhythmic agents will aid in the rational design of more potent antiarrhythmic drugs with improved therapeutic margin and enhanced specificity. It is doubtful that any single drug will be capable of preventing and curing all important types of arrhythmias and meet all the requirements put forward for the ideal antiarrhythmic drug. Thus, the next generation of antiarrhythmic agents will be directed toward selectively influencing a specific cardiac channel and will most likely be more effective and associated with fewer side effects than the present conventional drugs. It is relevant to mention, however, that the newer drugs should be compatible with implantable atrial defibrillators as well as effective in atrial tissue modified by catheter ablation. Both of these technologies are likely to be an integral part of management of patients with atrial fibrillation in the future.

Conclusions

Pharmacological therapy for atrial fibrillation is an active and evolving area of research. Changes in the clinical features and pathophysiology of atrial fibrillation have been paralleled by a dramatic increase in the number of therapeutic strategies and advances in our ability to assess the efficacy and safety of new interventions. However, despite such laudable achievements, important limitations remain, and empiricism still characterizes the treatment of this disorder. A great need exists for a more efficient characterization of patient subgroups to allow a more individualized and effective use of current and future therapeutic agents. The development of innovative remedies for this disorder is also highly auspicious, and insights into the basic pathophysiological mechanisms will certainly prove critical to indicate the direction to pursue. In addition, larger randomized comparative trials will provide the rationale for a more logical pharmacological approach. Finally, although our complete understanding of the drug substrate interaction at the molecular level is still in its infancy, as molecular cardiology continues to make advances, treatment beyond the imagination will unfold and change our outlook on this complex arrhythmia.

References

1. Bialy D, Lehmann MH, Schumacher DN, et al. Hospitalization for arrhythmias in the United States: importance of atrial fibrillation. *J Am Coll Cardiol.* 1991;19:41A. Abstract.
2. Kannel WB, Abott RD, Savage DD, et al. Epidemiologic features of chronic atrial fibrillation: the Framingham Study. *N Engl J Med.* 1982;306:1018–1022.
3. Moe GK. On the multiple wavelet hypothesis of atrial fibrillation. *Arch Int Pharmacodyn Ther.* 1962;140:183–188.
4. Wang W, Bourne G, Wang Z, et al. Comparative mechanisms of antiarrhythmic drug action in experimental atrial fibrillation. *Circulation.* 1993;88:1030–1044.
5. Coumel P. Neural aspects of paroxysmal atrial fibrillation. In: Falk RH, Podrid PJ, eds. *Atrial Fibrillation: Mechanisms and Management.* New York, NY: Raven Press Ltd: 1992:109–125.
6. Kadish A, Spear J, Levine J, et al. The effects of procainamide on conduction in anisotropic canine ventricular myocardium. *Circulation.* 1986;74:616–625.

 7. Sekiguchi M, et al. Experience of 100 atrial endomyocardial biopsy and the concept of atrial cardiomyopathy. *Circulation.* 1984;70(suppl II):II–118. Abstract.
 8. Guiraudon CM, Ernst NM, Klein GJ, et al. The pathology of intractable "primary" atrial fibrillation. *Circulation.* 1992;6(suppl I):I–662. Abstract.
 9. Reimold SC, Chalmers TC, Berlin JA, et al. Assessment of the efficacy and safety of antiarrhythmic therapy for chronic atrial fibrillation: observations on the role of trial design and implications of drug-related mortality. *Am Heart J.* 1992;124:924–932.
10. Coplen SE, Antman EM, Berlin JA, et al. Efficacy and safety of quinidine therapy for maintenance of sinus rhythm after cardioversion. *Circulation.* 1990;82:1106–1116.
11. Vitolo E, Tronci M, Larovere MT, et al. Amiodarone versus quinidine in the prophylaxis of atrial fibrillation. *Acta Cardiol.* 1981;36:431–444.
12. Martin A, Benbow LJ, Leach C, et al. Comparison of amiodarone and disopyramide in the control of paroxysmal atrial fibrillation and atrial flutter (interim report). *Br J Clin Pract.* 1986;44(suppl):52–60.
13. Syzszka A, Paluszkiewicz L, Baszynska H, et al. Prophylactic treatment after electroconversion of atrial fibrillation in patients after cardiac surgery: a controlled two-years follow-up study. *J Am Coll Cardiol.* 1993;21:201A. Abstract.
14. Zehender M, Hohnloser S, Muller B, et al. Effects of amiodarone versus quinidine and verapamil in patients with chronic atrial fibrillation: results of a comparative study and a 2-year follow-up. *J Am Coll Cardiol.* 1992;19:1054–1059.
15. Reimold S, Cantillon C, Friedman P, et al. Propafenone versus sotalol for suppression of recurrent symptomatic atrial fibrillation. *Am J Cardiol.* 1993;71:558–563.
16. Juul-Möller S, Edvardsson N, Rehnqvist-Ahlberg N. Sotalol versus quinidine for the maintenance of sinus rhythm after direct current conversion of atrial fibrillation. *Circulation.* 1990;82:1932–1939.
17. Marcel A, Crijns H, Van Gelder I, et al. Low-dose amiodarone for maintenance of sinus rhythm after cardioversion of atrial fibrillation or flutter. *JAMA.* 1992;267:3289–3293.
18. Singh BN, Nademanee NK. Control of arrhythmias by selective lengthening of cardiac repolarization: theoretical considerations and clinical observations. *Am Heart J.* 1985;109:421–430.
19. Flaker G, Blackshear J, McBride R, et al. Antiarrhythmic drug therapy and cardiac mortality in atrial fibrillation. *J Am Coll Cardiol.* 1992;20:527–532.
20. Singh B, Sarma J, Zhang Z, et al. Controlling cardiac arrhythmias by lengthening repolarization: rationale from experimental findings and clinical considerations. *Ann N Y Acad Sci.* 1992;644:187–209.
21. Echt DS, Black JN, Barbey JT, et al. Evaluation of antiarrhythmic drugs on defibrillation energy requirements in dogs: sodium channel block and action potential prolongation. *Circulation.* 1989;79:1106–1117.
22. Babbs CF, Yim GKW, Whistler SJ, et al. Elevation of ventricular defib-

rillation threshold in dogs by antiarrhythmic drugs. *Am Heart J.* 1979; 98:345–350.

23. Echt DS, Cato EL, Coxe DR. pH dependent effects of lidocaine on defibrillation energy requirements in dogs. *Circulation.* 1989;80: 1003–1009.

24. Fain ES, Lee JT, Winkle RA. Effects of acute and chronic amiodarone on defibrillation energy requirements. *Am Heart J.* 1987;114:8–17.

25. Guarnieri T, Levine JH, Veltri EP, et al. Success of chronic defibrillation and the role of antiarrhythmic drugs with the automatic implantable cardioverter-defibrillator. *Am J Cardiol.* 1987;60:1061–1064.

26. Guarnieri T, Datorre SD, Bondke H, et al. Increased pacing threshold after an automatic defibrillator shock in dogs: effects of class I and class II antiarrhythmic drugs. *PACE Pacing Clin Electrophysiol.* 1988;11: 1324–1330.

27. Singer I, Guarnieri T, Kupersmith J. Implanted automatic defibrillators: effects of drugs and pacemakers. *PACE Pacing Clin Electrophysiol.* 1988;11:2250–2262.

28. Hellestrand KJ, Burnett PJ, Milne JR, et al. Effect of the antiarrhythmic agent flecainide acetate on acute and chronic pacing thresholds. *PACE Pacing Clin Electrophysiol.* 1983;6:892–899.

29. Wang MJ, Dorian P. DL and D sotalol decrease defibrillation energy requirements. *PACE Pacing Clin Electrophysiol.* 1989;12:1522–1529.

30. Langberg JJ, Underwood T, Gallagher M, et al. The effects of ibutilide applied to the epicardium on defibrillation threshold. *J Am Coll Cardiol.* 1993;21(suppl):244A. Abstract.

31. Ayers GM, Alferness CA, Ilina M, et al. Ventricular proarrhythmic effects of ventricular cycle length and shock strength in a sheep model of transvenous atrial defibrillation. *Circulation.* 1994;89:413–422.

Chapter 16

Future Directions of Nonpharmacological Therapy

Mark E. Josephson, MD; Kevin M. Monahan, MD; and Mark J. Seifert, MD

Atrial fibrillation is the most common arrhythmia, afflicting 1% to 2% of our population. Its frequency increases with age, and it is the most common cause of hospital admission for an arrhythmia. Atrial fibrillation is often associated with sinus node dysfunction as part of the bradycardia tachycardia syndrome. It may occur paroxysmally or chronically and may be associated with a variety of cardiac diseases, but it may also be part of the "natural history" of the brady-tachy syndrome. The associated morbidity and mortality of atrial fibrillation are related to thromboembolic complications, heart failure, and palpitations or syncope associated with a rapid ventricular response. While anticoagulation can in large part prevent the thromboembolic phenomenon, pharmacological therapy has been rather disappointing in preventing the recurrence of paroxysmal atrial fibrillation, resulting in the high cost associated with recurrent hospitalizations. Moreover, the proarrhythmic effects of these agents, as well as other disabling side effects, have led physicians to consider nonpharmacological alternatives to manage various problems posed by atrial fibrillation. Four nonpharmacological approaches have been applied and will be discussed in this chapter. These include (1) pacing for the prevention and potential termination of atrial fibrillation, (2) atrioventricular (AV) junctional ablation for rate control with associated pacemaker implantation, (3) low-energy cardioversion of paroxysmal episodes of atrial fibrillation, and (4) surgery.

From DiMarco JP, Prystowsky EN (eds): *Atrial Arrhythmias: State of the Art.* Armonk, NY, Futura Publishing Company, Inc., © 1995.

Pacing for Atrial Fibrillation

Several retrospective observational studies have reported a high incidence of development of chronic atrial fibrillation in patients with sinus node dysfunction in whom VVI pacemakers have been implanted. Many of these studies[1-11] demonstrated that in patients with sick sinus syndrome treated with atrial or AV sequential pacing, there was a much lower incidence of development of chronic atrial fibrillation than when VVI pacemakers were used. The presence of ventriculoatrial (VA) conduction and failure to use rate-responsive ventricular pacing in these older studies may have been important contributors to the negative outcomes in patients treated with ventricular-based pacing systems. Rosenqvist et al[8,9] demonstrated that patients treated with VVI pacing had a 47% incidence of developing chronic atrial fibrillation, whereas those treated with atrial or AV sequential pacing had a 6.7% incidence of developing chronic atrial fibrillation with a 4-year follow-up. Moreover, they demonstrated marked reductions in congestive heart failure (37% vs 15%) and overall mortality (23% vs 8%) when atrial-based pacing systems were used. Sutton and Kenney[10] recently reviewed 18 studies evaluating permanent pacing in the sick sinus syndrome. The incidence of atrial fibrillation developing with atrial-based pacing was 4%, whereas that associated with VVI pacing was 22%. All of these studies were retrospective and not randomized and thus suffer from the potential for physician bias in patient selection. In addition, rate-responsive VVI pacing was not used in these studies. These problems were recently reviewed by Lamas et al,[11] who urged that a prospective randomized study be undertaken to assess the true value of atrial-based systems. Lamas proposed a study evaluating the various programming modalities available to prevent atrial fibrillation. Such a study would use VVIR pacing, AAIR pacing, DDIR pacing and DDDR pacing.

Ventricular pacing may induce atrial fibrillation in part through the presence of VA conduction, with the resultant continuous cannon A waves leading to atrial stretch and altered atrial refractoriness predisposing to the development of atrial fibrillation. With atrial-based systems, AV sequential pacing maintains AV synchrony, improved hemodynamics, and in instances of chronotropic insufficiency increases the heart rate and potentially reduces dispersion of atrial refractoriness, which may be related to the devel-

TABLE 1. Studies Comparing Atrial Fibrillation and Survival Rates in VVI vs Atrial or Dual-Chamber Pacing

Authors	Follow-up, months	No. of Patients		AF (%)		CHF (%)		Mortality (%)	
		VVI	A/AV	VVI	A/AV	VVI	A/AV	VVI	A/AV
Lemke et al[1]	60	—	100	—	11	—	—	—	15
Markewitz et al[3]	32	87	136	30	7	—	—	—	—
Hesselson et al[4]	96	100	303	80	20	—	—	—	—
Rosenqvist et al[8,9]	48	79	89	47	7	37	15	23	8
Santini et al[6]	54	125	214	47	7	—	—	30	14
Sasaki et al[2]	50	34	41	44	17	21	2	35	12
Sethi et al[5]	49	47	40	21	3	23	5	15	10
Stangl et al[7]	53	112	110	19	6	—	—	28	17
Sutton and Kenney[10]	38	651	410	22	4	—	—	—	—

AF=atrial fibrillation; CHF=congestive heart failure. Adapted from Lamas GA, et al. *PACE Pacing Clin Electrophysiol.* 1992;15:1109–1113.

opment of atrial fibrillation. DDD systems may be not optimal for patients with paroxysmal atrial fibrillation because they may track the atrial fibrillation, leading to a rapid ventricular response. Therefore, if such systems are used, some method of controlling atrial tracking is needed. Although this problem can be avoided by DDIR programming, improvements in current automatic mode switching will probably provide the optimal way to manage this disorder and prevent tracking of paroxysmal episodes when they occur.

A specific group of patients in whom pacing may be especially useful are those with bradycardia-dependent atrial fibrillation or those with so-called "vagally mediated" atrial fibrillation. Coumel and his colleagues[12–14] have been responsible for our recognizing this group of patients, in whom there was a strong male predominance, with onset of the syndrome occurring at middle age. Episodes frequently occur at night but also may be precipitated in the postprandial state. Sympathetic drive and emotion appear to play no role in the genesis of this arrhythmia. Analysis of events preceding the onset of these arrhythmias shows progressive sinus bradycardia and an increase in the high-frequency heart rate variability characteristic of vagal influence. Preliminary evidence in a small group of these patients suggests that atrial pacing above a critical rate may prevent occurrences of atrial fibrillation. Attuel et al[14] noted a paradoxical improvement of intra-atrial conduction delay associated with such atrial pacing in these patients. Although the follow-up has been short, these investigators have demonstrated a high incidence of freedom of recurrence of atrial fibrillation with atrial-based pacing. Thus, it seems at present that patients with paroxysmal atrial fibrillation, particularly those associated with sinus node dysfunction or vagally mediated atrial fibrillation, are appropriate candidates for atrially based pacing systems. While an AAI(R) pacing modality would seem logical, AV conduction problems, a common accompaniment of sinus node dysfunction, limits its utility. Although a prospective randomized control study is necessary, review of the literature suggests that the optimal pacing modality in such patients would be DDIR. Use of such pacemakers would be expected to decrease the incidence of atrial fibrillation, with attendant reduction in heart failure and overall mortality. Whether or not thromboembolic complications can be prevented is uncertain.

While overdrive pacing has been used to treat a variety of reentrant arrhythmias, including atrial tachycardia and atrial flutter, cardiac pacing techniques have not been used to treat atrial fibrillation because of the assumed inability to capture the atrium during atrial fibrillation. However, recent studies using high-resolution mapping in experimental animal models of atrial fibrillation and in experimental human atria have demonstrated multiple simultaneous small meandering wave fronts of activation as the mechanism of atrial fibrillation. For instance, Allessie et al[15,16] proposed that, for fibrillation to perpetuate, a critical number of wave fronts must be present, which in turn requires a critical mass of atrial tissue. Analysis of atrial electrograms in these studies,[15-17] as well as observations in humans,[18] showed variation of local atrial cycles, suggesting that an excitable gap is present during atrial fibrillation at many sites within the atrium at different times. This observation offers the potential to capture the atria during established atrial fibrillation and might serve as a potential mechanism for pace termination of atrial fibrillation. Allessie et al[17] attempted to stimulate areas of the atrium during an experimental model of atrial fibrillation. Although they were able to capture areas of up to 4 cm^2, fibrillation was never terminated. Preliminary data from our laboratory have demonstrated the ability to capture multiple areas of atrial tissue during atrial fibrillation, but as yet, only the acceleration of local atrial electrograms has occurred, and not the termination of established atrial fibrillation. However, further studies using multisite atrial pacing should be considered to evaluate termination of atrial fibrillation, particularly in the postoperative patient. In a similar vein, multisite atrial pacing may be used to capture large areas of the atrium simultaneously to prevent initiation of atrial fibrillation by limiting the amount of tissue available for reentry to occur in response to any atrial premature complex. Such studies will certainly commence in the next several years.

AV Junctional Ablation for Ventricular Rate Control

Pharmacological therapy directed toward rate control has been relatively successful for rate control in chronic atrial fibrillation but has been less effective in those with paroxysmal atrial fibrillation. Many patients require combinations of drugs that have potential side effects. In recognition of the problem of ventricular rate control, AV junctional ablation was developed as a means to control the ventricular response in atrial fibrillation by patient preference or in patients whose arrhythmia control was refractory to pharmacological agents or in whom pharmacological agents produced undesirable side effects.[19,20] Although AV junctional ablation was initially performed by direct surgical approaches,[21] the advent of catheter ablation has totally replaced this approach and has achieved high success rates (80% to 90%) for the production of complete heart block with relatively no morbidity.[20,22] A 2% to 5% incidence of sudden death after successful ablation by DC current has been reported, but most of these cases were compounded by the presence of serious organic heart disease and demonstrated proarrhythmic effects of antiarrhythmic agents used in the patients as adjunctive therapy.[23] The incidence of sudden death appears to be diminished with the use of radiofrequency ablation. Thus, it is unclear whether ablation itself carries a substantial risk.

This approach has been associated with improvement in congestive heart failure as well as subjective quality of life and appears to be cost-effective.[22] As acceptance of such a strategy for patients with drug-refractory atrial fibrillation grows, one must always be cognizant of the limitations of this strategy; ie, atrial systole is not restored in those patients with chronic atrial fibrillation, and the long-term risk of embolization is unaltered. Obviously, the production of complete heart block necessitates a pacemaker, and the choice of pacemaker depends on whether or not chronic atrial fibrillation is present. In the patient with chronic atrial fibrillation, VVIR pacemakers should be used, but as stressed above, in patients in whom intermittent sinus rhythm is present, the use of an atrial-based dual-chamber system with rate responsiveness (in the presence of chronotropic incompetence) should be used. Such pacemakers obviously will need some form of mode switching or upper rate control to prevent tracking of atrial arrhythmias should they occur spontaneously. We have frequently found AV nodal ablation to be a procedure of choice in elderly patients who find it difficult to take multiple drugs with their attendant side effects. This approach should probably be considered early in patients with bradycardia-tachycardia syndrome who are having pacemakers implanted for symptomatic bradycardia, especially if recurrent episodes of atrial fibrillation are observed. Whether or not radiofrequency or other energy sources can be used to alter the functional refractory period of the AV node without inducing complete heart block and eliminate the need for permanent pacing awaits further investigation.

Implantable Atrial Defibrillator

With success of the implantable cardioverter/defibrillator (ICD) in the treatment of ventricular tachycardia and fibrillation, interest has grown in the development of such a device for the detection and termination of atrial fibrillation. Such a system could potentially eliminate the need for costly hospital admissions, inpatient cardioversions, antiarrhythmic medications with proarrhythmic potential, and possibly chronic anticoagulation. Central to the discussion in the development of such a device are its feasibility, the potential problems associated with its use, and delineation of indications for its implantation. The ability of an atrial defibrillation system to restore sinus rhythm has been demonstrated in several animal models of atrial fibrillation. Using a talc-induced pericarditis model in the dog, Dunbar et al[24] were able to successfully cardiovert 26% of atrial tachyarrhythmic episodes with one 1.0-J shock. In their study, the defibrillation electrodes were confined to the right atrium or right atrium and superior vena cava, and energy was delivered with a monophasic pulse waveform. Histological sectioning after repeated cardioversion attempts revealed no pathological evidence of electrically induced injury. Powell et al[25], using a rapid atrial pacing model of atrial fibrillation in sheep, evaluated atrial defibrillation using a right atrial spring electrode and a left thoracic subcutaneous patch. They noted a dose-response curve that plateaued at 5 J, at which approximately 80% of atrial fibrillation episodes could be converted. At 1.5 J, approximately 50% of episodes were terminated. There was an incidence of ventricular fibrillation of 2.4%, which appeared to be related to poor synchronization to the R wave. Most recently, Cooper et al[26] reported the results of low-energy intra-atrial cardioversion in the rapid atrial pacing sheep model using a variety of atrial electrode configurations. They were able to terminate atrial fibrillation in 55% of animals by use of a transvenous configuration. The highest success rates were obtained with a transvenous right-to-left lead configuration (cathode positioned in the right atrial appendage and the anode in the biphasic waveform). Under these conditions, the successful energy requirement for 50% cardioversion was 1.3 ± 0.4 J.

These findings support the notion that low-energy cardioversion will be possible in humans and suggest that the incorporation of a critical mass of atrial tissue within the field of energy delivered, as well as the delivery of a biphasic waveform, may be an important determinant of success. It remains to be seen, however, whether these designs result in defibrillation thresholds in enlarged and diseased human atria as low as those observed in normal experimental animal models. Two human studies have been carried out.[27,28] As with the animal studies, biphasic waveforms were superior to monophasic waveforms delivered with epicardial paddles intraoperatively.[27] When endocardial catheter defibrillation was attempted using biphasic waveforms between the right atrium and coronary sinus, atrial defibrillation thresholds ranged from 3 to 8 J.[28] It remains to be seen what level of energy will be tolerable for the individual patient in terms of pain. In previous studies using low-energy cardioversion for ventricular tachycardia, severe pain was perceived at energy levels of ≤ 2 J.[29] Although this concern has become secondary in the progress of ICDs, it is likely to prove a major consideration in implantable atrial defibrillators. During an episode of ventricular tachycardia or ventricular fibrillation, consciousness is often impaired, and the life-threatening nature of the arrhythmia can justify imposition of a high degree of discomfort. On the other hand, the nonthreatening nature of atrial fibrillation, which in the vast majority of patients will necessitate multiple discharges, will require a nearly painless discharge of energy to gain general acceptance.

The ability to automatically and reliably detect atrial fibrillation through intracardiac electrograms is an additional consideration in assessment of the feasibility of an atrial defibrillator. In comparison with ventricular electrograms used in current ICD algorithms, atrial electrograms are smaller and more variable in amplitude. As such, the degree of sensitivity required for their detection may render the devices more prone to electromechanical interference as well as the potential for oversensing far-field ventricular electrograms. Despite these limitations, the ability to diagnose atrial fibrillation may prove less problematic, since early works using rate criteria, power spectral analysis, and probability density function appear promising in their ability to differentiate atrial fibrillation from sinus tachycardia with a high degree of specificity.[30] The proarrhythmic potential of transvenous atrial defibrillation has been noted in animal studies by Dunbar, Cooper, and Powell and their colleagues.[24-26] In both the dog model and the sheep model, ventricular fibrillation has been induced in up to 2.5% of defibrillation attempts. This phenomenon was correlated with high shock energies and the timing of delivery late after the QRS during ventricular repolarization. These data were similar in both the dog and sheep models regardless of configurations used. These findings emphasize the importance of achieving reliable synchronization to ventricular depolarization in the development of the atrial defibrillator. Therefore, it is likely that initial devices will be manually activated to ensure safety. Nevertheless, it is likely that devices with backup ventricular defibrillation will be required, since total freedom from induction of ventricular fibrillation during actual defibrillation cannot be guaranteed.

Ultimately, the clinical success of the atrial defibrillator will depend on appropriate patient selection. Ideally, these devices would be used in the treatment of sustained (>1 minute), recurrent atrial fibrillation occurring with a frequency high enough to make such devices relevant and cost-effective. If episodes occurred too frequently, the inconvenience of potentially painful discharges and limited battery life would render such therapy inappropriate. How frequent or disabling the arrhythmia would be needs to be determined. This highlights the need for establishing a method to assess the presence of asymptomatic short runs of atrial fibrillation not

predicted by the incidence of symptomatic episodes in those patients with paroxysmal atrial fibrillation. If short-lived, asymptomatic episodes were present, they could lead to a much higher incidence of painful shocks than is currently predicted by "clinically
symptomatic" recurrent episodes. Such shocks would clearly be undesirable and limit the utility of this device. This may require the
presence of several minutes of sensed atrial fibrillation before the
delivery of defibrillation shocks.

Surgical Approaches to Atrial Fibrillation

The ideal surgical operation to treat atrial fibrillation would
prevent its occurrence while maintaining normal sinus and AV
nodal function and removing the risk of embolization. Approaches
to achieve this are based on the observation that maintenance of
atrial fibrillation requires a critical mass of tissue through which independent wavelets of deploarization can propagate.[15,16] One of the
early procedures developed was left atrial isolation,[31] in which the
mass of atrial tissue available for fibrillation would be essentially divided by two. While this procedure met with some success in canine
experimental models of fibrillation, it failed to produce atrial synchrony and reduce the potential risk of embolization. Another isolation procedure, known as the corridor procedure, was developed
by Guiraudon et al in 1985.[32] In this procedure, the right atrium was
divided into three components, the center of which would be an isolated corridor containing the sinus node and the AV node in a strip
of atrial tissue. However, the remainder of the atria could continue
to fibrillate. Thus, anticoagulation would still be necessary, and the
optimal effects of atrial contraction or overall hemodynamic function would not be achieved. The major effect of this procedure
would therefore be prevention of rapid, irregular rhythms, preclud-
ing palpitations and heart failure. Thus, there are limited advantages of the corridor procedure over catheter ablation of the AV
node and rate-responsive pacemaker implantation. While one is
spared the implantation of the pacemaker, the operative mortality
is greater, and a significant number of patients will later require
pacemakers. Moreover, catheter ablation is much less complex a
procedure and can be more widely applied. As such, the corridor
procedure has been largely abandoned even by Dr Guiraudon as a

method of treating atrial fibrillation (G.M. Guiraudon, personal communication).

Over the past decade, Cox and his colleagues[33-36] have systematically studied the mechanisms of atrial flutter and fibrillation and developed a surgical procedure, the "maze" procedure, aimed at preventing atrial fibrillation while maintaining sinus rhythm, AV synchrony, and atrial transport functions (Fig 1). This difficult procedure entails multiple atriotomies, which allow narrow routes of atrial activation between the sinus node and AV node but eliminate the possibility of impulses reentering an area previously activated. The critical mass of atrial tissue required for reentry is limited by the suture lines. Between 1987 and 1992, Cox and his colleagues operated on 75 patients.[36] Only 1 patient died, although the perioperative period was fraught with recurrent episodes of atrial flutter/fibrillation and massive fluid retention (thought to be due to loss of atrial natriuretic factor secondary to the atriotomies). Following this initial period, atrial fibrillation was eliminated with (6 of 65) or without (58 of 65) antiarrhythmic agents, with only 1 recurrence. Atrial transport has been documented in all but 1 patient by transesophageal echocardiography and magnetic resonance imaging; however, nearly 40% of patients required atrial or dual-chamber pacing because of preoperative or perioperative sinus node dysfunction. Thus, while the procedure seems to achieve the desired success of rendering the atrial myocardium refractory to the development of atrial fibrillation (in the absence of a perioperative situation), a significant minority of patients still require pacemakers. The preservation of sinus rhythm or atrial paced rhythm and AV synchrony appears to optimize ventricular function. However, the importance of this augmentation of ventricular function with respect to quality of life has not been established in any sort of controlled clinical trial. Moreover, the assumption that the risks of thromboemboli are totally eliminated by this procedure has yet to be validated, since the multiple atriotomies and persistent scar tissue that forms may serve as a nidus for thrombus even though the atria can contract. Further modification of the maze procedure is required to ensure the preservation of sinus node function; however, the presence of sinus node dysfunction in a significant number of patients before they undergo the maze procedure will always ensure that at least 25% require pacemakers. This detracts somewhat from the claim that this procedure is a "cure." In addition, in patients with a very dilated diseased atrium, additional strips of atrial my-

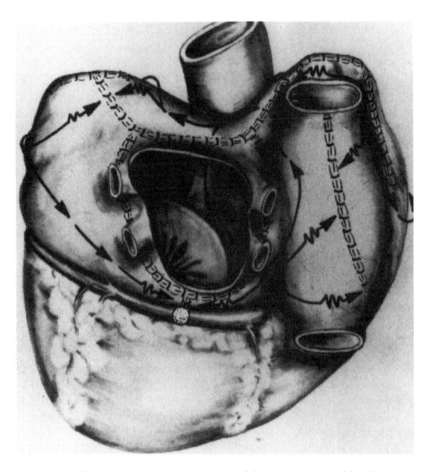

FIGURE 1. *Three-dimensional depiction of the incisions used for the maze procedure. The multiple incisions guide the impulses through narrow pathways preceding atrial fibrillation and maintaining sinus rhythm. Arrows show pattern of propagation of sinus impulse. Adapted from Cox JL, et al.* J Thorac Cardiovasc Surg. *1991;101:569–583.*

ocardium may need to be removed to limit the mass of tissue between suture lines. Thus, one must be cautiously optimistic about the ultimate value of this extremely complex procedure.

The maze procedure has also been applied to patients undergoing surgery for other reasons, such as atrial septal defects and mitral valve repair, and in such instances seems reasonable, although it increases morbidity in those procedures.[34] The major question that remains is who should undergo such a procedure. Until now, it has been reserved for patients with medically refractory atrial fibrillation who cannot tolerate the presence of atrial fibrillation for a variety of reasons. Cox et al[34,36] suggest that a single thromboembolic phenomenon is an indication for the procedure. While the former may be a reasonable criterion to consider undergoing open-heart surgery, I do not agree that the latter is an absolute indication. Although anticoagulation does not reduce the incidence of thromboemboli to zero, persistence of thromboemboli in the presence of anticoagulation may reflect extracardiac sources of emboli, and in such instances the maze procedure would not be expected to improve on that incidence. Thus, until patients with persistent atrial fibrillation and rate control with either pacemaker or drugs who are anticoagulated are compared with those undergoing the maze operation for quality-of-life issues and cost-effectiveness issues, one cannot strongly advocate one approach over the other. However, as our knowledge of the basic mechanisms underlying atrial fibrillation improves and catheter techniques evolve, it may be possible to achieve results similar to those of the maze procedure by use of catheter ablation techniques. This is a goal of the future that will certainly be actively pursued in the next decade.

Conclusions

Although chronic atrial fibrillation and many episodes of atrial fibrillation can be managed by pharmacological means, a significant proportion of patients remain symptomatic and/or intolerant of the drugs that are necessary to keep them controlled. In such instances, the role of nonpharmacological therapies is expanding. The ability to prevent atrial fibrillation by pacing techniques and the development of an implantable atrial cardioverter/defibrillator may be important additions soon to be applied for patients with atrial fibrillation. Surgical intervention may theoretically be the best way to treat atrial fibrillation; however, in the absence of definitive data demonstrating that the results of the procedure are better than other forms of nonpharmacological or pharmacological therapies, the complexity of the procedure and the limited number of centers capable of performing the procedure suggest that further studies are necessary before one can recommend surgery as an early procedure at this time. The appropriate use of these nonpharmacological approaches is expected to evolve over the next decade as clinicians, basic scientists, and industry work together to address this most common of arrhythmias.

References

1. Lemke B, Holtman BJ, Selbach H, et al. The atrial pacemaker: retrospective analysis of complications and life expectancy in patients with sinus node dysfunction. *Int J Cardiol.* 1989;22:185–193.
2. Sasaki Y, Shimotori M, Akahane K, et al. Long term follow-up of patients with sick sinus syndrome: a comparison of clinical aspects among unpaced, ventricular inhibited paced, and physiologically paced groups. *PACE Pacing Clin Electrophysiol.* 1988;11:1575–1583.
3. Markewitz A, Schad N, Hemmer W, et al. What is the most appropriate stimulation mode in patients with sinus node dysfunction? *PACE Pacing Clin Electrophysiol.* 1986;9:1115–1120.
4. Hesselson AB, Parsonnet V, Perry G. Progression to atrial fibrillation from the DDD, DVI, and VVI pacing modes. *PACE Pacing Clin Electrophysiol.* 1990;13:564. Abstract.
5. Sethi KK, Bajaj V, Mohan JC, et al. Comparison of atrial and VVI pacing modes in symptomatic sinus node dysfunction without associated tachyarrhythmias. *Indian Heart J.* 1990;42:143–147.
6. Santini M, Alexidou G, Ansalone G, et al. Relation of prognosis in sick sinus syndrome to age, conduction defects and modes of permanent cardiac pacing. *Am J Cardiol.* 1990;65:729–735.
7. Stangl K, Seitz K, Wirtzfeld A, et al. Difference between atrial single chamber pacing (AAI) and ventricular single chamber pacing (VVI) with respect to prognosis and antiarrhythmic effect in patients with sick sinus sydnrome. *PACE Pacing Clin Electrophysiol.* 1990;13: 2080–2085.
8. Rosenqvist M, Brandt J, Schuller H. Atrial versus ventricular pacing in sinus node disease: a treatment comparison study. *Am Heart J.* 1986;11:292–297.
9. Rosenqvist M, Brandt J, Schuller H: Long-term pacing in sinus node disease: effects of stimulation mode on cardiovascular morbidity and mortality. *Am Heart J.* 1988;116:16–22.

10. Sutton R, Kenney RA. The natural history of sick sinus syndrome. *PACE Pacing Clin Electrophysiol.* 1986;9:1110–1113.
11. Lamas GA, Estes NAM, Schneller S, et al. Does dual chamber or atrial pacing prevent atrial fibrillation? The need for a randomized controlled trial. *PACE Pacing Clin Electrophysiol.* 1992;15:1109–1113.
12. Coumel P. Neural aspects of paroxysmal atrial fibrillation. In: Falk R, ed. *Atrial Fibrillation Mechanisms and Management.* New York, NY: Raven Press; 1992;109–126.
13. Coumel P, Friocourt P, Mugica J, et al. Long term prevention of vagal arrhythmias by atrial pacing at 90/minute: experience with 6 cases. *PACE Pacing Clin Electrophysiol.* 1983;6:552.
14. Attuel P, Pellerin D, Mugica J, et al. DDD pacing: an effective treatment modality for recurrent atrial arrhythmias. *PACE Pacing Clin Electrophysiol.* 1988;11:1647.
15. Allessie MA, Lammers WJEP, et al. Experimental evaluation of Moe's multiple wavelet hypothesis of atrial fibrillation. In: Zipes DP, Jalife J, eds. *Cardiac Arrhythmias.* New York, NY: Grune & Stratton; 1985.
16. Allessie MA, Rensma PL, et al. Pathophysiology of atrial fibrillation. In: Zipes DP, Jalife J, eds. *Cardiac Electrophysiology: From Cell to Bedside.* Philadelphia, Pa: WB Saunders; 1990;548–559.
17. Allessie MA, Kirchof CJ, Scheffer GJ, et al. Regional control of atrial fibrillation by rapid pacing in conscious dogs. *Circulation.* 1991;84:1689.
18. Josephson ME. *Clinical Cardiac Electrophysiology Techniques and Interpretations.* Philadelphia, Pa: Lea & Febiger; 1993:117–149.
19. Gonzales R, Scheinman M, Margaretten W, et al. Closed chest electrode-catheter technique for His bundle ablation in dogs. *Am J Physiol.* 1981;241:283.
20. Scheinman MM, Laks MM, DiMarco J, et al. Current role of catheter ablative procedures in patients with cardiac arrhythmias: a report for health professionals from the Subcommittee on Electrocardiography and Electrophysiology, American Heart Association. *Circulation.* 1991;83:2146.
21. Klein GJ, Sealy WC, Pritchett, ELC, et al. Cryosurgical ablation of the atrioventricular node-His bundle: long term follow-up in properties of the junctional pacemaker. *Circulation.* 1980;61:8.
22. Evans T, Huang WH, CAR Investigators. Comparison of direct current RF energy for catheter ablation of the atrioventricular junction: results of a prospective multicenter study. *Circulation.* 1990;82(suppl III):III–719. Abstract.
23. Evans GT Jr, Scheinman MM, Bardy G, et al. Predictors of in-hospital mortality after DC catheter ablation of atrioventricular junction: results of a prospective, international, multicenter study. *Circulation.* 1991;84:1924–1937.
24. Dunbar DN, Tobler HG, Fetter J, et al. Intracavitary electrode catheter cardioversion of atrial tachyarrhythmias in the dog. *J Am Coll Cardiol.* 1986;7:1015.
25. Powell AC, Garan H, McGovern BA, et al. Low energy conversion of atrial fibrillation in sheep. *J Am Coll Cardiol.* 1992;20:707–711.

26. Cooper RA, Alferness CA, Smith W, et al. Internal cardioversion of atrial fibrillation in sheep. *Circulation.* 1993;87:1673.

27. Keane D, Boyde E, Robles A, et al. Biphasic versus monphasic waveform in epicardial atrial fibrillation. *PACE Pacing Clin Electrophysiol.* 1992;15:570.

28. Keane D, Sulke N, Cooke R, et al. Endocardial cardioversion of atrial flutter and fibrillation. *PACE Pacing Clin Electrophysiol.* 1993;16:928.

29. Saksena S, Chandran P, Shah Y, et al. Comparative efficacy of transvenous cardioversion and pacing in patients with sustained ventricular tachycardia: a prospective, randomized, crossover study. *Circulation.* 1985;72:153.

30. Slocum J, Sahakian A, Swiryn S. Computer discrimination of atrial fibrillation and regular atrial rhythms from intra-atrial electrograms. *PACE Pacing Clin Electrophysiol.* 1988;11:610.

31. Williams JM, Ungerleider RM, Lofland GK, et al. Left atrial isolation: new technique for the treatment of supraventricular arrhythmias. *J Thorac Cardiovasc Surg.* 1980;80:373–380.

32. Defauw J, Guiraudon GM, van Hemel MN, et al. Surgical therapy of paroxysmal atrial fibrillation with the "corridor" operation. *Ann Thorac Surg.* 1992;53:546–571.

33. Cox JL. The surgical treatment of atrial fibrillation, IV: surgical technique. *J Thorac Cardiovasc Surg.* 1991;101:584–592.

34. Cox JL. Evolving applications of the maze procedure for atrial fibrillation. *Ann Thorac Surg.* 1993;55:578–580.

35. Cox JL, Boineau JP, Schuessler RB, et al. Successful surgical treatment of atrial fibrillation: review and clinical update. *JAMA.* 1991;266:1976–1980.

36. Cox JL, Boineau JP, Schuessler RB, et al. Five-year experience with the maze procedure for atrial fibrillation. *Ann Thorac Surg.* 1993;56:814–823.

Index